Toxicological Aspects of Drug-Facilitated Crimes

Toxicological Aspects of Drug-Facilitated Crimes

Edited by

Pascal Kintz PhD

Consultant in Forensic and Analytical Toxicology,
X-Pertise Consulting, Oberhausbergen, France

AMSTERDAM • BOSTON • HEIDELBERG • LONDON
NEW YORK • OXFORD • PARIS • SAN DIEGO
SAN FRANCISCO • SINGAPORE • SYDNEY • TOKYO
Academic Press is an imprint of Elsevier

Academic Press is an imprint of Elsevier
32 Jamestown Road, London NW1 7BY, UK
225 Wyman Street, Waltham, MA 02451, USA
525 B Street, Suite 1800, San Diego, CA 92101-4495, USA

Notice
No responsibility is assumed by the publisher for any injury and/or damage to
persons or property as a matter of products liability, negligence or otherwise, or from
any use or operation of any methods, products, instructions or ideas contained in the
material herein. Because of rapid advances in the medical sciences, in particular,
independent verification of diagnoses and drug dosages should be made.

British Library Cataloguing-in-Publication Data
A catalogue record for this book is available from the British Library

Library of Congress Cataloging-in-Publication Data
A catalog record for this book is available from the Library of Congress

ISBN: 978-0-12-416748-3

For information on all Academic Press publications
visit our website at elsevierdirect.com

Typeset by MPS Limited, Chennai, India
www.adi-mps.com

14 15 16 17 18   10 9 8 7 6 5 4 3 2 1

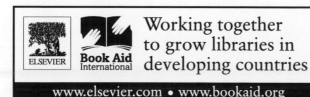

Working together
to grow libraries in
developing countries

www.elsevier.com • www.bookaid.org

Contents

3. Drugs Involved in Drug-Facilitated Crime— Pharmacological Aspects

Anne-Sophie Lemaire-Hurtel and Jean-Claude Alvarez

4. Ethanol- and Drug-Facilitated Crime

Christian Staub and Aline Staub Spörri

5. Memory Impairment after Drug-Facilitated Crimes

Elodie Saussereau, Michel Guerbet, Jean-Pierre Anger
and Jean-Pierre Goullé

6. Cannabis and Drug-Facilitated Crimes

Bertrand Brunet and Patrick Mura

7. Drugs Involved in Drug-Facilitated Crimes (DFC). Analytical Aspects: 1—Blood and Urine

Luc Humbert, Guillaume Hoizey and Michel Lhermitte

8. Drugs Involved in Drug-Facilitated Crimes (DFC). Analytical Aspects: 2—Hair

Marjorie Chèze and Jean-Michel Gaulier

9. Case Reports in Drug-Facilitated Crimes. From A for Alprazolam to Z for Zopiclone

Véronique Dumestre-Toulet and Hélène Eysseric-Guérin

10. The Specific Problem of Children and Old People in Drug-Facilitated Crime Cases

Pascal Kintz

11. Clinical Aspects of Drug-Facilitated Sexual Assault

A.L. Pelissier and J.S. Raul

In the last few years, considerable information about drug-facilitated crimes (DFCs) (rape, sexual assault, robbery, sedation of elderly persons) has accumulated. In these situations, the victims are subjected to non-consensual acts while they are incapacitated through the effects of a drug. This impairs their ability to resist or to give consent to the act. In a typical scenario, a predator (rapist, robber) surreptitiously spikes the drink of an unsuspecting person with a hypnotic drug. Victims, both women and men, usually report loss of memory during and after the event. For the perpetrator, the ideal substance is one that is readily available, is easy to administer, rapidly impairs consciousness and causes anterograde amnesia (i.e. it prevents the recall of events that occurred while under the influence of the drug but not general memory).

The most commonly encountered drugs in alleged DFCs are ethanol (alcohol) and cannabis. Pharmaceuticals are also largely used, with sedation as a common activity. Drugs involved can be benzodiazepines (flunitrazepam, lorazepam, etc.), hypnotics (zopiclone, zolpidem), sedatives, neuroleptics, and some histamine III-antagonists or anesthetics (gamma hydroxybutyrate or GHB, ketamine). In some complicated cases, even clonidine or tetrahydrozoline have been detected. Due to their low dosage, except for GHB, a surreptitious administration into beverages such as coffee, soft drinks (e.g. Cola) or even better alcoholic cocktails is relatively simple.

Blood and urine are the conventional specimens to document drug exposure. The narrow window of detection of GHB, 6 and 10 hours in blood and urine, respectively, is an example of the current limitation of these specimens to demonstrate exposure after late sampling. For all compounds involved in DFC, the detection times in blood and urine depend mainly on the dose and sensitivity of the method used. Prohibiting immunoassays and using only hyphenated techniques, substances can be found in blood from 6 hours to 2 days and in urine from 12 hours to 5 days. Sampling blood or urine has little impact 48 hours after the offense occurred. To address a response to this important caveat, hair was suggested as a valuable specimen. Hair sampling is a useful complement to these analyses to increase the window of detection and to permit differentiation of a single exposure from chronic use of a drug by segmentation. Moreover, due to the long delays that are frequently encountered between the event and the matter being reported to the police, hair can often be the only matrix capable of providing corroborative evidence of a committed crime.

This book will compile numerous case reports, as I wanted the authors to discuss in depth the practical aspects of DFCs and how interpretation was achieved.

A drug-facilitated offense is not a new phenomenon and has been known since Homer's *Odyssey*: Kirke (or Circe) was a goddess *pharmakeia* (witch or sorceress) who lived with her nymph attendants on the mythical island of Aeaea. She was skilled in the magic of metamorphosis, the power of illusion, and the dark art of necromancy. When Odysseus landed on her island she transformed his men into pigs. The drug used was *Datura stramonium*!

Many years later, in 2003, I published my first paper about chemical submission (Kintz, P. (2003) Soumission chimique: quels produits, quels prélèvements, quelles analyses? *J Méd Lég Droit Méd* 45, 158−160). Since that time, I know that the imagination of the perpetrators has no limit, including the chemical nature of the compound that is administered and the manner to administer it to the victim.

Special thanks must go to all the authors who have agreed to write a chapter to what, I hope, is a worthwhile book. Various opinions, sometimes controversial, have emerged among the different authors. I find it helpful to define the areas of agreement among the active investigators and what issues require further efforts to reach a consensus.

Pascal Kintz
X-Pertise Consulting, France

List of Contributors

Pr. Jean-Claude Alvarez Service de Pharmacologie-Toxicologie, Faculté de Médecine PIFO, Université Versailles Saint-Quentin

Jean-Pierre Anger Université de Rennes 1 – Scolarité médecine et pharmacie, Rennes

Bertrand Brunet Service de Toxicologie et Pharmacocinétique, Centre Hospitalier Universitaire, Poitiers

Marjorie Chèze Directrice Scientifique, Laboratoire Toxlab, Paris

Marc Deveaux Directeur Général, Laboratoire Toxlab, Paris

Samira Djezzar Directrice du CEIP Ile de France-Centre, Hôpital Fernand Widal, Assistance Publique-Hôpitaux de Paris, Paris

Véronique Dumestre-Toulet Laboratoire Toxgen, Bordeaux

Hélène Eysseric-Guérin Responsable toxicologie médico-légale, Laboratoire de Pharmacologie et Toxicologie, CHU de Grenoble

Jean-Michel Gaulier Service de pharmacologie, toxicologie et pharmacovigilance, Limoges

Jean-Pierre Goullé Departement de pharmacie, Université de Rouen Mont-Saint-Aignan, Haute-Normandie

Michel Guerbet Guerbet Groupe, Villepinte

Guillaume Hoizey Directeur général adjoint, Laboratoire Toxlab, Paris

Luc Humbert Laboratoire de Toxicologie & Génopathies, Centre de Biologie Pathologie, Lille

Pascal Kintz X-Pertise Consulting, Oberhausbergen

Dr. Anne-Sophie Lemaire-Hurtel Praticien Hospitalier, Laboratoire de pharmacologie-toxicologie, Service de Pharmacologie Clinique, Amiens

Michel Lhermitte Service Toxicologie et Génopathies, Centre de Biologie Pathologie Génétique, CHRU de Lille

Patrick Mura Service de Toxicologie et Pharmacocinétique, Centre Hospitalier Universitaire, Poitiers

A.L. Pelissier Faculté de Médecine, Service de Medecine Légale, Marseille

Gilbert Pépin Directeur fondateur, Laboratoire Toxlab, Paris

Jean-Sébastien RAUL Institut de Médecine Légale, Strasbourg

Nathalie Richard Directrice adjointe, Direction des médicaments en neurologie, psychiatrie, antalgie, rhumatologie, pneumologie, ORL, opthtalmologie, stupéfiants; ANSM, Saint Denis

Elodie Saussereau Laboratoire de pharmacocinétique et de toxicologie cliniques, Groupe hospitalier, Le Harvre

Christian Staub Centre Universitaire Romand de Medecine Legale (CURML), Unite de Toxicologie et Chimie Forensiques, Geneve

Aline Staub Spörri Official Food Control Authority and Veterinary Affairs of Geneva, Geneva

Chapter 1

The History of Drug-Facilitated Crimes in France

Gilbert Pépin

During the month of June 1982, three identical incidents were reported to the Poison Control Center of Marseille, France. They involved young girls, victims of sexual assault, who had experienced amnesia and were found by the roadside in the Aix countryside. During police questioning, they said they had been hitchhiking. One of them reported having flashbacks, describing one in which she sees a vehicle stop and the driver offer her a can of soda which she partially drinks and then throws into the street. Informed of the facts, the police find a can by the roadside. The toxicological analysis of the content revealed the presence of triazolam. The man in the vehicle is found shortly after and confessed that he would pierce a hole in the bottom of the can, then introduce a crushed triazolam tablet, seal it with a patch, and offer his victims the undamaged can. These first cases observed in France were reported in September 1983 by Poyen, Arditti and Jouglard during the 21st Annual Conference of French Poison Control Centers.[1] The term "drug-induced submission" was proposed by the authors at that time. This term was later replaced with "chemical submission." The crimes committed in this way were called "drug facilitated crimes" (DFCs) and included "drug facilitated sexual assaults" (DFSAs). In his presentation, Poyen stated that the well-known amnesiac effects of benzodiazepine tranquilizers cause those who have ingested them unknowingly to be easily swayed, losing all capacity to judge and resist. At that time, he also spoke about children "beaten" with drugs and stated that the populations at risk were young women, the elderly and adolescents who were "robbed of their dignity as well as their money."

A second publicized case dates from May 15, 1993, when a hostage-taker in a kindergarten in Neuilly, France, was killed by security forces. At the request of the police, a doctor prepared a cup of coffee with Gamma-OH®

Toxicological Aspects of Drug-Facilitated Crimes. DOI: http://dx.doi.org/10.1016/B978-0-12-416748-3.00001-3

and Hypnovel®. The nurse who gave the coffee to the kidnapper stated that the man in question began to drink it and then spat it out, clearly suspicious of such an action. In order to prove to the public that the hostage-taker had not been killed while out of commission, toxicological tests were conducted to verify the absence of incapacitating substances in the criminal's blood. The analyses showed a physiological concentration of gammahydroxybutyric acid (GHB) (<2 μg/mL) and the absence of midazolam (<0.1 ng/mL). In other words, there was clear evidence of an attempt at "legal" drug-induced submission by slipping midazolam into a cup of coffee. Nevertheless, given that the person ingested just one sip and then spat it out could not be considered murder. The person in question was not under the influence when he was killed by police gunfire.

In 1994, Bismuth[2] published clinical case studies of drug-induced submission, which at that time already demonstrated the importance of detection techniques. Indeed, the immunochemical methods used by hospital emergency services gave negative results even when prior analyses (shown by a highly indicative chart) by gas chromatography/mass-spectrometry (GC-MS) revealed the presence of triazolam. The first case was that of a 45-year-old man robbed after Halcion® was slipped into his coffee. The second was that of a man whose wife regularly administered sodium bromide to limit his sexual inclinations—it was a car accident that brought this story to light, but the husband did not wish to press charges.

In 1997, Bismuth published eight cases of what she denounced as psychological manipulation.[3] The products in question were Halcion® (triazolam), Rohypnol® (flunitrazepam) and Temesta® (lorazepam).

In 1997, Pépin and coworkers also cited the case of a 50-year-old man who died of hypothermia. He was found in a doorway without a jacket on a very cold winter night. The evening before, in a nearby bar, he had consumed a beer in the company of another man. The investigation revealed that the victim's credit card was used after his death. The toxicological analysis showed the presence in the victim's urine of midazolam (15 ng/mL) which was administered by the SAMU (mobile emergency unit). A concentration of 13 pg/mL of 7-aminoflunitrazepam was also noted. The perpetrator, who was subsequently arrested, admitted to having added a tablet of Rohypnol® to his victim's beer. This was his fortieth victim over the last 10 years. He said he was living off the proceeds of his crimes, but this was the first case of death among his "clients." However, this case was not published until 2001.[4] It was the first French case involving repeated chemical-induced submission for the purpose of stealing credit cards.

Given the increasing number of cases concerning drug-induced submission through the use of hypnotics or tranquilizers, the head of the Agence du Médicament (French health authority) decided to set up a multidisciplinary exploratory committee within the agency. It would be chaired by Professor Lagier and would meet from May to July 1997. The group published a report entitled "Thoughts on the Criminal Use of Psychoactive Substances".[5]

Pharmacists, analysts, judicial experts (among others: Ghysel of the Police Laboratories; Kintz of the Société Française de Toxicologie Analytique, SFTA; and Pépin of the Compagnie Nationale des Biologistes et Analystes Experts, CNBAE), representatives from the three medical orders (doctors, pharmacists, dentists), representatives from the Direction Générale de la Santé (DGS), as well as clinicians (among them Mallaret, Diamant-Berger, Bismuth and Jouglard) participated in this group. Officials from the Agence du Médicament, including Alexandre, Gatignol, Guiton, Andrieu and Castot, also attended.

The group wanted to make concrete proposals, including facilitating the dissemination of information and cooperation between the different professionals involved, to ensure that cases were diagnosed under the best possible conditions and in a timely manner. Its aim was to prevent the criminal use of these products or, at the very least, to make such crimes as difficult as possible. The group also emphasized the need for medical and medico-legal care of the victims, and from the outset insisted that the toxicological analyses by immunochemistry routinely performed in hospital emergency rooms were inadequate and insufficient for the detection of the products in question, considering their short half-life and low therapeutic concentration. The report insisted that the medical profession was generally unaware of this problem, and did not take into account the medico-legal aspect of drug-induced submission, and therefore legal errors were made resulting in the release of the perpetrators.

In 1998, Ghysel, Pépin and Kintz[6] specified the nature of the products involved, how the samples should be taken from the victims, how to preserve the samples, and which toxicology tests should be performed with the proper equipment in order to expose drug-induced submission, which they then called "chemical submission." Dr. Samira Djezzar also set up in 1998 consultations in Paris for victims of drug-induced submission who did not wish to press charges. These victims could either go directly to his office during his shift at the Fernand Widal Hospital, or they could be sent to him by the Hôtel Dieu Hospital emergency service.

The following year, Djezzar and Dally published an article[7] concerning the seizure of 4 kg of GHB manufactured illegally in a Paris laboratory. The press then highlighted the misuse of this synthetic molecule in the United States, where it was nicknamed the "date-rape drug," and how it was being administered without the victims' knowledge due to its euphoric effects. However, no cases of the possible misuse of GHB had been reported in France in the scientific journals at that time.

In 2000, Questel et al. characterized chemical-induced submission as a major public health issue.[8] The authors reviewed a number of cases previously reported over a 4-year period in the Urgences Médico Judiciaires (UMJ) at Hôtel Dieu Hospital in Paris. Only 82 of the 128 cases of alleged chemical-induced submission were used in their study. Clinical cases showed four predominant symptoms: amnesia or partial memory loss, impaired ability to react (sedation), asthenia and anxiety proportional to amnesia. Urinary research showed 57% of the tests to be positive with 47% detecting benzodiazepines (in order of frequency: oxazepam, flunitrazepam, clobazam, lorazepam, bromazepam, chlordiazepoxide, nordazepam), and much less frequently 4.7% detected phenothiazines (levomepromazine, aceprometazine), barbiturates and tricyclic antihistamines (doxylamine). Alcohol was found in 20% of the cases. Vasseur reported a clinical case from the UMJ at Hôtel Dieu Hospital with the use of doxylamine detected by GC-MS.[9] On June 30, 2000, the *Quotidien du Médecin* began to publicize the problem within the medical community in an article entitled "Tranquilizers involved in crimes."

In 2001, Pépin and co-workers, published the case of the repeat offender mentioned above, who was the offender in 40 DFC cases.[4] Also in 2001, Kintz presented a synthesis of his experiences as a legal expert in the domain of chemical-induced submission.[10] His observations identified zolpidem as the most frequently used substance, followed by benzodiazepines (lorazepam, bromazepam, fluitrazepam), neuroleptics (haloperidol, prometazine) and narcotics (cannabis, MDMA, LSD and ketamine). He did not identify any cases of GHB.

At the 9th Annual SFTA meeting in March 2001,[11] nine papers addressing the clinical, toxicological and analytical aspects of benzodiazepines were presented. In addition, eight other papers were presented specifically focusing on chemical-induced submission by use of benzodiazepines, the main authors of whom were Mallaret, Kintz, Questel, Diamant-Berger, Lagier, Pépin, Gaillard, Ghysel, Goullé and Danel. A large number of cases were cited and their pharmacological, clinical and analytical aspects were discussed. At the conference, Questel and Diamond-Berger reported the cases identified in Paris following the creation of a network of clinical services including Poison Control Centers (CAP), Centre d'Evaluation et d'Informations sur la Pharmacodépendance (CEIP) and the Centre Regional de Pharmacovigilance (CRPV). One hundred and thirty-seven cases were noted between 1993 and 2001 where psychoactive products were identified. Benzodiazepines or the like were the most often found in the toxicological analysis of 102 cases (74%). All types of benzodiazepines were found, but the main ones cited were bromazepam, lorazepam, flunitrazepam and zolpidem. Using Temesta®, which had been crushed into the victims' food, the clinical services also reported a series of 19 attacks by the same perpetrator whose motive was theft. The other products detected were: sedating antihistamines (doxylamine, hydroxyzine, buclizine) in 12 cases, neuroleptics (cyamemazine, loxapine) in seven cases, a barbiturate (phenobarbital) in five cases, trihexyphenidyl in two cases, and tramadol in one case. As Dr. Questel said:

This study clearly underlines the importance of the quality of the analytical method used for the detection of these molecules. Immunological detection must be carried out through the use of chromatographic techniques, which are the most reliable. The present results show that current analytical techniques used for detecting toxic substances, such as immunochemistry, have proven to be completely inadequate and inappropriate in detecting substances linked to chemical-induced submission. It is essential that only experienced laboratories equipped with GC-MS technology perform these analyses. These laboratories will be required to conform to the specifications established by the Agence Française de Sécurité Sanitaire des Produits de Santé (AFSSAPS, French health agency).

Indeed, although some scientific associations such as the SFTA had already set up a quality control program for toxicology analysis laboratories, control by an official body appeared essential. As a result of the study, the expert concluded that the victims' medico-legal care must be improved. Therefore, it appeared crucial that the appropriate information and recommendations be disseminated to both the general public and to those involved in supporting the victims, primarily the police and the medico-legal emergency hospital services.

On January 24, 2001, a meeting was held at the Inter-ministerial Mission for the Fight against Dependency and Addiction (MILDT) to determine the actions to be taken by the various structures involved. They included[1]: drafting a protocol describing procedures for taking samples and analysis to be performed (AFSSAPS)[2]; elaborating procedures aimed at instructing and orienting the justice system (MILDT), the police and the gendarmerie; and[3] writing a document to educate emergency services about the problem of chemical-induced submission (Direction Générale de la Sante/Direction des Hôpitaux et de l'Offre de Soins (DGS/DHOS)). Chemical-induced submission was then publicized in the press: "These Tranquilizers Involved in Crimes," *Le Parisien* July 2, 2002, "The Date Rape Drug in Three Clicks of the Mouse," *Journal du Dimanche* October 2, 2002, "The Date Rape Drug Wreaks Havoc," *Le Parisien* July 1, 2002 and "Beware of the Date Rape Drug," *L'Express* August 22, 2002.

On September 19, 2002, the AFSSAPS' Narcotics and Psychotropic Drugs Unit set up a survey which would systematically collect data involving cases where psychoactive products were used. The CEIP Paris (Dr. Djezzar) was responsible for the implementation of the study and coordinating it with different CEIP, CRPV and Poison Control Centers. In late 2002, the SFTA published a special issue of the *Annales de Toxicologie Analytique* devoted to chemical-induced submission[12] consisting of 10 articles by 32 authors, mainly toxicological analysts. The journal stressed the absolute necessity of using a separation method coupled with a mass spectrometer if possible, in tandem with hair analysis in order to achieve conclusive results. Indeed, Pépin and Chèze[13] showed that hair analysis was the only reliable method of detection when the victim pressed charges several days after the event took place, when the drug in question had little chance of appearing in biological fluids.

Hair testing also had the advantage of being able to materialize the absence of the substance administered without the victim knowing, before and after the fact, which is crucial in proving that chemical-induced submission occurred in a single dose. Just as for fingerprinting, the authors wanted a few specialized, well-equipped laboratories to receive national accreditation after qualified testing. These labs would be in charge of analyzing blood, urine and especially biological tissue (skin, nail, hair) in order to look for the substances involved in chemical-induced submission.

Under the leadership of Kintz, Goullé, Mura and Pépin, the SFTA decided to create a special committee on chemical-induced submission. The first meeting was held on January 16, 2003 with Kintz appointed as its first and only chairman. It would meet regularly once or twice a year until 2011.

On October 16, 2002, on behalf of the Interior Minister, Mr. Gaudin, General Director of the National Police, addressed a memo to the Paris Prefect of Police and the directors and heads of the central services of the national police concerning the emergency medico-legal treatment of victims of criminally administered psychoactive substances.[14] On November 26, 2002, Mr. Barrau, the State Prosecutor in Créteil, in collaboration with Dr. Pépin and in conjunction with the urgences médico-judiciaires at the hospital in Créteil, organized a conference on chemical-induced submission intended for all the judges in the High Court and all the judicial police officers in their jurisdiction.

The DHOS/DGS No. 2002/626 circular was published on December 24, 2002.[15] It addressed the authorized emergency treatment of victims of chemical-induced submission who unknowingly ingest psychoactive substances. Effective immediately, the circular stated that toxicology screening was essential in detecting a substance administered without the victim's knowledge for criminal purposes. The circular outlined methods for drawing blood, obtaining urine and hair samples, a list of psychoactive substances to look for, and a nationwide list of laboratories recommended by the AFSSAPS. This list was regularly updated after organized quality control checks and after ensuring the labs had available the specific, appropriate techniques required for analysis. Medical findings and toxicology tests could only be carried out when requested in the course of an investigation and samples stored under lock and key, as stated by law.

On February 6, 2003, Ms. Monteil, Director of the Judicial Police, organized a conference presented by Professor Ricordel and Dr. Pépin to over 200 official judicial police officers on the "proper handling of material findings during an investigation and the analyses which may be requested by experts, particularly in terms of chemical-induced submission." On February 7, 2003, Mr. Duneton, General Director of the AFSSAPS, informed hospital emergency wards of the nationwide study put into place to identify cases of chemical-induced submission as well as the chemical substances most frequently found in order to adapt and update the database of cases and ensure their prevention. In a memo dated February 11, 2003, Mr. Marin, Director of Criminal Affairs at the Ministry of Justice, addressed the general prosecutors and heads of the Courts of Appeal, informing them of their obligation to apply the measures stipulated in the circular dated December 24, 2002 and providing models of analysis for legal requisition. The memo stated: "In these situations, the prosecution should take all necessary measures in favor of the victim. From this viewpoint, it is necessary to develop the intervention of special services designed to assist victims in their jurisdiction in accordance with the provisions stated in paragraph 7, article 41 of the French Penal Code."

On April 7, 2003, Professor Trouvin, in collaboration with Mrs. Castot (AFSSAPS, Director of Medicine Evaluation) and Mmes. Richard and Gatignol (AFSSAPS, Narcotics and Psychotropic Drug Unit), organized a meeting for all of those concerned by the implementation of a nationwide monitoring of chemical-induced submission cases. This monitoring was to be conducted by the CEIP in collaboration with the CRPV and the CAP. This agreement included a list of laboratories approved for the detection of chemical-induced submission.

Dr. Pépin, Vice-President of the CNBAE, met with Mr. Bot, General Prosecutor in Paris, on April 16, 2003 to ask that in cases of chemical-induced submission for which a complaint has been filed, that the hospital emergency laboratory no longer be legally required to perform the analyses via immunochemistry. Indeed, in proven cases, their generally negative results were inconsistent with the findings of the forensic toxicologist experts appointed by a judge. These experts used the separation method combined with mass or tandem mass spectrometry, which is much more specific and sensitive. The discrepancy between the hospital laboratory results and those of expert forensic toxicologists has been the subject of debate during trials in the Criminal Court leading to the wrongful release of the accused. This proposal was accepted.

As part of the SFTA's "chemical submission" committee, a study protocol was coordinated by Kintz and written up in May 2003. Thirteen toxicologist analysts participated. The five most commonly used molecules in chemical-induced submission (lorazepam, bromazepam, flunitrazepam, zolpidem, clonazepam) were absorbed in a single dose by five healthy volunteers. Urine samples and hair were collected and sent for blind testing to the 13 laboratories that agreed to participate in the study. The hair analysis was conducted by laboratories only in Paris and Strasbourg.

Given the results of this study, and at the request of the board of directors of the SFTA, a consensus document entitled "Chemical Submission: Analytical Aspects" was written and adopted at an SFTA general meeting, and then published in the *Annales de Toxicologie Analytique*.[16]

Chemical-induced submission was officially recognized as a crime by the following relevant authorities in 2003: hospitals, scientific associations, the

Ministry of Justice, the Ministry of Interior, the Ministry of Health (DGAS-DHOS, MILDT, AFSSAPS, CEIP, CRPV, CAP) and the SFTA.

Like that in 2003, Pépin and Chèze presented seven oral communications and conferences on the topic of DFC and DFSA, in France and abroad. They also published three papers. Kintz and coworkers presented for their part eight oral communications. Kintz published four papers during the same year. They were the most active scientists on this subject in France. Members of the SFTA and the CNBAE were and still are the essential components in analyzing and assessing the psychoactive agents present. This is key both medically and judicially in the fight against this type of criminality.

At the end of 2012, the problem is still relevant. On November 13, 2012, Mr. Maraninchi (General Director of the Agence Nationale de Sécurité du Médicament (ANSM) (French health agency), at the suggestion of Mrs. Richard, Head of the Narcotics and Psychotropic Drug Unit, has just renewed the convention concerning the nationwide study of chemical-induced submission with the CNBAE for a period of three years. This agreement has provided for the participation and financial compensation of 41 legal toxicologist expert members to identify the maximum amount of chemical-induced submission cases and their conditions (nature of the products used, mode of administration, information about the victim, circumstances of the aggression) to improve the fight against this particular form of criminality. It seems that France is one of the only countries to have set up this type of organized data collection at the national level.

ACKNOWLEDGMENT

I would like to thank Mrs. Jocelyne Arditti, Mrs. Samira Djezzar, Mrs. Nathalie Richard and Mrs. Marjorie Chèze for the documents transmitted.

REFERENCES

1. Poyen B, Jouglard J. [The drug-induced submission]. Abstracts of the 21th Annual Conference of French Poison Control Centers Association, Paris, France; 1983.
2. Bismuth C, Dally S. Drug-induced submission. In: *Cas cliniques en toxicology*. Paris: Flammarion; 1994. pp. 82−3.
3. Bismuth C, Dally S, Borron SW. Chemical submission: GHB, benzodiazepines and other knock out drops. *J Toxicol Clin Tox* 1997;**35**:595−8.
4. Pépin G, Gaillard Y. Original chemical submission: report of 2 cases. *Ann Toxicol Anal* 2001;**13**:122.
5. Lagier G. [Thoughts on criminal use of psychoactive substances]. Report to the French Health Agency (Agence du Médicament), 1997. 52 pp.
6. Ghysel MH, Pépin G, Kintz P. Drug-induced submission. *Toxicorama* 1998;**10**:126−7.
7. Djezzar S, Dally S. Misappropriate use and drug-induced submission. *Med Leg Hosp* 1999;**2**:37.

8. Questel F, Bécour B, Dupeyron JP, Galliot-Guilley M, Diamant-Berger O. Drug-induced submission. *J Med Leg Droit Med* 2000;**13**:459−65.

9. Vasseur P. Sexual assault after drug-induced submission. *Med Leg Hosp* 2000;**3**:94.

10. Kintz P, Villain M, Cirimele V, Goulé JP, Pépin G. Criminal use of psychoactive substances. *Acta Clin Belg* 2002;(Suppl. 1):24−30.

11. 9th SFTA Annual Congress. [Abstracts] *Ann Toxicol Anal* 2001;**13**: 113−54.

12. [Chemical submission]. *Ann Toxicol Anal* 2002;**14**: 359−425 [special issue].

13. Pépin G, Chèze M, Duffort G, Vayssette F. Interest of hair analysis by tandem mass spectrometry in DFC cases: a report of 9 cases. *Ann Toxicol Anal* 2002;**14**:395−406.

14. Ministère de l'Intérieur, de la Sécurité Intérieure et des Libertés Locales [Ministry of Interior]. Circulaire Int C 02 00185 C, October 16, 2002.

15. Ministère de la Santé, de la Famille et des Personnes Handicapées [Ministry of Health]. Circulaire DHOS/DGS 2002/626, December 24, 2002.

16. [Chemical submission: analytical aspects]. Consensus of the French Society of Analytical Toxicology (SFTA). *Ann Toxicol Anal* 2003;**15**:239−42.

Chapter 2

Epidemiology of Drug-Facilitated Crimes and Drug-Facilitated Sexual Assaults

Samira Djezzar, Nathalie Richard and Marc Deveaux

1. INTRODUCTION

Drug-facilitated crime (DFC) is a general term that includes robbery, money extortion, deliberate maltreatment of vulnerable people (children, including Munchausen by proxy syndrome; the elderly; the disabled; and/or mentally ill people), rape and sexual assault: drug-facilitated sexual assault (DFSA) is a subset of DFC.[1−3]

DFCs are criminal acts carried out by means of administering covertly a psychotropic substance to a person with the intention of impairing behavior, state of awareness, perceptions, degree of consciousness, judgment, decision-making capacity or anterograde memory.

Substances used in DFCs are usually odorless or tasteless, dissolve readily in beverages (alcoholic or non-alcoholic), are fast acting, effective at a low dose, have a short plasma half-life, are potent central nervous system (CNS) depressants, mimic severe alcohol intoxication or sedation, and cause anterograde amnesia.

The most frequently used drugs (a total of ≈ 100 molecules are described to be potentially active in DFC) are prescription and over-the-counter medications: benzodiazepines and Z-drugs, antihistamines, non-benzodiazepine sedatives, some neuroleptics and gammahydroxybutyric acid (GHB). All these drugs have to be considered alone or in conjunction with alcohol, cannabis, 3,4-methylenedioxy-N-methylamphetamine (MDMA), cocaine and other drugs of abuse. The key is that the drugs assist or facilitate the crime or the sexual assault. A list of substances which have been encountered at least once in DFC/DFSA cases is give in Table 2.1, according to refs.[1,4,5]

While the covert use of drugs to facilitate crime has occurred over the centuries, this phenomenon has developed during the past 20 or so years,

Toxicological Aspects of Drug-Facilitated Crimes. DOI: http://dx.doi.org/10.1016/B978-0-12-416748-3.00002-5

TABLE 2.1 Substances Encountered at Least Once in DFC/DFSA Cases, in Alphabetical Order

Antihistamines and Others

Antihistamines

brompheniramine	diphenhydramine
cetirizine	doxylamine
chlorpheniramine	hydroxyzine
cyclobenzaprine	niaprazine

Others

acepromazine	haloperidol
aceprometazine	imipramine
alimemazine	loxapine
amitriptyline	meprobamate
chloral hydrate	mequitazine
clomipramine	methoximeprazine
clonidine	new antidepressants (SSRI, NASRI)
clozapine	oxomemazine
cyamemazine	propericiazine
desipramine	tianeptine
dextromethorphan	trihexylphenidine
doxepine	trimebutine
droperidol	valproic acid

Barbiturates

amobarbital	pentobarbital
barbital	phenobarbital
butalbital	secobarbital

Benzodiazepines and Z-drugs

alprazolam	lormetazepam
bromazepam	medazepam
chlordiazepoxide	midazolam
clobazam	nitrazepam
clonazepam	nordiazepam
clorazepate	oxazepam
clotiazepam	phenazepam
cloxazolam	prazepam
diazepam	temazepam
estazolam	tetrazepam
flunitrazepam	triazolam
loprazolam	zaleplon zolpidem zopiclone
lorazepam	
Ethanol (alcoholic beverages)	

Opioids (licit narcotic analgesics)

buprenorphine	dihydrocodeine
codeine	fentanyl
dextropropoxyphene	hydrocodone

(Continued)

TABLE 2.1 (Continued)

hydromorphone	pethidine
methadone	pholcodine
morphine	tramadol
oxycodone	

Street drugs and traditional drugs of abuse

Cannabinoids

natural (cannabis, THC)	synthetic cannabinomimetics (spice, etc.)

Opiates

heroin	morphine

Cocaine

cocaine and crack cocaine	

Amphetamines

amphetamine	MDEA
PMA	MDMA
MBDB	methamphetamine
MDA	

GHB

GHB, GBL, 1,4-BD, valerolactone	

Others

atropine	organic solvents (chloroform, n-decane,
ayahuasca	ether, toluene)
cathinone and cathinone derivatives	phencyclidine (PCP)
kawa-kawa	piperazine group
ketamine	poppers
LSD, LSA	salvinorine A
mescaline	scopolamine
mushrooms (hallucinogenic)	

Adapted from Refs (1,4,5).

and DFCs (including DFSAs) have been highlighted by an increase in the reporting of these crimes by victims worldwide and by an increase in positive analytical results. The upsurge in adjudication by the legal system has also increased awareness.

Because of the large number of unreported rapes, the prevalence of sexual assaults is underreported. This is why the prevalence of DFSAs is unlikely ever to be recognized.

As stated in the UNODC guidelines from 2011,[1] information available on DFC is primarily based on anecdotes and the data collection procedures may be very different from one country to another. It could be national or regional surveys (by toxicologists, psychiatrists, emergency units), responses to charity helplines, governmental (Ministry of Justice, Ministry of Health) statistics, or local or regional data published sporadically by scientists in scientific journals or presented in national or international meetings. The international scientific associations where DFC cases are regularly and actively presented during their annual meetings are: French Society of Analytical Toxicology (SFTA); The International Association of Forensic Toxicologists (TIAFT); Society of Forensic Toxicologists (SOFT); International Association of Therapeutic Drug Monitoring and Clinical Toxicology (IATDMCT); European Association of Poisons Centers and Clinical Toxicologists (EAPCCT); American Academy of Forensic Sciences (AAFS); and Society of Hair Testing (SoHT). This list is not comprehensive. Unfortunately forensic scientists do not always publish their results and numerous oral or poster presentations in different meetings are not immediately published or not published at all in scientific journals, and this can lead to some of the collected data being lost. However, one must be aware of the publication of the abstracts of national meetings in international peer-reviewed journals: for example, the abstracts of the French annual meeting of pharmacovigilance are published in *Fundamental Clinical Pharmacology* and are easily accessible.[6]

In this chapter, the authors develop how the prevalence of DFC is evaluated, focusing on DFSA. As this aspect is well studied in France, the focus will be on French organizations, together with data from other countries in the world (Europe, America, Australia). It appears that little information and statistics are available in these countries and none at all in Asia.

2. EPIDEMIOLOGICAL DATA ON DRUG-FACILITATED CRIME IN FRANCE

2.1 Introduction

The sedative and amnesic effects of benzodiazepines (BZD) are well known and are the basis for their use as anaesthetic premedication. However, in 1982, Poyen[7] reported first in France the possibility of criminal behavior under the influence of these molecules. Other pharmacological effects of benzodiazepines are also used for DFCs, such as decreased resistance or defense reactions, poor assessment of danger and emotion modification.

The first clinical descriptions in France date from the early 1980s.[7,8] Subsequent publications of sporadic cases or small series of DFCs failed to accurately reflect the reality and extent of the problem,[9] especially as these publications were often based on the same cases, mostly in the Ile-de-France region.[10,11] These publications describe the same modi operandi, the same victim profiles and use of the same substances. In 2000, Marc et al.[12] reported a series of 23 cases of sexual assault in the context of DFC using BZD in the eastern Ile-de-France region; 22% of these cases had voluntarily consumed alcohol, thereby potentiating the effects of benzodiazepines. Unfortunately, BZD was only detected in urine by immunochemistry, an imprecise method. A growing number of publications have also reported the use of benzodiazepines, particularly flunitrazepam, which has been called the "date-rape drug," and more rarely other psychoactive substances.[13]

DFC has become a major problem in France, leading to increased awareness of public authorities that have set up surveys and studies to evaluate the extent and seriousness of the problem, especially in order to improve the management of victims by proposing protocols and procedures to guide healthcare professionals. The first study conducted by health and justice working parties involved in all steps of DFC led to a consensus definition and the initiation of a national survey in 2003.[14]

French epidemiological data on DFCs are derived from two sources: the national survey initiated in 2003 and data from the French scientific literature. Some data are duplicated, as most authors of published studies also participated in this survey.

2.2 Methods of the French National Survey

This prospective multicenter study is designed to identify cases of DFC, the substances used and the modi operandi. The study is based on data collected from victims claiming suspected assault in the context of amnesia suggestive of DFC, or subjects claiming to have been drugged without their knowledge, in contrast with other studies based on screening for psychoactive substances in sexual assault victims.[15] Not all victims of DFC are sexually assaulted, as they may also be victims of theft, sedation or abuse, psychological manipulation and other offenses. Infractions may also appear to be trivial, e.g. in a party setting (the use of space cake).

This study also includes victims who did not file a complaint, at least initially, but who wanted to know whether or not they had been drugged without their knowledge.

The management of DFC victims especially comprises the collection of biological fluid samples for toxicological analyses whether or not the victims have filed a complaint. In some cases of delayed management, the victim's hair may be analyzed.

Toxicological analyses were performed with appropriate techniques, such as high performance liquid chromatography, coupled to either diode array detection (LC-DAD), mass spectrometry (LC-MS), tandem mass spectrometry (LC-MS/MS) or electrospray mass spectrometry (LC-ES/MS), and gas chromatography coupled to mass spectrometry (GC-MS) or tandem mass spectrometry, according to the consensus established by the French Society of Analytical Toxicology (SFTA).[16] Samples were collected by health professionals. They were in duplicate in the event of a counter-appraisal. Blood had to be collected (3×10 mL) in a container with preservatives (EDTA to avoid *in vitro* GHB formation) within 24 to 72 hours after ingestion of the psychoactive substances, accompanied by a urine specimen (30 mL). Forensic toxicology laboratories and forensic toxicology judicial experts were actively involved in this study, as their skill and experience are essential for these assessments.

All data were recorded on an anonymous case report form, completed by the physician or the toxicologist who examined the victim or who performed toxicological analyses in the context of a complaint, respectively. The following information was recorded on this form:

- Detailed information on the victim's drug treatments and substance use (alcohol, illicit drugs) before and after the events.
- Dates and exact times of the events and management of the victim, especially any biological samples taken for laboratory tests, to allow comparison with the half-life of the substance(s) detected.
- The type of offense (theft, burglary, psychological manipulation, etc.) or crime (rape, child sexual abuse, sexual assault).
- A brief description on the offender (gender, known or unknown to the victim, acting alone or as part of a group, etc.), when the victim does not present amnesia.
- Description of the context of the assault, indicating the place (bar/night club or public place, home, etc.) and the consumption of any food or drink that could have contained psychoactive substances.
- Clinical findings, looking for signs of anterograde amnesia, the victim's mental state and physical and gynecologic injuries, etc.

Assessment is based on comparison of the findings of clinical examination of the victim following the assault and pharmacological and pharmacokinetic data of the substance(s) administered without the victim's knowledge.

As indicated above, this study distinguishes various methods of assault according to whether the victim voluntarily consumed the psychoactive substances or whether these substances were administered without the victim's knowledge. A diagnosis of chemical vulnerability was adopted when toxicological analyses eliminated the presence of psychoactive substances other than those voluntarily consumed by the victim.

The criteria for likely DFC, defined by a steering committee under the direction of ANSM, comprise:

- Assault or attempted assault documented by clinical examination, a complaint or eyewitness reports.

- An identified psychoactive substance, especially by toxicological analysis using a chromatographic method, not part of the victim's usual treatment.
- Compatible clinical findings and chronology.
- Offender's confession or conviction (when this information is available).

2.3 Survey Results

Between 2003 and the end of 2011, 2144 case files for victims of assault under the influence of a psychoactive substance were collected and reviewed, and 890 (42%) of these case files were sufficiently documented to allow detailed assessment. The difficulty of comprehensive documentation to allow an accurate diagnosis of DFC was observed at a fairly early stage of the survey,[17] as investigations are based on the victims' allegations, which must be verified. Detection of a psychoactive substance does not always correspond to DFC when the victims' substance consumption before and after the events cannot be precisely determined at clinical interview.

Case reports were derived from various sources and 44 duplicate cases were identified, allowing cross-checking and completion of case reports. More than one-half of cases (507 cases/54%) were derived from forensic toxicology laboratories, 266 cases (28%) were derived from forensic medicine departments, 125 cases (13%) were derived from a hospital outpatient or private practitioner, and 39 cases (4%) were derived from the victims themselves or legal authorities.

The prevalence of cases of DFC increased during the survey period (Figure 2.1). This increasing prevalence was probably related to the growing

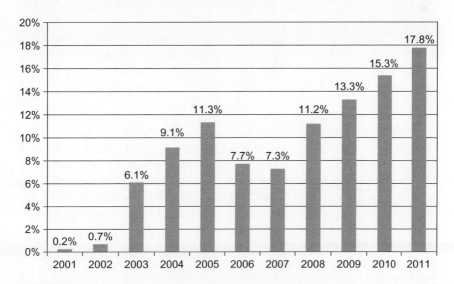

FIGURE 2.1   Prevalence of drug-facilitated crime over a 9-year period.

awareness of the general public, health professionals and legal authorities concerning the risks of DFC. This increased awareness is the result of media coverage of surveys, allowing improved knowledge and management by the professionals concerned.[17,18] Several cases dating back to 2002 were included as investigations were completed during the survey period. Almost one-half of cases (404 cases/45%) occurred in the Ile-de-France region, the most densely populated region of France (11.9 million inhabitants in 2012).[19]

Data concerning filing of a complaint were available for 747 victims (84%). The great majority of victims (701/79%) filed a complaint, while 5% (46 cases) decided not to file a complaint. Victims consulted sufficiently early after the assault, allowing laboratory samples to be taken within 16 hours after ingestion in 46% of cases. Identification of the substances used in this study was based on the result of toxicological analysis and sometimes on the offenders' confessions. Toxicological analyses were performed on plasma and urine samples in 77% and 69% of victims, respectively. Hair tests were required in 203 cases (23%). In some cases, substances were detected in vectors found in the bottom of a glass (nine cases), vomit or gastric fluid (eight cases). The laboratory test results were confirmed for several victims by analyzing powder or tablets (six cases) found at the site of the assault or at the offenders' home. Identification of psychoactive substances was also based on the offenders' confessions in 24 cases.

Analysis of the data collected distinguished the numerous cases of "chemical submission" (473 cases/53%) from cases of "chemical vulnerability" with the use of non-therapeutic substances (280/31%) and "chemical vulnerability" with the use of therapeutic substances and non-therapeutic substances (137/15%) (Table 2.2).

In the case of chemical submission, the victim is under the influence of a psychoactive substance consumed unwittingly, while, in cases of chemical vulnerability, psychoactive substances are consumed voluntarily by the victim, placing them in a more vulnerable and therefore dangerous state.

2.3.1 Drug-Facilitated Crimes

Over a 9-year period, 473 cases meeting the criteria of probable chemical submission or DFC, defined by the steering committee, were identified. Chemical submission is characterized by a premeditated choice of substance by the offender. Cases of forced ingestion of the substance, in which the offender may act alone or as part of a group, are also included in this category. Victims submitted to forced ingestion represented 8% of cases in this series (29 women and 11 men).

Victims were predominantly female (295/62%) with a sex ratio of 0.6, and were aged between two months and 90 years with a mean age of 29.76 years for the 452 victims over the age of 1 year for whom age was reported

TABLE 2.2 Summary of Cases of Chemical Submission and Chemical Vulnerability in France

	Chemical Submission	Vulnerability Using Non-Therapeutic PAS	Vulnerability Using All PAS
N (%)	473 (53%)	280 (31%)	137 (15%)
Female	295 (62%)	249	123
Male	178 (38%)	31	14
Minors	87 (18%)	67	18
Mean age (years)	29.7	22.7	32.6
Place of assault			
Home/hotel	222 (47%)	61 (21%)	47 (34%)
Party place	101 (21%)	104 (37%)	26 (20%)
Public place	66 (14%)	27 (10%)	10 (7%)
NI	84 (18%)	88 (31%)	53 (39%)
Aggressions			
Sexual assault	219 (46%)	235 (84%)	117 (86%)
Sexual assault + theft	21 (4%)	7 (3%)	7 (6%)
Theft/burglary	104 (22%)	14 (5%)	8 (6%)
Attempted DFC	83 (18%)	23 (8%)	1
Simple sedation	20 (4%)		
Sedation for the purposes of murder	17 (4%)		
Inheritance theft	1		1
Physical assault	5	1	
Psychological manipulation	1		1
Kidnapping	2		1

(two infants aged two months and eight months were not included in calculation of the mean age) (Table 2.2). The sex and age distribution of the cases shows that females between the ages of 15 and 39 years constituted the group most frequently submitted to DFC, with a peak of 36% in the 20–29-year age group. Male victims were predominantly between the ages

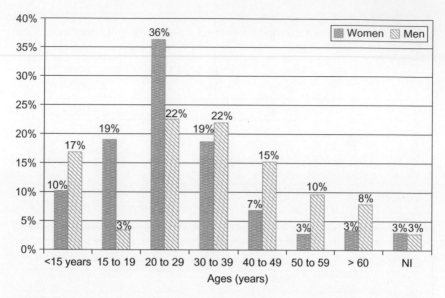

FIGURE 2.2 Drug-facilitated crime: age and sex distribution of the victims (NI = not informed).

of 20 and 39 years (two peaks of 22%). However, a peak of 17% was observed for males under the age of 15 years, corresponding to a high proportion of very young victims of DFC (Figure 2.2).

Voluntary alcohol ingestion was reported in 46% of subjects of legal age or old enough to use another non-therapeutic substance (435 cases over the age of 12 years), while this information was not available for 132 cases (30%). Cannabis use was reported less frequently, by only 16% of victims. Administration of a substance without the victim's knowledge requires the use of a vector to mask this substance. In this survey, the vector was suspected in 324 cases (68%) and no information concerning the vector was available for 109 cases (23%), bearing in mind that 40 victims (8%) were submitted to forced administration. This vector was an alcoholic beverage in 142 cases (44%), a soft drink in 70 cases (22%) and a drink not otherwise specified in 40 cases (12%). Food was suspected in 38 cases and direct administration of the substance was reported in 28 cases (substitution of a medicinal product or other substance by a different type of molecule). Infusion of a molecule in physiological saline in hospital (three cases) or use of a cigarette containing the substance responsible (three cases) were seldom reported.

Victims generally met their assailant in a party context in 101 cases (21%), while 222 victims (47%) met their assailant at home or in an equivalent setting (hotel, prison). The exact site of administration of the substance was often difficult to determine: the place where the victim met the assailant and unwittingly consumed the substance or the site of the actual assault.

Presumably, the victim usually meets the offender in a party context, at which the assault generally takes place in a more intimate setting. Other places were also described, such as a public place (not a bar or night club) in 14% of cases (67 cases occurred at work, in hospital, in a nursing home, in a car park, etc.). The site of chemical submission was not reported for 87 cases (18%).

A wide range of crimes were reported or observed, but DFCs were dominated by sexual assault. Rape or sexual assault, according to the legal definition, accounted for more than one-half (51%) of cases. Isolated sexual assault was reported in 219 cases (46%), followed by isolated theft in 104 cases (22%), or more rarely both crimes simultaneously in 21 cases (4%). Sedation for the purposes of abuse or homicide was reported in 37 cases (8%). Homicide used another, generally violent, means. Cases of repeated abuse predominantly concerned children and the elderly. Various other forms of assault were reported in nine cases (2%), such as physical assault, kidnapping or mental manipulation in a context of inheritance theft. Attempted DFC was considered to have occurred in 83 cases (18%) on the basis of either severe amnesia (sexual assault could not be confirmed or excluded by an adult victim) or abnormal symptoms or behavior reported by persons caring for the victim (the assailant did not complete the crime).

2.3.2 Particular Case of Children and the Elderly

Children under the age of 15 years represent 13% (60 cases) of all DFC victims. These young children, who are vulnerable because of their age, can be victims of various types of abuse. The apparently most harmless and most frequent form of abuse consists of sedation to make the child sleep, and can be considered to be a form of chemical child abuse. Twenty-one children (35%) were victims of repeated sedation in this setting, with one death. Four other children were sedated for the purposes of subsequent homicide. Sexual assault was reported in 22 children (37%), in an incestuous setting in eight cases. More rarely, attempted DFC (nine cases) and kidnapping (two cases) were also reported. In some cases, hair analyses indicated repeated administration of the substance over time, using the same or different psychoactive substances. Hair analysis can provide a major contribution because the diagnosis is very often suspected after a long time in the absence of any acute complications, and hair analysis can also be used to establish a history of consumption over a fairly long period depending on the length of the hair.

This practice of chemical child abuse was underdiagnosed for a long time due to the difficulty of understanding how parents could perform such reprehensible acts. However, certain complications such as respiratory distress and even death have been reported, due to poor evaluation of the dose or the toxic nature of the substances used. Several sporadic cases, not included in the national survey, have been published in France. Various substances are used in this context, such as benzodiazepines,[20,21] neuroleptics or H1

antihistamines[22,23] or even methadone in infants with serious consequences.[24] Sexual assault is not uncommon and, despite the child's young
age, psychoactive substances have the same effect as in adults.[21]

Subjects over the age of 65 years represented only 2% of all victims (16
cases) in this survey. They were mostly victims of theft (including inheritance theft) in four cases, while sedation in a context of abuse was described
in five cases. Chemical sedation of the elderly, like chemical child abuse, is
underreported due to failure to recognize this practice. It is often difficult to
distinguish between a medically justified indication and an abusive prescription. Detailed medical records are required to assess such cases.

Kintz et al. reported a series of cases of DFC in the elderly,[25] involving
various crimes, motivated by material gain in some cases. One or several
psychoactive substances were used concomitantly or alternately during
repeated abuse.

The proportion of reported cases of chemical abuse in children and the
elderly is clearly underestimated, as many of these victims are not seen in
hospital and the few cases in this survey were detected in the context of a
complication leading to a report to the police.

2.3.3 Clinical Features

The symptom most commonly reported and which remains fairly anxiogenic
is amnesia. Amnesia was described in more than one-half of cases (57%;
270 cases). It was anterograde, either partial or complete with flashes that
often revealed sexual assault. A lowered level of consciousness was reported
less frequently, in 184 cases (39%), generally drowsiness or sleep, or more
rarely coma. Physical injuries were reported in 80 cases (17%), consisting of
bruising essentially on grip zones and genital lesions, which were less common among sexually active adults.

2.3.4 Psychoactive Substances

A wide range of psychoactive substances were used by DFC offenders, but
some substances were used much more frequently than others. Table 2.3
gives a list of substances encountered in France in this study. Seventy
molecules were used without the victims' knowledge or were forcibly administered in 612 cases. These substances were grouped into families of psychoactive substances and predominantly consisted of benzodiazepines and
Z-drugs (BZD) in 63% of cases, followed by sedative H1 antihistamines and
other substances in 12% of cases (Figure 2.3). These results confirm those
reported in other series in the Paris area.[10,11] Non-therapeutic substances
represented 16% of all psychoactive substances reported.

More specifically, three BZD and analogs were more frequently used:
clonazepam (26%), followed by zolpidem (16%) and bromazepam (15%).
The use of these three molecules varied over time, probably because of a

TABLE 2.3 Psychoactive Substances Involved in DFC in France (number)

Benzodiazepines and Z-drugs	Adults	Children	All Victims
clonazepam	92	9	101
zolpidem	54	6	60
bromazepam	45	13	58
nordiazepam	21	6	27
zopiclone	18	9	27
alprazolam	16	3	19
diazepam	16		16
oxazepam	16		16
flunitrazepam	13	1	14
lorazepam	11	4	15
tetrazepam	10		10
lormetazepam	5	1	6
prazepam	3	2	5
loprazolam	3		3
midazolam	3		3
clobazam	2		2
triazolam	1	1	2
acepromazine	1		1
clotiazepam	1		1
temazepam	1		1
Antihistamines and sedatives			
doxylamine	19	4	23
hydroxyzine	12	2	14
cyamemazine	11	2	13
alimemazine	5	2	7
cetirizine	5		5
niaprazine		3	3
haloperidol	2		2
propericiazine		2	2

(*Continued*)

TABLE 2.3 (Continued)

Benzodiazepines and Z-drugs	Adults	Children	All Victims
phenobarbital	2		2
diphenhydramine	1		1
loxapine		1	1
droperidol	1		1
mequitazine	1		1
trihexyphenidyl	1		1
Opioids			
dextropropoxyphene	5		5
pholcodine	5		5
buprenorphine	2	2	4
morphine	4		4
codeine	2	1	3
tramadol	1	1	2
oxycodone	1		1
methadone	1		1
trimebutine	1		1
Miscellaneous			
ether		4	4
amitriptyline	3		3
ketamine	2		2
mianserine	2		2
citalopram	1	1	2
tianeptine	1		1
fluoxetine	1		1
venlafaxine	1		1
imipramine	1		1
clomipramine	1		1
ketoprofen	1		1
ibuprofen	1		1

(*Continued*)

TABLE 2.3 (Continued)

Benzodiazepines and Z-drugs	Adults	Children	All Victims
propranolol	1		1
ephedrine / pseudo-ephedrine	1		1
lidocaine	1		1
Non-therapeutic substances			
cannabis	22	4	26
MDMA /amphetamine	23	1	24
cocaine	12		12
alcohol	12	3	15
GHB / GBL	14		14
GBL	1		1
LSD	2		2
chloroform	1	1	2
toluene	1		1
pesticide	1		1
n-decane	1		1
scopolamine	1		1

non-systematic and irregular collection bias (Figure 2.4). Zolpidem, which has a very short half-life, was detected in biological fluids well after the events (up to 4 days in our study) by skilled analysts using sophisticated assay techniques.[26]

Flunitrazepam, called the "date-rape drug" in the USA,[15] was detected in 14 cases (4%) despite the blue color of the tablet, which was specifically modified in order to avoid this type of abuse.[27] However, this color change has not had any real impact in France. The substances most commonly used were also those misused in a context of substance abuse or off-label use.[28]

The main molecules in the group of antihistamines and other sedatives (14 molecules and 76 cases) were doxylamine (30%), hydroxyzine (18%) and cyamemazine (17%).

Volatile substances were used in children and adolescents between the ages of 7 and 13 years for the purposes of sexual assault. Chloroform was used in two cases, resulting in death due to overdose in one case, in which

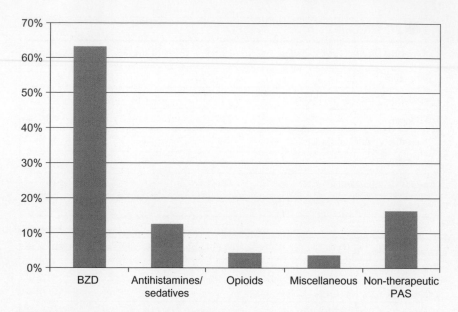

FIGURE 2.3　Distribution of psychoactive substances used in cases of DFC.

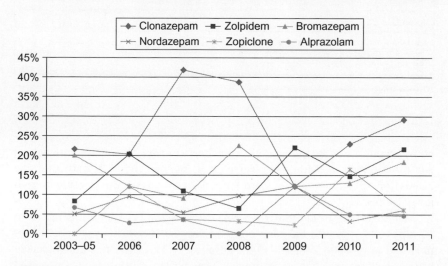

FIGURE 2.4　Time-course of the benzodiazepines most commonly used for DFC.

chloroform was detected in bodily fluids,[29] while the use of ether was reported in police records in four cases of incest.

Non-therapeutic substances mainly corresponded to delta-9-tetrahydrocannabinol in 26% of cases, administered without the victim's knowledge in the form of space cake in a series of eight cases in the context of an after-work drink. The eight victims filed a complaint on the grounds of DFC. Delta-9-tetrahydrocannabinol was also used in a context of forced inhalation or child abuse.

The next most common substance after cannabis was MDMA, which was detected in 24% of cases, a molecule commonly used for its emotion-modifying effects. The exacerbated empathy associated with hedonistic effects of MDMA induces compulsively pleasure-seeking behavior, thereby facilitating the victim's participation in his or her own rape.[30–32] Forced alcohol ingestion was reported in 15% of cases.

GHB and its precursor gammabutyrolactone (GBL) were used in 14 cases and one case, respectively. GBL is detected in the metabolized form of GHB and information concerning the use of GBL is provided by confiscation of the bottle and analysis of its content. The very small number of cases of GHB use in the present series can be explained by the illicit drug status of GHB and its very short half-life which prevents detection in delayed laboratory samples.[33]

The choice of one molecule rather than another is not dictated by the victim's gender or age, as, with a few exceptions (volatile substances), children in this series received the same substances as adults, regardless of the risk of overdose complications. The use of several psychoactive substances was not uncommon.

Information concerning the offenders was missing from this survey. Except for cases in which the offender was a family member or close friend and therefore identified, the other offenders, whether or not they were known to the victims, were not identified either because of amnesia or because they were part of a large crowd. Police investigation often constitutes an obstacle to documentation of these cases. However, several situations are particularly interesting. Chèze et al.[34] reported three examples of serial offenders with a fairly unusual modus operandi with crime-free periods corresponding to periods of imprisonment. Victim hair analyses (two, eight and 22 cases, respectively) identified the molecules used by the assailants for their thefts and were used to establish a history of their offenses. The offender who robbed 22 victims of their bank card used a psychoactive substance cocktail prepared in advance in a bottle, containing flunitrazepam, clonazepam, doxylamine, cyamemazine, zolpidem and lorazepam. Some of these victims were included in the present survey. This example also illustrates that DFC offenders do not always use the same molecule, but take the risk of preparing mixtures that could be life-threatening.

2.3.5 Chemical Vulnerability Due to Voluntary Consumption of Psychoactive Substances

The slightly less numerous (417 cases) victims of this group were consulted under similar conditions and for the same reasons as victims of chemical submission. Cases of vulnerability due to consumption of non-therapeutic substances (280 cases; 67%) were distinguished from cases of vulnerability due to consumption of the victim's usual psychotropic treatment together with consumption of non-therapeutic substances (137 cases; 33%). The first group predominantly reported consumption of alcohol in 256 cases (91%), followed by cannabis in 104 cases (37%). Cocaine use was reported more rarely, in five cases. Victims often did not incriminate alcohol because they considered that they had consumed the usual quantities.

The group of patients taking psychotropic treatment, and consequently vulnerable as a result of their mental illness and their drug therapy, were even more susceptible to the effects of occasional use of alcohol (62%) or cannabis (29%). These two groups were essentially composed of female victims, in 89% and 90% of cases, respectively (Table 2.2).

The age distribution of the victims showed that non-therapeutic substances were more frequently used in subjects between the ages of 15 and 29 years, while the use of psychotropic treatments mainly concerned older subjects, aged 20 to 39 years (Figure 2.5).

As most victims were female, sexual assault was the predominant offense, in 86% and 91% of cases, respectively. Other offenses were less common (Table 2.2).

Within these three groups, victims of chemical vulnerability using non-therapeutic substances were younger (mean age: 22.7 years vs. 27.7 for DFC and 32.6 years for cases involving all psychoactive substances), are more frequently assaulted in a party setting (87% vs. 21% and 20%) and they

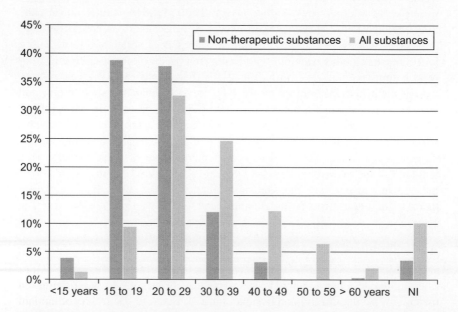

FIGURE 2.5 Chemical vulnerability: age distribution of the victims (NI = not informed).

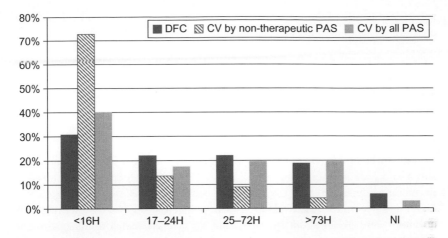

FIGURE 2.6 Distribution of victims according to time prior to collection of laboratory samples (NI = not informed).

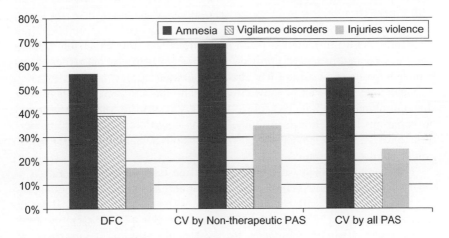

FIGURE 2.7 Distribution of the most common signs in the three groups.

predominantly consulted in less than 16 hours (72%) (Figure 2.6). The elimination kinetics of the substances could possibly provide a logical explanation. The effects of alcohol fade more rapidly than those of other psychoactive substances either administered alone or in combination with alcohol in the other two groups, which encourages these subjects to consult or file a complaint earlier. This group also presented the highest rate of amnesia (69% vs. 57% and 56%) and physical injuries, related to the effects of alcohol (Figure 2.7). The use of alcohol or other non-therapeutic psychoactive substances is one of the major risk factors for young people, exposing them to a risk of physical assault and especially sexual assault.[35–38]

2.4 Aspects of the Regulations

The results of the successive studies show that medicines rather than illicit drugs are substances mostly incriminated, especially benzodiazepines and Z-drugs; even voluntarily consumption of alcohol and cannabis is quite frequent and is a predisposing factor of vulnerability.

French health authorities (ANSM, French medicine agency) set up measures to prevent the criminal use of drugs. The risk of chemical submission in the medicinal product (psychotropic substances) is now systematically taken into account in the evaluation of new medicine. For example, negative opinions were given about the marketing of effervescent lormetazepam and zolpidem tablets.

In December 2012, the liquid clonazepam formulation was modified by addition of a blue coloring following the request of French health authorities.

A specific working group linked to the French marketing authorization committee "Drug formulation recommendations and drug diversion prevention" was created in order to provide guidelines to help pharmaceutical companies in the development of new drug formulations.

Guidelines should allow the victim's watchfulness to increase when he or she is drinking or eating. To achieve these goals, specific formulations could be based on the addition of excipients which could contain specific properties, for example excipients that allow for visible detection or a taste detection of the drug, like bittering agent.

The risk of chemical submission should be taken into consideration in the evaluation of a medicinal product (pre- and post-marketing authorization). This concern will be taken into account at the international level: Recommendation 1777 from the Parliamentary European Assembly 2007 urges "pharmaceutical companies to develop methods of making relevant drugs more identifiable when added to liquid," and the Commission on Narcotic Drugs adopted two resolutions in 2009 and 2010 (Commission on Narcotic Drugs, March 2009: resolution 52/8: Use of pharmaceutical technology to counter drug-facilitated sexual assault ("date rape"), and Commission on Narcotic Drugs, March 2010, resolution 53/7: International cooperation in countering the covert administration of psychoactive substances related to sexual assault and other criminal acts). These resolutions urge states to combat the phenomenon of drug-facilitated sexual assault and to consider making recommendations about formulations to the pharmaceutical industries. In fact, most of the substances (except alcohol) implicated in DFC cases are under international control and scheduled under the UN Single Convention on Narcotic Drugs 1961 and the

Convention on Psychotropic Substances 1971.[1] Unfortunately psychotropic substances such as GBL and some over-the-counter drugs (notably antihistamines) used in DFSA cases remain outside international controls. However, controls may exist at the national level in some countries. Such disparities allow trafficking through different countries, often via the Internet and couriers: it is difficult to obtain accurate data on the nature and the extent of the problem.[1]

3. EPIDEMIOLOGICAL DATA ON DRUG-FACILITATED CRIME IN THE USA

The US Department of Justice publishes annually the Uniform Crime Report (UCR) which itemizes the number of forcible rapes reported to law enforcement agencies throughout the United States. However, these statistics are limited[3] because they exclude forcible rape, copulation and sodomy, statutory rapes and rapes accomplished without force when victims are incapacitated.[39] It appears that the number of incidents is possibly 10 times higher[3] and that about one in six women in the United States is a victim of rape or attempted rape. These data are provided by national victimization surveys sponsored by the National Institute of Justice (NIJ) and Centers for Disease Controls and Prevention (CDC). Regarding the specific DFSA case, it is observed in most interviews that the victims are reluctant to make police reports. Like acts of sexual violence against women, crimes against males are highly underreported to the police.[3,4]

In 1999, ElSohly and Salamone published the first comprehensive study attempting to evaluate the incidence of DFSA.[40] They reported the results of 1179 urine sample analyses from 49 states, Puerto Rico, and the District of Columbia. The states sending the most samples were California, Texas, Florida, Pennsylvania, New York, Minnesota, Illinois, Indiana, Michigan, Maryland, Virginia, and Massachusetts. Methods used were immunoassays, GC-MS (especially for flunitrazepam and GHB) and GC-FID (ethanol). Over 61% of all samples were positive for one or more drugs, including ethanol. ElSohly and Salamone's paper was severely criticized[5,41] because: a) the urine specimens were screened by a laboratory funded by Hofmann-La Roche for flunitrazepam metabolites (coming from Rohypnol®, Hofmann-La Roche Laboratories) at a very low concentration and other benzodiazepines were not screened at such low levels, and so their prevalences could have been underestimated, and b) the cut-off used to differentiate endogenous from exogenous GHB was too low, so the prevalence of GHB was also underestimated.[42] Despite this bias, this study first demonstrated at a large scale that DFSA involves a wide range of drugs, not just those that were popularized by the media (i.e. GHB and Rohypnol®). The prevalence of ethanol was very high (38%), followed by cannabis, cocaine, benzodiazepines, amphetamines and GHB.

In 2001, the ElSohly combined his results with those from Hindmarch[43] and updated their database in order to obtain an up-to-date database containing 3303 urine samples collected over a 4-year period (1996—2000)[44]. Seventy-three percent of samples were reported to have been collected within the first 24 hours after the incident. Alcohol, either alone or in combination with other drugs, was by far the commonest substance found, being present in 67% of samples. Cannabis was the second most prevalent drug, present in 30.3% of samples. The remaining positive drugs findings were composed of benzodiazepines (4.8%), cocaine (2.8%), amphetamines (1.9%), opiates (0.7%) and propoxyphene (0.3%).

Another study reported of a total of 2003 urine specimens from victims of sexual assaults.[37] Analyses were conducted by GC-MS (1997—1999). Nearly two-thirds of the samples contained alcohol and/or drugs; the predominant substances found were alcohol, present in 63% of cases, and marijuana, present in 30%. A substantial subset of the specimens was found to contain other illicit substances, frequently in combination. GHB and flunitrazepam were each detected in less than 3% of the positive samples.

After the publication of important papers on analytical developments,[45—47] Juhascik estimated the occurrence of DFSA cases in the USA.[15] Specimens collected from individuals, who presented in four clinics (Texas, California, Minnesota and Washington) with complaints of being sexually assaulted, were tested for 45 different drugs and alcohol. Overall, 43% of 144 subjects (7% of 859 complainants) could be classified as DFSA cases.

Important conclusions were a) that subjects underreported their use of drugs, and b) that the true proportion of DFSA cases is underreported because of the frequently large timespan between the incident and reporting.

In 2007, interviews conducted at the National Crime Victims Research and Treatment Center on 5001 women drew the conclusion that, more specifically in term of DFSA, the vast majority of cases involved alcohol (>95%), while drugs alone were involved in less than 5% of cases. Alcohol combined with drugs was estimated at a level of 15—25% of the cases.[5]

As stated by Arbanel earlier,[3] there is currently no systematic effort under way to measure exactly the prevalence and incidence of DFCs/DFSAs at a nationwide scale in the USA. Moreover, in most survey research designed to measure the scope of sexual violence, DFSAs have not been included.[3,39] The FBI laboratory collects data and adds them the Uniform Crime Report. Unfortunately, it seems that DFSAs are lumped with all rapes and DFCs with robberies (M. LeBeau, FBI laboratory. Personal communication). However, papers from McCauley, Kilpatrick et al. (Department of Psychiatry and Behavioral Sciences at the Medical University of South Carolina, Charleston) together with the National Crime Victims Research and Treatment Center attempted to identify the scope, nature and consequences of rape of a number of women in the USA and in college settings.[48—50]

These surveys are conducted at a national level and this may help largely to improve the knowledge of prevalence of DFSAs. A national protocol for sexual assault medical forensic examination (adults/adolescents) has just been published by the Office on Violence Against Women from the NDJ.[51] Moreover, the clinical report from the American Academy of Pediatrics on "The Evaluation of Sexual Abuse in Children" states that data collected must include patient history of DFSA: this may help also to evaluate the prevalence of such crimes.[52]

4. EPIDEMIOLOGICAL DATA ON DRUG-FACILITATED CRIME IN CANADA

In Canada, the Royal Canadian Mounted Police (RCMP) and the federal agency Statistics Canada keep national statistics on DFCs and DFSAs, but these data are not so easy to obtain. Two papers deal with the prevalence of DFSA cases: one from British Columbia[53] and a most comprehensive one from Ontario.[54] The period studied in the retrospective population base from British Columbia was wide (1993 to 2002), but gave only demographics data and no data were provided regarding alcohol and the different drugs used in DFCs/DFSAs. The most important conclusion was the demonstration that the incidence of hospital-reported DFSAs has shown a marked and sustained increase since 1999 and that young women in their teens are particularly vulnerable to this form of sexual assault. The study from DuMont was also a prospective study in seven hospital-based sexual assault treatment centers in Ontario (2005−2007). One hundred and seventy-nine urine samples were suitable for analysis for CNS-active substances most commonly implicated in the literature as facilitating sexual assault: alcohol, cannabinoids, cocaine, opiates, GHB, amphetamines, benzodiazepines (flunitrazepam, diazepam, nordiazepam, lorazepam, clonazepam, alprazolam), MDMA, ketamine and others (antidepressants, cough suppressants, muscle relaxants, anticonvulsants). All specimens were analyzed in a toxicology laboratory according to a predetermined blind protocol, but details were not given on the analytical methods.

A total of 184 of 882 eligible participants met suspected DFSA criteria. Urine samples were positive for drugs in 45% of cases, alcohol in 13%, and both drugs and alcohol in 18%. The drugs found on toxicological screening were unexpected in 87 of the 135 (64%) cases with a positive drug finding and included cannabinoids (40%), cocaine (32%), amphetamines (13%), MDMA (9%), ketamine (2%) and GHB (1%). Unexpected drugs are defined as not reported as being voluntarily consumed. Alcohol was present in 31% of the cases (alcohol alone in 13%, both alcohol and drugs in 18%, neither alcohol nor drugs in 24%). No data are given on the urine alcohol concentrations and on a possible back-calculation or estimation of the blood alcohol concentration. However, the authors point out that there is a need to

warn young people that there can be no consent to sexual activity while
intoxicated.

5. EPIDEMIOLOGICAL DATA ON DRUG-FACILITATED CRIME IN AUSTRALIA

We found only two papers reviewing cases of alleged DFSA.[55,56] The files
of the Victorian Institute of Forensic Medicine were reviewed from May
2002 to April 2003. Seventy-six cases of suspected DFSA were identified
from a total of 434 cases (17.5%) of adult sexual assault. The median delay
from alleged event to examination was 20 hours (mean 23 hours).
Toxicological analysis in blood and/or urine confirmed the presence of alcohol in 37% of cases. Toxicological analysis was performed in all cases
($n = 22$) where covert administration was suspected by any party: subject,
doctor or police. Unexpected toxicology was found in 15 cases (20%). In 10
cases the known consumption of at least one psychoactive drug was confirmed (in five cases this was two drugs): cannabis, antidepressants, amphetamines, BZD and opiates.

6. EPIDEMIOLOGICAL DATA ON DRUG-FACILITATED CRIME IN THE UNITED KINGDOM

Over a 3-year period (2000–2002), the Forensic Science Service (FSS) studied 1014 cases of alleged DFSA cases.[57,58] The cases were submitted from
33 of the 43 police forces in England and Wales, and two of the police
forces in Scotland. In 39% of cases, the samples (blood and/or urine) were
collected within 12 hours of the incident. Analyses were conducted for alcohol, common drugs and usual drugs of abuse. Methods were GC-FID,
enzyme immunoassay and confirmation using GC-MS in SIM mode. The
majority (81%) of the samples (blood and/or urine) contained alcohol.
Nearly 50% of the cases were positive for alcohol and/or other incapacitating
drugs. Illicit drugs were detected in more than one-third (35%) of the cases,
with cannabis being the most commonly detected (26% of cases) followed
by cocaine (11%). In only 2% of cases ($n = 21$) a sedative or a disinhibiting
drug was detected when its presence could not be explained by the complainant (by taking the drug on prescription). These drugs were, in decreasing
order: BZD ($n = 12$), MDMA ($n = 3$), antihistamines ($n = 2$), GHB ($n = 2$),
zopiclone ($n = 1$), mirtazapine ($n = 1$). These results were confirmed by
Beynon a few years later.[59]

The authors agree that the low number of positive cases detected ($n = 21$)
may have underestimated the true number of deliberate DFSA cases that
occurred over this period.

To our knowledge, only the FSS published results of epidemiological
studies. But what will happen now, since this laboratory was closed? We

may suspect that these data are not being collected except by scientists in different laboratories, which will vary from region to region.

Equivalent data are available from Northern Ireland: Hall published two papers in 2008 giving extensive results for alcohol and drugs.[60,61] Data were identified from the Forensic Science Northern Ireland (FSNI) database from 1999 up to and including 2005. Blood and/or urine were analyzed, but the methods were not detailed. The results for 2005 are summarized: the percentage of cases containing alcohol was 65%, and 78% contained alcohol, drugs or both. By 2005, drugs were identified in 20 cases among 51 (39%). The analgesic group was the commonest drug group identified ($n = 11$). Recreational drugs (cannabis, MDMA) were found in eight samples. Six samples tested positive for BZD. Almost half of the cases contained more than one drug.

Papers from the UK after 2006 cite Operation Matisse.[62] This was a 12-month study into the nature of DFSA for the period 2004–2005. One hundred and twenty individuals reported to the police that they had been drugged and assaulted. Reporting occurred within 72 hours of the sexual assault. Controlled or prescription drugs were detected in 48% of cases. Cannabis was the most common (20%) followed by cocaine (17%). GHB was detected in two cases, but flunitrazepam was not detected in any of the cases.

7. EPIDEMIOLOGICAL DATA ON DRUG-FACILITATED CRIME IN IRELAND

As in other western countries, there is a large degree of underreporting of rapes and DFSAs to the National Police Service of the Republic of Ireland. In his recent review, McBierty explains that reports from both the police (Rape Crisis Network National Statistics) and the Central Statistics Office (CSO) would suggest that less than one in five victims of rape reported the offense. This is very low.[63]

Despite the Sexual Assault and Violence in Ireland Report (SAVI report, 2002; cited by McBrierty[63]) and the follow-up SAVI revisited from 2005 providing invaluable sources of information regarding the prevalence of sexual abuse and violence in Ireland, no data are provided regarding alcohol and the different drugs used in DFCs/DFSAs.

Irish legislation and case law concerning DFSA is complex, with much of the case law regarding the key concept of capacity to consent to sexual intercourse. Few specifics guided the judges and juries, but since 2005, a victim of DFSA may be considered a vulnerable adult with regard to their potential lack of capacity to consent, according to the Law Reform Commission, Consultation Paper on Vulnerable Adults and the Law.[63]

8. EPIDEMIOLOGICAL DATA ON DRUG-FACILITATED CRIME IN THE NETHERLANDS

Data from the Netherlands Forensic Institute (NFI) were published in 2011 by Bosman.[64] Cases were selected over a 3-year period (January 2004 through December 2006), including those with an indication of sexual assault and the presence of blood and/or urine for analysis. General screening for the drugs listed by SOFT[65] was performed using ELISA, GC-MS and LC-DAD. The determination of any detected molecule was performed using GC-MS, LC-DAD, GC-MS/MS and LC-MS/MS. Alcohol and GHB were determined by specific methods. A total of 134 cases of alleged DFSA were screened for drugs of abuse, prescription drugs and GHB, and 108 for alcohol. Most of the victims were women (94%). Twenty-seven percent of the cases were negative. Alcohol alone or together with other drugs was the most common finding (51 cases of 108). A wide range of drugs was found, in descending order: cocaine (14%), BZD (10%), MDMA and MDA (10%), THC (10%), amphetamine (4%), GHB (detected in only two cases) and ketamine (detected in one case). Different sedative therapeutic drugs were found each for one case: amitriptyline, codeine, methadone and zolpidem. A combination of drugs often occurs. The authors could not discriminate between proactive (involuntary ingestion) and opportunistic (voluntary ingestion) DFSA. As far as the authors know, it is obvious that the cases described at the NFI for toxicological analysis are an underestimation. The numbers seem not to be registered properly and there is no mention of a national agency to collect the data and to publish them (I. Bosman, NFI. Personal communication).

9. EPIDEMIOLOGICAL DATA ON DRUG-FACILITATED CRIME IN GERMANY

In a recent review of the prevalence of drugs used in DFC, Madea discussed that in Germany most of the crimes committed in association with drugs (so-called knock-out drugs) are of a sexual nature, occurring in the setting of the disco and rave scenes (DFSA).[66] A few papers deal with epidemiological data, only on a regional basis and not regularly, and most of them are unfortunately in German. However, the main results we found in the literature are as follow, summarized by Madea[66]:

- From 1995 to 1998, the Munich department of forensic medicine (Bavaria) registered a total of 92 DFC cases in which the administration of a knock-out drug was suspected—13% were DFSA.
- From 1997 to 2006, the Bonn department of forensic medicine (North Rhine-Westphalia) registered a 10-fold increase in the number of investigations of possible intoxicating substances in sexual assaults, currently reaching 40 to 50 cases per year.

In the paper published in 2009,[66] the authors stated that in this study, as in their own experience (data from Bonn area), benzodiazepines were the most commonly used type of substance, followed by other hypnotic agents (zopiclone, GHB >10 mg/mL in urine), antihistamines (diphenhydramine), sedating antidepressants and other illegal drugs (MDMA).

These data are not provided by a regional or a federal agency. The provisions of the German criminal code regarding sexual assaults, including DFSA as an aggravating circumstance, are extensively described in English in refs.[66,67]

10. EPIDEMIOLOGICAL DATA ON DRUG-FACILITATED CRIME IN DENMARK

As in many other western countries, DFC and DFSA cases were perceived to have increased in Denmark. However, in 2012, Birkler et al. stated that no information exists on how widespread the phenomenon is in this country.[68] Using UPLC-TOF-MS instrumentation, they developed and validated a general screening method capable of detecting a broad range of medicinal drugs and drugs of abuse. Forty-six of the most prevalent drugs were targeted. Alcohol, barbiturates and cannabis were analyzed by in-house diagnostic methods.

One hundred and sixty-seven blood samples obtained from victims of sexual assault in the Aarhus area were studied over a two and half-year period. Twenty (12%) of the victims suspected they had been exposed to a DFSA. The average timespan between sexual assault and medical examination was 23.5 hours (SD 11.5, median 22), fairly later than the whole study population (15 hours longer). Seventeen of the 20 victims reported they had consumed alcohol prior to the assault, but only four (20%) were analyzed positive for alcohol. BZD were identified in 25% of the cases, either alone or in combination with other drugs. Meprobamate, phenobarbital, oxycodone, methylphenidate and amphetamine were each detected once. THC and/or THC-COOH were detected in three cases. The authors note that in some of the cases where no sedative drugs had been observed, a rather high amount of alcohol had been ingested. As seen in other studies, alcohol is the most prominent substance encountered in sexual assault cases, and therefore is a high risk factor.[58,66]

There is no mention of a national agency to collect the data and to publish them.

11. EPIDEMIOLOGICAL DATA ON DRUG-FACILITATED CRIME IN NORWAY

In Norway, only one paper[69] describes the results of a retrospective, descriptive study of 730 female patients who were examined at the Sexual Assault

Center in Trondheim, Norway (a precinct of 280,000 inhabitants), from July 2003 to December 2010. A total of 264 patients among 730 could be included because urine and/or blood were obtained for toxicological analyses. Fifty-seven (22%) of the 264 victims suspected a proactive DFSA. If available, urine samples were screened for a predefined selection of substances likely to be used in DFSAs[1] and included ethanol, benzodiazepines/benzodiazepine-like drugs, cannabinoids, opioids, central stimulants, GHB and ketamine. If the urinary screening test was positive for one or more of these substances, the corresponding substances were also quantified in serum (the limits of detection in urine are given extensively by the authors). In cases with only serum available, specific analyses were prioritized according to the characteristics of the individual case. The analytical methods employed were LC/MS, GC/MS and immunoassay.

The average timespan between sexual assault and medical examination was 29.6 hours (median 12.5 hours, range 1 hour to 16 days); mainly because of the relatively long time interval, short-acting drugs such as GHB could not be detected. Twenty-two of the 57 patients (38%) were positive for alcohol only; 13 (22%) were positive for at least one drug other than alcohol. The results are fully detailed by the authors: five patients were positive for benzodiazepines (diazepam and/or oxazepam, clonazepam), one was positive for morphine and oxycodone, two were positive for cannabis and four were positive for amphetamines (some tested positive for more than one drug).

An important result is given regarding alcohol ingestion and self-reporting by the victims: among the 57 patients suspecting proactive DFSA, only three did not report intake of alcohol/drug(s), while 36 reported intake of alcohol only, 17 reported intake of alcohol and drug(s), and one reported intake of drug(s) only. The proportions were similar to those in the group not suspecting proactive DFSA.

Hagemann[69] concludes that one bias in epidemiological studies is the relatively small sample size, especially concerning cases of suspected proactive DFSA. However, her findings are very similar to findings in Scandinavian studies, which probably reflect the low prevalence of recreational drugs in Scandinavia as compared to other western countries.[68–72]

12. EPIDEMIOLOGICAL DATA ON DRUG-FACILITATED CRIME IN SWEDEN

As forensic toxicology in Sweden is centralized to only one accredited laboratory (Department of Forensic Genetics and Forensic Toxicology, Linköping, Sweden), the results of analysis from both the living and the dead are entered into a forensic database (Toxbase) along with age and gender of the victims/suspects.[70] A total of 1806 cases registered between 2003 and 2007 from female victims of sexual assault were included in the study published in 2008.[70] Another paper studied the cases registered as sexual assault and rape, including date rape, for which the police had requested the analysis of ethanol and other drugs between 2008 and 2010.[71] Unfortunately, the DFSA cases were not described separately.

Blood samples were available for toxicological analysis in a total of 1638 (91%) of all cases of sexual assault over the 5-year period of the first investigation, and 1460 cases in the second 2-year period. In both studies, analyses were performed in blood by immunoassay, GC-MS, GC-NPD, GC-FID for ethanol, GHB, a large number of prescription drugs and their metabolites and illicit drugs.

Jones[71] stated that the proportion of drug-positive to drug-negative cases, the predominance of ethanol positive cases as well as the types of other drugs show a remarkably good agreement in the two studies (2008/2010) spanning a period of 8 years. In one-third of the cases, ethanol and other drugs were not detected. In 12−13% of the cases, ethanol occurred together with at least one other drug. The mean and median concentrations of ethanol in blood ($n = 806$ and 658) were 1.24 and 1.23 g/L respectively and 1.19 and 1.22 g/L, respectively. One or more other drugs alone were found in $n = 210−262$ cases (15−14%). Cannabis (marijuana) and amphetamines were the major illicit drugs, whereas diazepam, alprazolam, zopiclone as well as various analgesic opiates and SSRI antidepressants were the major prescription drugs identified. Jones[70,71] concluded his papers by a very practical statement: "Interpreting the analytical results in terms of voluntary vs. surreptitious administration of drugs and the degree of incapacitation in the victim as well as ability to give informed consent for sexual activity is fraught with difficulties."

Sweden seems to be the only country in Scandinavia where a national agency is able to collect the data and to publish them (not systematically, but in peer-reviewed journals).

13. EPIDEMIOLOGICAL DATA ON DRUG-FACILITATED CRIME IN POLAND

In a paper published in a Polish journal, Adamowicz[73] described a 15-fold increase in DFSA cases in 2003−2004 compared to 2000−2002. Data where obtained in one laboratory in the Krakow region. The most common substances detected in blood and/or urine by LC-DAD, NCI-GC-MS and GC-EI-MS were amphetamine and cannabis, while alcohol, MDMA, benzodiazepines, propranolol and lidocaine were detected only in a few cases. The same author recorded a total of 133 victims analyzing urine and mainly blood samples.[74,75] However, no precise data were given. There is no mention of a national agency to collect the data and to check the proven DFC/DFSA cases at a nationwide scale.

14. EPIDEMIOLOGICAL DATA ON DRUG-FACILITATED CRIME IN BELGIUM

In Belgium, there is absolutely no mention of a regional or federal agency to collect and publish data. Only scientists from the National Institute for Forensic Sciences (INCC) and some others from different universities publish specific, highly sensitive and fully validated methods together with a few examples.[76–79] These methods may be very helpful to any forensic scientist in DFC/DFSA cases, but no comprehensive data are published actually in Belgium.

15. EPIDEMIOLOGICAL DATA ON DRUG-FACILITATED CRIME IN ITALY

A very few cases are reported from Italy and the teams from universities and university hospitals from Pavia, Padua, Verona and Rome seem to be the more active in this field, but only case reports were found in the literature[80,81]: barbiturates, morphine and GHB were involved in isolated cases. Bertol[82] drew attention to the problem of careless use of immunoassay tests for DFC, as they may provide false-negative results due to the low responses presented by 3-hydroxy-flunitrazepam and 7-amino-nitrazepam.Unfortunately, no epidemiological data were provided.

In Italy there is no organization that collects data on DFC or DFSA in a systematic way, either globally or regionally, but a procedure for epidemiological identification of the DFC/DFSA cases is now being set up. In 2011, the Department of Antidrug Policies of the Presidency of the Council of Ministers implemented a project at national level to develop a national network aimed at collecting these kinds of data. The project has been assigned to the Pavia Poison Control Centre and involves about 30 emergency rooms throughout the country. The project states that when the assaulted patient decides to adhere to the survey, and after signing the informed consent, under the normal procedures used for diagnostic and therapeutic treatment of cases of sexual assault or other suspicion of crime (robbery/scam), blood and urine samples are taken for toxicological analysis. If the assault occurred more than two weeks earlier, a sample of hair is also taken and brought to the Institute of Forensic Medicine of the Catholic University of Rome, or to the Pavia Poison Control Centre. Analyses on biological samples are performed by these two centers. Data are meant to be collected and included into the database of the National Observatory of the Department of Antidrug Policies (see C. Rimondo, Italian Early Warning System Coordinator; S. Pichini, Istituto Superiore di Sanita, Roma; and A. Polettini, University of Verona. Personal communications). The provisions of the Italian criminal code regarding sexual assaults, including DFSA as an aggravating circumstance, are described in English in ref. [67]

16. EPIDEMIOLOGICAL DATA ON DRUG-FACILITATED CRIME IN SPAIN

In 2008, a paper in Spanish stated that no epidemiological data existed in Spain.[83] Only one unusual case was published, describing a DFSA using aromatic solvent.[84] However, in 2005, Lopez-Rivadulla et al. proposed a protocol for multicentric surveys of chemical submission[85] and finally, in 2012, a protocol was published by the Ministry of Justice.[86] This protocol is followed by all the laboratories involved in judicial toxicological expertise. The National Institute of Toxicology and Forensic Sciences (INT-CF), several university laboratories like the University Institute of Forensic Sciences in Santiago de Compostela, and other Institutes of legal medicine notably from Catalonia and the Basque Country must follow the protocol. Unfortunately, there have been no published data until now. In Spain all issues related to DFSA and DFC are currently collected by judicial system, and private organizations are not allowed to collect the data (M. López-Rivadulla, University of Santiago de Compostela, C. Jurado, INT-CF, Sevilla. Personal communications).

17. CONCLUSION

Chemical submission is a phenomenon as old as humanity. This type of crime may affect children, the elderly, the disabled and young females, as well as men. Despite chemical submission, now well known through the press and women's magazines, the true extent of DFC and DFSA remains unknown as only reported data are used.

National data from poison control centers, hospital emergency rooms, national or regional surveys published in scientific journals, and law enforcement seizures must be used to evaluate the relative magnitude of problems and illicit availability of different classes of drugs. These data need to have a high degree of certainty and must be the result of cooperation between all the counterparts involved, the police, medical staff, forensic toxicologists, judicial experts and judicial authorities.

After this review of the data collected on DFC and DFSA, it is clear that victims of sexual assault should have easy and fast access (less than 48 hours) to emergency healthcare with trained staff, and should be encouraged to seek immediate help. Toxicological screening and analysis should be routinely offered according a strict protocol to achieve a comprehensive assessment in each individual case. Blood, urine and hair should be analyzed in order to achieve a high degree of certainty. Based on the current study, it should be pointed out that the perceived dangers of surreptitious drugging with so-called "date-rape drugs" such as GHB and flunitrazepam is most likely overrated, and that BZD and recreational drugs like cannabis and amphetamines are the most often used drugs. The dangers of voluntary excessive intake of alcohol (and drugs) should be emphasized further.

REFERENCES

1   UNODC laboratory and scientific section, Vienna. *Guidelines for the forensic analysis of drugs facilitating sexual assault and other criminal acts.* New York: United Nations; 2011.

2. Chemical submission. *Ann Toxicol Anal (special issue)* 2002;**14**:359−425.

3. Arbanel G. The victim. In: LeBeau MA, Mozayani A, editors. *Drug-facilitated sexual assault: a forensic handbook.* San Diego: Academic Press. <http://refhub.elsevier.com/6978-0-12-416748-3.00002-5/sbref2>

4. LeBeau M, Mozayani A. *Drug-facilitated sexual assault. a forensic handbook.* San Diego: Academic Press; 2001.

5. LeBeau MA, Montgomery MA. The frequency of DFSA investigations. *Forensic Sci Rev* 2010;**22**:7−14.

6. Rédaction Prescrire. Drugs and memory lost. *Rev Prescrire* 2009;**29**:827.

7. Poyen B, Rodor F, Jouve-Bestagne MH, Galland MC, Lots R, Jouglard J. Amnesia and behavior disorders of criminal appearance after ingestion of benzodiazepines. *Thérapie* 1982;**11**:675−8.

8. Poyen B, Jouglard J. The drug submission. *Abstracts of 21st Annual Conference of French Antipoison Centers Association.* Paris; 1983.

9. Bismuth C, Dally S, Borron SW. Chemical submission: GHB, benzodiazepines and other knock out drops. *J Toxicol Clin Tox* 1997;**35**:595−8.

10. Questel F, Lagier G, Fompeydie D, Djezzar S, Dally S, Elkharrat D, et al. Criminal use of psycho-active drugs: analysis of a cohort in Paris. *Ann Toxicol Anal* 2002; **14**:371−80.

11. Djezzar S, Questel F, Gourlain H, Fompeydie D, Richard N, Gatignol C, et al. Chemical submission: study of case reports. Porto Rico: San Juan; 2004. Abstracts of 66th Annual Scientific Meeting of the College on Problems of Drug Dependence.

12. Marc B, Baudry F, Vaquero P, Zerrouki L, Hassnaoui S, Douceron H. Sexual assault under benzodiazepine submission in a Paris suburb. *Arch Gynecol Obstet* 2000;**263**:193−7.

13. Anglin D, Spears KL, Hutson HR. Flunitrazepam and its involvement in date or acquaintance rape. *Acad Emerg Med* 1997;**4**:323−6.

14. The French National Agency for Medicines and Health Products Safety. *National chemical submission survey protocol.* <http://ansm.sante.fr/var/ansm_site/storage/original/application/8be07abe84b74f041208b50c7570be65.pdf>; [accessed 07.13].

15. Juhascik MP, Negrusz A, Faugno D, Ledray L, Greene P, Lindner A, et al. An estimate of the proportion of drug-facilitation of sexual assault in four U.S. localities. *J Forensic Sci* 2007;**52**:1396−400.

16. Chemical submission: analytical aspects, consensus of the French Society of Analytical Toxicology (SFTA). *Ann Toxicol Anal* 2003;**15**:239−42.

17. Djezzar S, Questel F, Burin E, Dally S, French Network of Centers for Evaluation and Information on Pharmacodependence. Chemical submission: results of 4-year French inquiry. *Int J Legal Med* 2009;**123**:213−9.

18. The French National Agency for Medicines and Health Products Safety. *National chemical submission survey.* <http://ansm.sante.fr/Activites/Pharmacodependance-Addictovigilance/Soumission-chimique/%28offset%29/5#paragraph_574>; [accessed 31.07.13].

19. National Institute of Statistics and Economic Studies. *Demographic database.* <http://www.insee.fr/fr/ppp/bases-de-donnees/recensement/populations-legales/france-regions.asp?annee = 2010>; [accessed 07.13].

20. Kintz P, Villain M, Chèze M, Pépin G. Identification of alprazolam in hair in two cases of drug-facilitated incidents. *Forensic Sci Int* 2005;**153**:222−6.

21. Rey-Salmon C, Pépin G. Drug-facilitated crime and sexual abuse: a pediatric observation. *Arch Pediatr* 2007;**14**:1318−20.

22. Kintz P, Villain M, Cirimele V. Determination of trimeprazine-facilitated sedation in children by hair analysis. *J Anal Toxicol* 2006;**30**:400−2.

23. Kintz P, Evans J, Villain M, Salquebre G, Cirimele V. Hair analysis for diphenhydramine after surreptitious administration to a child. *Forensic Sci Int* 2007;**173**:171−4.

24. Kintz P, Villain M, Dumestre-Toulet V, Capolaghi B, Cirimele V. Methadone as a chemical weapon: two fatal cases involving babies. *Ther Drug Monit* 2005;**27**:741−3.

25. Kintz P, Villain M, Cirimele V. Chemical abuse in the elderly: evidence from hair analysis. *Ther Drug Monit* 2008;**30**:207−11.

26. Kintz P, Villain M, Dumestre-Toulet V, Ludes B. Drug-facilitated sexual assault and analytical toxicology: the role of LC-MS/MS: a case involving zolpidem. *J Clin Forensic Med* 2005;**12**:36−41.

27. New color-releasing formulation of Rohypnol announced at national NCASA meeting. Change welcomed by rape crisis community. *National coalition against sexual assault.* Enola, PA: Press release; 1997.

28. The French National Agency for Medicines and Health Products Safety. *National survey of clonazepam.* <http://ansm.sante.fr/Activites/Surveillance-des-stupefiants-et-des-psychotropes/Medicaments-a-risque-d-usage-detourne-ou-de-dependance/Medicaments-a-risque-d-usage-detourne-ou-de-dependance/RIVOTRIL/%28language%29/fre-FR>; [accessed 31.07.13].

29. Gaillard Y, Masson-Seyer MF, Giroud M, Roussot JF, Prevosto JM. A case of drug-facilitated sexual assault leading to death by chloroform poisoning. *Int J Legal Med* 2006;**120**:241−5.

30. Jansen L, Theron L. Ecstasy (MDMA), methamphetamine, and date rape (drug-facilitated sexual assault): a consideration of the issues. *J Psychoactive Drugs* 2006;**38**:1−12.

31. Eiden C, Cathala P, Fabresse N, Galea Y, Mathieu-Daudé JC, Baccino E, et al. A case of drug-facilitated sexual assault involving 3,4-methylenedioxy-methylamphetamine. *J Psychoactive Drugs* 2013;**45**(1):94−7.

32. Chèze M, Deveaux M, Martin C, Lhermitte M, Pépin G. Simultaneous analysis of six amphetamines and analogues in hair, blood and urine by LC-ESI-MS/MS. Application to the determination of MDMA after low Ecstasy intake. *Forensic Sci Int* 2007;**170**:100−4.

33. Chèze M, Hoizey G, Deveaux M, Muckensturm A, Vayssette F, Billault F, et al. Series of new cases of intoxication by GHB or GBL. Determination in blood, urine, hair and nails. *Ann Toxicol Anal* 2012;**24**:59−65.

34. Chèze M, Muckensturm A, Hoizey G, Pépin G, Deveaux M. A tendency for re-offending in drug-facilitated crime. *Forensic Sci Int* 2010,**20**(196).14−7.

35. Wolitzky-Taylor KB, Ruggiero KJ, Danielson CK, Resnick HS, Hanson RF, Smith DW, et al. Prevalence and correlates of dating violence in a national sample of adolescents. *J Am Acad Child Adolesc Psychiatry* 2008;**47**:755−62.

36. Rickert VI, Wiemann CM. Date rape among adolescents and young adults. *J Pediatr Adolesc Gynecol* 1998;**11**:167−75.

37. Slaughter L. Involvement of drugs in sexual assault. *J Reprod Med* 2000;**45**:425−30.

38. Resnick HS, Walsh K, Schumacher JA, Kilpatrick DG, Acierno R. Prior substance abuse and related treatment history reported by recent victims of sexual assault. *Addict Behav* 2013;**38**:2074−9.

39. Russel DEH, Bolen RM. *The epidemic of rape and child sexual abuse in the United States.* Thousand Oaks: Sage Publications; 2000.

40. ElSohly MA, Salamone SJ. Prevalence of drugs used in cases of alleged sexual assault. *J Anal Toxicol* 1999;**23**:141−6.

41. LeBeau MA, Montgomery MA. Challenges of drug-facilitated assault. *Forensic Sci Rev* 2010;**22**:2−6.

42. LeBeau MA, Christenson RH, Levine B, Darwin WD, Huestis MA. Intra- and interindividual variations in urinary concentrations of endogenous GHB. *J Anal Toxicol* 2002;**26**:340.

43. Hindmarch I, Brinkmann R. Trends in the use of alcohol and other drugs in cases of sexual assault. *Hum Psychopharmacol Clin Exp* 1999;**14**:225−31.

44. Hindmarch I, ElSohly MA, Gambles J, Salamone S. Forensic urinalysis of drug use in cases of alleged sexual assault. *J Clin Forensic Med* 2001;**8**:197−205.

45. Negrusz A, Gaensslen RE. Analytical developments in toxicological investigation of drug-facilitated sexual assault. *Anal Bioanal Chem* 2003;**376**:1192−7.

46. Juhascik M, Le NL, Tomlinson K, Moore C, Gaensslen RE, Negrusz A. Development of an analytical approach to the specimens collected from victims of sexual assault. *J Anal Toxicol* 2004;**28**:400−6.

47. ElSohly MA, Gul W, Murphy TP, Avula B, Khan IA. LC-(TOF) MS analysis of benzodiazepines in urine from alleged victims of drug-facilitated sexual assault. *J Anal Toxicol* 2007;**31**:505−14.

48. McCauley JL, Conoscenti LM, Ruggiero KJ, Resnick HS, Saunders BE, Kilpatrick DG. Prevalence and correlates of drug/alcohol-facilitated and incapacitated sexual assault in a nationally representative sample of adolescent girls. *J Clin Child Adolesc Psychol* 2009;**38**:295−300.

49. McCauley JL, Ruggiero KJ, Resnick HS, Kilpatrick DG. Incapacitated, forcible, and drug/alcohol-facilitated rape in relation to binge drinking, marijuana use, and illicit drug use: a national survey. *J Trauma Stress* 2010;**23**:132−40.

50. McCauley JL, Kilpatrick DG, Walsh K, Resnick HS. Substance use among women receiving post-rape medical care, associated post-assault concerns and current substance abuse: results from a national telephone household probability sample. *Addict Behav* 2013;**38**:1952−7.

51. US Department of Justice, Office on violence against women. 2nd ed. *A national protocol for sexual assault medical forensic examinations. Adults/adolescents*, 228119. NCJ; April 2013107−110.

52. Gavril AR, Kellog ND, Nair P. Value of the follow-up examinations of children and adolescents evaluated for sexual abuse and assault. *Pediatrics* 2012;**129**:282−9.

53. McGregor MJ, Ericksen J, Ronald LA, Janssen PA, Van Vliet A, Schulzer M. Rising incidence of hospital-reported drug-facilitated sexual assault in a large urban community in Canada. Retrospective population-based study. *Can J Public Health* 2004;**95** (441−445).

54. Du Mont J, Macdonald S, Rotbard N, Bainbridge D, Asllani E, Smith N. Drug-facilitated sexual assault in Ontario, Canada: toxicological and DNA findings. *J Forensic Leg Med* 2010;**17**:333−8.

55. Moreton R, Bedford K. *Spiked drinks: a focus group study of young women's perception of risk and behavior.* Central Sydney Area Health Service Camperdown, NSW; 2002.

56. Hurley M, Parker H, Wells DL. The epidemiology of drug facilitated sexual assault. *J Clin Forensic Med* 2006;**13**:181−5.
57. Scott-Ham M, Burton FC. Toxicological findings in cases of alleged DFSA in the United Kingdom over a 3-year period. *J Clin Forensic Med* 2005;**12**:175−86.
58. Scott-Ham M, Burton FC. A study of blood and urine alcohol concentrations in cases of alleged drug-facilitated sexual assault in the United Kingdom over a 3-year period. *J Clin Forensic Med* 2006;**13**:107−11.
59. Beynon CM, McVeigh C, McVeigh J, Leavey C, Bellis MA. The involvement of drugs and alcohol in drug-facilitated sexual assault: a systematic review of the evidence. *Trauma Violence Abuse* 2008;**9**:178−88.
60. Hall J, Goodall EA, Moore T. Alleged drug facilitated sexual assault (DFSA) in Northern Ireland from 1999 to 2005. A study of blood alcohol levels. *J Forensic Leg Med* 2008;**15**:497−504.
61. Hall JA, Moore CBT. Drug facilitated sexual assault—a review. *J Forensic Leg Med* 2008;**15**:291−7.
62. Gee D, Owen P, McLean I, Brentha K, Thundercloud C. *Operation Matisse: investigating DFSA. Association of Chief Police Officers of England.* London: Wales and Northern Ireland; 2006.
63. McBrierty D, Wilkinson A, Tormey W. A review of drug-facilitated sexual assault evidence: an Irish perspective. *J Forensic Leg Med* 2013;**20**:189−97.
64. Bosman IJ, Verschraagen M, Lusthof KJ. Toxicological findings in cases of sexual assaults in the Netherlands. *J Forensic Sci* 2011;**56**:1562−8.
65. LeBeau MA. Guidance for improved detection of drugs used to facilitate crimes. *Ther Drug Monit* 2008;**30**:229−33.
66. Madea B, Musshoff F. Knock-out drugs: their prevalence, modes of action, and means of detection. *Dtsch Arztebl Int* 2009;**106**:341−7.
67. Dorandeu AH, Pagès CA, Sordino MC, Pépin G, Baccino E, Kintz P. A case in southeastern France: a review of DFSA in European and English-speaking countries. *J Clin Forensic Sci* 2006;**13**:253−61.
68. Birkler RID, Telving R, Ingemann-Hansen O, Charles AV, Johannsen M, Andreasen MF. Screening analysis for medicinal drugs and drugs of abuse in whole blood using ultraperformance liquid chromatography time-of-flight mass spectrometry (UPLC-TOF-MS)—toxicological findings in cases of alleged sexual assault. *Forensic Sci Int* 2012;**222**:154−61.
69. Hagemann CT, Helland A, Spigset O, Espnes KA, Ormstad K, Schei B. Ethanol and drug findings in women consulting a Sexual Assault Center—associations with clinical characteristics and suspicions of drug-facilitated sexual assault. *J Forensic Leg Med* 2013;**20**:777−84.
70. Jones AW, Fredrik C, Kugelberg FC, Holmgren A, Ahlner J. Occurrence of ethanol and other drugs in blood and urine specimens from female victims of alleged sexual assault. *Forensic Sci Int* 2008;**18**:40−6.
71. Jones AW, Holmgren A, Ahlner J. Toxicological analysis of blood and urine samples from female victims of alleged sexual assault. *Clin Toxicology (Philadelphia, Pa)* 2012;**50**:555−61.
72. Bogstrand ST, Normann PT, Rossow I, Larsen M, Morland J, Ekeberg O. Prevalence of alcohol and other substances of abuse among injured patients in a Norwegian emergency department. *Drug Alcohol Depend* 2011;**117**:132−8.
73. Adamowicz P, Kala M. Date-rape drugs scene in Poland. *Przegl Lek* 2005;**62**:572−5.

74. Adamowicz P, Kala M, Lechowicz W. Date-rape drugs in Poland-An eight year review. *Ann Toxicol Anal* 2008;**20**:S1−38.

75. Adamowicz P, Kala M. Simultaneous screening for and determination of 128 date-rape drugs in urine by gas chromatography-electron ionization-mass spectrometry. *Forensic Sci Int* 2010;**198**:39−45.

76. Del Mar Ramirez Fernandez M, Laloup M, Wood M, De Boeck G, Lopez-Rivadulla M, Wallemacq P, et al. Liquid chromatography-tandem mass spectrometry method for the simultaneous analysis of multiple hallucinogens, chlorpheniramine, ketamine, ritalinic acid, and metabolites, in urine. *J Anal Toxicol* 2007;**31**:497−504.

77. Laloup M, Del Mar Ramirez Fernandez M, Wood M, Maes V, De Boeck G, Vanbeckevoort Y, et al. Detection of diazepam in urine, hair and preserved oral fluid samples with LC-MS-MS after single and repeated administration of Myolastan and Valium. *Anal Bioanal Chem* 2007;**388**:1545−56.

78. Del Mar Ramirez Fernandez M, Wille SM, Kummer N, Di Fazio V, Ruyssinckx E, Samyn N. Quantitative analysis of 26 opioids, cocaine, and their metabolites in human blood by ultra-performance liquid chromatography-tandem mass spectrometry. *Ther Drug Monit* 2013;**34**:510−21.

79. Ingels AS, Neels H, Lambert WE, Stove CP. Determination of gamma-hydroxybutyric acid in biofluids using a one-step procedure with "in-vial" derivatization and headspace-trap gas chromatography-mass spectrometry. *J Chromatogr A* 2013;**1296**:84−92.

80. Frison G, Favretto D, Tedeschi L, Ferrara SD. Detection of thiopental and pentobarbital in head and pubic hair in a case of DFSA. *Forensic Sci Int* 2003;**133**:171−4.

81. Rossi R, Lancia M, Gambelunghe C, Oliva A, Fucci N. Identification of GHB and morphine in hair in a case of drug-facilitated sexual assault. *Forensic Sci Int* 2009;**186**:1−3.

82. Bertol E, Vaiano F, Furlanetto S, Mari F. Cross-reactivities and structure-reactivity relationship of 6 benzodiazepines to Emit® immunoassay. *J Pharm Biomed Anal* 2013;**84**:168−72.

83. Cruz-Landeira A, Quintela-Jorge O, Lopez-Rivadulla M. Chemical submission: epidemiology and keys for the diagnosis. *Med Clin (Barc)* 2008;**131**:783−9.

84. Martinez MA, Ballesteros S. An unusual case of DFSA using aromatic solvent. *J Anal Toxicol* 2006;**30**:449−53.

85. López-Rivadulla M, Cruz A, Quintela O, De Castro A, Concheiro M, Bermejo A. Chemical submission: past, present and future. Instructions for multicentric surveys. *Rev Toxicol* 2005;**22**(Suppl. 1). Available at: <http://tox.umh.es/aetox/Revista/e-revistas/analit/ana03>; [accessed 09.13].

86. Ministerio de Justicia. *Instructions in case of sexual assault with suspicion of intoxication.* Available from "noticias" at: <http://institutodetoxicologia.justicia.es>; 2012 [accessed 09.13].

Chapter 3

Drugs Involved in Drug-Facilitated Crime— Pharmacological Aspects

Anne-Sophie Lemaire-Hurtel and Jean-Claude Alvarez

Drugs involved in drug-facilitated crime (DFC) include pharmaceutical drugs such as benzodiazepines and derivatives (zolpidem, zopiclone or zaleplon), which are involved in more than 60% of the cases of DFC (see Chapter 2), the most frequently used being clonazepam (26%), zolpidem (16%) and bromazepam (15%), sedatives like histamine antagonists (8.2%), neuroleptics (3.9%) or anesthetics (GHB and ketamine, together accounting for 2.8% of the cases). These drugs are used in DFC due to their pharmacodynamic properties. Pharmacokinetic properties are also important to the toxicologist, since they determine which compound has to be searched for and for how long it remains in the biological sample after administration.

1. BENZODIAZEPINES

1.1 Pharmacological Properties

The benzodiazepines typically share various activities like hypnotic, anxiolytic, skeletal muscle relaxant and anticonvulsant activity, and since their efficiency and tolerability are generally good, they are extensively used for hypnotic, antianxiety, anticonvulsant and myorelaxant treatments and as anesthetics. The use of the different marketed benzodiazepines according to their main pharmacodynamic properties is shown in Table 3.1.

The mechanism of action of all the benzodiazepines remains unclear; however, it has been shown that benzodiazepines facilitate gamma-aminobutyric acid (GABA)-mediated neurotransmission in the brain.[1] Benzodiazepines most likely facilitate the inhibitory presynaptic and/or postsynaptic reactions of GABA via an allosteric mechanism on the GABA receptor complex by changing the kinetics of the opening and closing of the

Toxicological Aspects of Drug-Facilitated Crimes. DOI: http://dx.doi.org/10.1016/B978-0-12-416748-3.00003-7

TABLE 3.1 Indications of Benzodiazepines According to their Main Pharmacodynamic Activity

Compound	Trade Name	Forms	Hypnotic	Antianxiety	Anticonvulsant	Anesthetic Adjunct	Skeletal Muscle Relaxant
Alprazolam	Xanax Niravam	VO		x			
Bromazepam	Lexomil Lectopam Lexotan	VO	x	x			
Chlordiazepoxide	Librax Librium	VO IM		x			
Clobazam	Urbanyl Frisium	VO	x	x	x		
Clonazepam	Rivotril Clonopin	VO Inj		x	x x		
Clotiazepam	Veratran	VO	x				
Diazepam	Valium Diazemuls Valrelease	VO Rectal Inj		x	x x x	x	x
Estazolam	Nuctalon Prosom	VO	x				

Flunitrazepam	Rohypnol	VO	x		
		IM	x		x
		Rectal	x		x
		Sublingual			
Flurazepam	Dalmadorm Dalmane	VO	x		
Loflazepate	Victan	VO	x		
Loprazolam	Havlane Dormonoct Somnovit	VO	x		
Lorazepam	Temesta Ativan	VO	x		x
		Inj		x	
Lormetazepam	Noctamide Loramet Minias N-methyllorazepam	VO	x	x	
Medazepam	Nobrium	VO	x		
Midazolam	Buccolam Dormicum Hypnovel versed	VO	x		x
		Inj			

(Continued)

TABLE 3.1 (Continued)

Compound	Trade Name	Forms	Hypnotic	Antianxiety	Anticonvulsant	Anesthetic Adjunct	Skeletal Muscle Relaxant
Nitrazepam	Mogadon Somnite	VO	x	x	x		
Nordiazepam	Nordaz Calmday Madar Stilny Vegesan	VO		x			
Oxazepam	Seresta Serax Seraprax Sobril	VO		x			
Prazepam	Lysanxia Centrax Verstran	VO		x			
Temazepam	Normison Methyloxazepam Euhypnos Restoril	VO Rectal	x	x			

Tetrazepam	Myolastan Epsipam Megavix Musaril Panos	VO		x
Triazolam	Halcion Novodorm Trilam	VO	x	
Zaleplon	Sonata Zerene Starnoc Andante	VO	Sublingual	x
Zolpidem	Stilnox Ambien Edluar Stilnoct	VO	Sublingual	x
Zopiclone	Imovane Noctirex Ximovane Zimovane	VO	Sublingual	x

GABA-activated chloride ion channels, but not their conductants.[2] The regional distribution of benzodiazepine receptors parallels that of GABA receptors in the brain, suggesting interaction. Benzodiazepines do not alter the synthesis, release, reuptake or enzymatic degradation of GABA.[3]

Increased GABA activity can explain most of the pharmacologic effects of benzodiazepines. Increased presynaptic inhibition at the spinal level may be one site of skeletal muscle relaxation. They also appear to have a direct peripheral action on the contractile process of muscle. Enhancement of GABA activity in the limbic area and mesencephalic reticular formation may be responsible for anticonvulsant properties. Finally, it seems that an endogenous protein ligand exists which normally binds to the benzodiazepine receptor producing anxiety. This endogenous ligand may also serve as a natural inhibitor for the regulatory site of GABA receptors. When benzodiazepines occupy the sites, the affinity of GABA receptors is increased. When the natural ligand occupies the site, GABA affinity is decreased.[4]

Pharmacologically, zolpidem, zaleplon and zopiclone bind to the omega-1 subclass of benzodiazepine receptors in the brain without binding to peripheral benzodiazepine receptors. This has been corroborated by the observation that these compounds have little or no muscle relaxant properties.[5]

The most frequent adverse effect occurring in at least 30% of patients is drowsiness. Memory impairment, loss of insight and transient euphoria are also common. These effects are one of the reasons why benzodiazepines are the most commonly used compounds in DFC. Moreover, in DFC, benzodiazepines are frequently dissimulated in an alcoholic drink, and it has been shown that memory deficits are more important when benzodiazepine and alcohol were associated.[6] Paradoxical reactions such as irritability or aggressive behavior have been documented[7] and appear to occur more often in patients with a history of impulsiveness or with a personality disorder.[8] However, aggressive reactions to benzodiazepines are rare, and may occur with a rate of 0.3% to 0.7%.[8]

1.2 Pharmacokinetics (PK) Aspects

The main PK parameters sought in DFC are described for each benzodiazepine in Table 3.2.[9−11]

Benzodiazepines generally present a good and rapid absorption. They are metabolized by oxidation via CYP3A alone or with CYP2C19 (clobazam and diazepam), or via glucuronidation (lorazepam, oxazepam, temazepam). Metabolism varies considerably between individuals, and inter-subject variation in concentration of both parent compounds and metabolites (actives or inactives) is common. Unchanged drugs are generally not found or are at very low concentration in urine, and many metabolites are conjugated. For these reasons, urine samples may be hydrolyzed with glucuronidase prior to

TABLE 3.2 Main Pharmacokinetic Parameters of Benzodiazepines Helpful in Drug-Facilitated Crimes[9–11]

Compound	Bioavailability	Metabolites and Urinary Excretion %	Peak Time	Half-Life $T_{1/2}$	Mean Peak Blood Concentration (after single dose)
Alprazolam	Oral: readily absorbed Oral: extended-release tablets: 90%	80% excreted in urine in 72 h as unchanged drug (10–20%) and metabolites, alpha-hydroxy-alprazolam, (active), 17%	Oral: disintegrating tablet: 1.5–2.5 h Oral: extended-release tablet: 5–11 h	Normal subjects: 10.6–12.5 h Elderly subjects: 16.3 h liver disease: 19.7 h Obese subjects: 21.8 h	10–30 µg/L (1 mg) Plasma levels are proportionate to the dose given
Bromazepam	Oral: solution or capsule: 84%	70% excreted in 72 h in urine, 2 to 3% excreted as unchanged drug, 27% as glucuronide of OH-bromazepam	1–2 h	8–20 h	10 µg/L (3 mg) 80 µg/L (6 mg) 100–170 µg/L (12 mg)
Chlordiazepoxide	VO: nearly complete IM: poor and slowly absorbed	Desmethyl-chlordiazepoxide, demoxepam, norcazepam and oxazepam all actives 60% excreted in urine: 1% unchanged, 6% demoxepam	1–2 h	Chlordiazepoxide: 10–30 h Demoxepam: 14–95 h	700–1200 µg/L (20 mg) 1600 µg/L (30 mg)
Clobazam	Oral: 90%	Clobazam metabolized in the liver primarily via N-demethylation by CYP3A4 to the	Tablets: 0.5–4 h, suspension: 0.5–2 h	Clobazam 10–50 h (mean = 25 h) N-desmethylclobazam 30–80 h (mean = 40 h)	173 µg/L clobazam and 27 µg/L for desmethylclobazam (10 mg)

(*Continued*)

TABLE 3.2 (Continued)

Compound	Bioavailability	Metabolites and Urinary Excretion %	Peak Time	Half-Life T$_{1/2}$	Mean Peak Blood Concentration (after single dose)
		active metabolite N-desmethylclobazam; 90% excreted in urine in 17 days, 5% as unchanged drug			730 µg/L clobazam (40 mg)
Clonazepam	90–100%	Extensive metabolism in 7-amino clonazepam (CYP3A4); 49–69% excreted in urine in 8 days, mainly as free and conjugated 7-aminoclonazepam, 0.5% as unchanged drug	Oral: 1–4 h Rectal, 10–30 min	20–60 h Serum half-lives ranged from 22 to 33 h (mean 28.7 h) in children	15 µg/L clonazepam, VO and 27 µg/L, IV (2 mg). Similar for 7-aminoclonazepam
Clotiazepam	–	Metabolites: Hydroxyclotiazepam (active) Desmethylclotiazepam (active)	Oral: tablets and drops: 0.6–1.5 h	4.6–10 h	100–160 µg/L (5 mg)
Diazepam	Oral: slow release: 98%	Metabolites: Nordiazepam, active N-methyloxazepam (temazepam), active. Both are converted to oxazepam which is then conjugated	Oral: immediate release: 0.5–1.3 h Oral, slow release: 3.8 h IM: 1 h Rectal: 1.5 h	Diazepam, 20 to 40 h Increases with age to 79 h (37–169 h) In newborn infants, diazepam more slowly metabolized to nordiazepam with a prolonged half-life of	140–190 µg/L for diazepam, 29 µg/L for nordiazepam (10 mg)

	IV, emulsion: 8 min	with glucuronic acid before excretion 75% eliminated in urine, primarily oxazepam glucuronide (33%) and 20% as conjugates of nordiazepam and temazepam; unchanged drug not detected	22–54 h and minimally if at all, hydroxylated to oxazepam Nordiazepam, 40–100 h In obese patients, markedly delayed (95 h as compared to 40 h in controls) and until 182 h for nordiazepam	
Estazolam	Oral: rapid (20 min)	87% of a dose is excreted renally in 5 days as 4-hydroxyestazolam and 1-oxo-estazolam; unchanged drug <4%	Oral: 2 h	10–30 h	55 μg/L (42–70 μg/L) (1 mg); 98 μg/L (75–137 μg/L) (2 mg); 121 μg/L (4 mg)
Flunitrazepam	Intramuscular, sublingual, conventional tablet: well absorbed Oral: 80% to 90% Rectal: 50%	87% of the dose excreted in urine in 7 days as metabolites (>11 identified): 7-amino Flu (10%), active; 3-hydroxy Flu (4%); unchanged drug: <0.2%	Oral: 1–2 h Intramuscular: 30–45 min	10–35 h	0.5–3.0 μg/L for Flu and 50–500 μg/L for 7-amino Flu (2 mg)
Flurazepam	Oral: capsule: rapidly absorbed	60–90% of the dose excreted in urine in 48 h: N-1-hydroxy-ethylflurazepam, active 29–55% (as conjugate);	Oral: 30–60 min; N-1-hydroxy-ethylflurazepam, 1 h	1–3 h; N-1-hydroxy-ethylflurazepam, 16 h; N-1-desalkylflurazepam, 47–100 h	<2 μg/L; N-1-hydroxy-ethylflurazepam, 6 μg/L;

(Continued)

TABLE 3.2 (Continued)

Compound	Bioavailability	Metabolites and Urinary Excretion %	Peak Time	Half-Life T$_{1/2}$	Mean Peak Blood Concentration (after single dose)
		N-1-desalkylflurazepam, active; unchanged drug: trace amount	N-1-desalkyl-flurazepam, 12 h		N-1-desalkylflurazepam, 18 µg/L (15 mg); 2.1 µg/L; N-1-hydroxy-ethylflurazepam, 18 µg/L; N-1-desalkylflurazepam, 23 µg/L (30 mg)
Loflazepate ethyl	Parent drug undergoes an important first-pass effect	Metabolized to descarboxyloflazepate, which is the active metabolite, and loflazepate; 63% excreted in urine as loflazepate, 3-hydroxyloflazepate, 3-hydroxy-descarboxyloflazepate	1.5 h	77 h	40–65 µg/L loflazepate (2 mg)
Loprazolam	Oral: tablet: 80% Food significantly reduces the rate of absorption, time to peak concentration, and peak plasma concentration of loprazolam	39% excreted in urine in 2 weeks: Loprazolam-N-oxide (18%), unchanged drug <1%	Oral: tablet: 1.6–5.5 h	Loprazolam: 12 h (3.3–19.8 h) and 16 h in elderly Loprazolam-N-oxide: 11.6–16.7 h	6 µg/L (1 mg) 11 µg/L (2 mg)

Lorazepam	Oral: 90% to 93% Intramuscular: 83% to 100%	90% eliminated in 5 days, 75% as lorazepam glucuronide, inactive and 14% as conjugates of minor metabolites; unchanged drug <1%	Oral: 2 h (0.5–3 h) Intramuscular: 1–3 h Sublingual: 1 h	Lorazepam: 12 h. In newborn infants, 3 to 4 times that of adults Pediatrics: 16.8 h Lorazepam glucuronide: 16 h	18 µg/L (2 mg)
Lormetazepam	Oral: 80%	86% eliminated in urine in 7 days, as lormetazepam glucuronide (70%), lorazepam glucuronide (6%), and unchanged drug (<1%)	Oral: 2 h	10 h (7–17 h) In elderly patients, seems to be increased to about 20 h Lormetazepam glucuronide, 13 h	5.6 µg/L (1 mg) and 7.0 in elderly patients 16 µg/L (2 mg)
Medazepam	Oral: 49% to 76%	Metabolized in diazepam, active; then in nordiazepam (major compound) and oxazepam; also normedazepam 55–75% excreted in urine over 8 days, primarily as oxazepam glucuronide	Oral: 1–2 h	1–2 h for medazepam; nordiazepam, 40–100 h	140–260 µg/L medazepam (10 mg) 520 µg/L medazepam, diazepam and nordiazepam not detected (20 mg); 980 µg/L medazepam, 30 µg/ L diazepam (50 mg)
Midazolam	Oral: 36–50% Intranasal: 50% Rectal: 52% Buccal: 74.5% IM: 90% A standard meal resulted in a slower	1-hydroxy-midazolam, major and active, 4-hydroxy-midazolam, 1,4-dihydroxy-midazolam 45% to 57% excreted in urine, mainly as glucuronides of the	Oral: 20–50 min; oral syrup in children 6 months–15 years old: 0.17–2.65 h	1–2 h; pediatric patients (6 months–15 years): 2.9–4.5 h Prolonged in the elderly (5.6 h), obese subjects, cardiac surgery patients	8.7 µg/L midazolam, 5.0 1-hydroxy-midazolam (2 mg) 69 µg/L (men) and 53 µg/L (women) midazolam (10 mg)

(Continued)

TABLE 3.2 (Continued)

Compound	Bioavailability	Metabolites and Urinary Excretion %	Peak Time	Half-Life T$_{1/2}$	Mean Peak Blood Concentration (after single dose)
	rate of oral midazolam absorption and a small reduction in the extent of absorption	metabolites; unchanged drug <1%	Intramuscular: 45 min Rectal: 20–50 min Buccal: 30 min Intranasal: 25 min; 1-hydroxy-midazolam 30 min	(10 h), critically ill patients (7.6 h), and patients with liver disease (7.4 h in cirrhotic) or conditions which may diminish cardiac output and hepatic blood flow Alpha-hydroxy-midazolam, 1 h	Elderly: 85 μg/L (men) and 96 μg/L (women) (10 mg)
Nitrazepam	Oral: 53% to 97%	7-aminonitrazepam, inactive; 7-acetamidonitrazepam, inactive 50% to 70% excreted in urine in 5 days, mainly as free and conjugated 7-aminonitrazepam (31%), free and conjugated 7-acetamidonitrazepam (21%); unchanged drug: 1%	Oral: 1–2 h	18–38 h (mean 28 h)	35 μg/L (25–50 μg/L) (5 mg) 84 μg/L (10 mg)
Nordazepam	Oral: 50%	Hydroxylation to oxazepam, which is conjugated with glucuronic acid Excreted in urine as oxazepam glucuronide; unchanged drug: 1%	2–4 h	40–100 h Prolonged in elderly and in patients with liver disease	118 μg/L (5 mg) 228 μg/L (10 mg)

Drug	Absorption	Metabolism/Excretion	Time to peak	Half-life	Concentrations
Oxazepam	Oral: 93%	50% excreted in urine in 48 h, as oxazepam glucuronide, inactive, 90% and trace of unchanged drug	Oral: 1–3 h	4–15 h (mean 8 h)	310 µg/L (15 mg); 520 µg/L (30 mg); 1060 µg/L (45 mg)
Prazepam		Nordazepam (active); 3-hydroxyprazepam (inactive), oxazepam (active) 38% excreted in urine in 48 h and 60% after 7 days, primarily as oxazepam glucuronide (30–60%) and 3-hydroxyprazepam glucuronide (3–35%); unchanged drug and nordazepam not found	Oral: 30 min for prazepam, 4–13 h for nordazepam	1.3 h for prazepam, 40–100 h for nordazepam	Prazepam not detected, nordazepam 138 µg/L (20 mg); 7 µg/L prazepam, 321 µg/L nordazepam (30 mg); 218 µg/L nordazepam (40 mg)
Temazepam	Oral: well absorbed Rectal: 60% to 90%	Inactive metabolites 80% to 90% excreted in urine as conjugated temazepam (73%) and free (1%), conjugated oxazepam (6%), unchanged drug (1–2%)	Oral, 0.3–1.4 h	3–15 h (mean 7–8 h)	205–430 µg/L (10 mg); 363–856 µg/L (20 mg); 873 µg/L (30 mg)
Tetrazepam	Oral tetrazepam is rapidly and completely absorbed (90% to 100%)	Metabolites: Nortetrazepam, active; 3-hydroxytetrazepam, active; 3-hydroxy-nortetrazepam, diazepam and nordazepam	Oral: 0.5–2 h, nortetrazepam, 4 h	13–45 h Nortetrazepam, 25–51 h	512 (men) and 558 (women) µg/L for tetrazepam, 6.0 (men) and

(Continued)

TABLE 3.2 (Continued)

Compound	Bioavailability	Metabolites and Urinary Excretion %	Peak Time	Half-Life T$_{1/2}$	Mean Peak Blood Concentration (after single dose)
		57% excreted in urine in 3 days, largely as hydroxylated and conjugated metabolites; unchanged drug: 2%			7.2 (women) µg/L for nortetrazepam (50 mg)
Triazolam	Oral: rapid and complete Sublingual: well absorbed	1-hydroxy-methyl-triazolam (or α-hydroxy-triazolam), active; 4-hydroxy-triazolam 80% excreted in urine in 48 h, as conjugated 1-hydroxy-methyl-triazolam (44%) and free (0.5%); unchanged drug: trace	0.5–3 h 0.7–2.5 h for α-hydroxy-triazolam 1.5–5 h for 4-hydroxy-triazolam	1.5–3 h 1-hydroxy-methyl-triazolam, 3.9 h 4-hydroxy-triazolam, 3.8 h	3.0 µg/L (2.3–3.7 µg/L) (0.25 mg); 4.4 µg/L (1.7–9.4 µg/L) (0.50 mg) 2.3 µg/L (0.25 mg sublingual) 8.7 µg/L triazolam, 6.1 µg/L for α-hydroxy-triazolam, 6.1 µg/L for 4-hydroxy-triazolam (0.88 mg)
Zaleplon	Oral: 30% Food prolongs absorption	5-oxo-zaleplon, inactive Desethylzaleplon, inactive conversion to this metabolite appears minimal: 5-oxo-N-desethylzaleplon, inactive Glucuronides, inactive	Oral: 1 hour	1 h	15 µg/L (5 mg) 26 µg/L (10 mg) 49 µg/L (20 mg)

	71% excreted in urine in 5 days, as conjugated and free 5-oxo-zaleplon (major compound) and N-desethylzaleplon; unchanged drug: <0.1%				
Zolpidem	Oral: tablets: 70%	Zolpidem is metabolized to inactive metabolites which are mostly excreted renally 48–67% excreted in urine in 4 days, as metabolite I (33–48%) and metabolite II (6–10%); unchanged drug: around 10%	Extended-release tablets oral, healthy male subjects: 1.5 h Oral: elderly subjects: 2 h Immediate-release tablets oral, healthy male subjects: 1.6 h Oral: elderly subjects: 2.9 h Sublingual tablets 35–75 min Oral spray: 0.9 h	Extended-release tablets oral, healthy male subjects: 2.8 h elderly subjects: 2.9 h Immediate-release tablets, healthy male subjects: 1.7–2.6 h, elderly subjects: 2.9 h Cirrhotic patients: 9.9 h End-stage renal failure patients on hemodialysis: 2.5 h	Extended-release tablets Oral, single-dose, healthy male subjects: 134 µg/L Oral, female subjects: 50% greater than males (12.5 mg) Immediate-release tablets Oral, single-dose, healthy male subjects: 59 µg/L (5 mg); 121 µg/L (10 mg) Oral spray, single-dose, healthy subjects: 114 µg/L (5 mg); 210 µg/L (10 mg)

(Continued)

TABLE 3.2 (Continued)

Compound	Bioavailability	Metabolites and Urinary Excretion %	Peak Time	Half-Life $T_{1/2}$	Mean Peak Blood Concentration (after single dose)
Zopiclone	80% rapidly absorbed from the gastrointestinal tract	At least 13 metabolites, all inactives, two majors: zopiclone-N-oxide (11% to 15% of a dose) and N-desmethyl zopiclone (15% to 20%) 84% excreted in urine in 24 h, zopiclone-N-oxide: 11%, N-desmethyl zopiclone: 15%, and unchanged drug: 4% to 5%	Oral: tablet: 1–1.5 h	3.5–6.5 h, increased by 59% in elderly subjects, and by 65% in patients with hepatic disease Zopiclone-N-oxide, 3.5–6 h N-desmethyl-zopiclone, 7–11 h	76 µg/L (7.5 mg) 131 µg/L (15 mg)

(according to 9–11)

analysis and the toxicologist may search preferentially for the metabolite of the benzodiazepine rather than for the parent drug.

2. GHB: GAMMA-HYDROXYBUTYRATE, SODIUM OXYBATE, 4-HYDROXYBUTYRATE, XYREM

2.1 Pharmacological Properties[9]

Sodium oxybate is the sodium salt of gamma-hydroxybutyrate (GHB), an endogenous compound present in most mammalian tissues at nanomolar concentration, and a metabolite of the neurotransmitter GABA.

It is a central nervous system (CNS) depressant. It binds to GABA-B receptors and to specific receptors. At low doses, it leads to a reduction in dopaminergic activity in the basal ganglia and, at high doses, it can stimulate dopamine release; it also interacts with other central mediators such as serotonin, opiates and cholinergic pathways.

Sodium oxybate may produce anesthesia by a general suppressant action on the entire cerebrospinal axis, and muscular relaxation by an action on the spinal cord.

The effects are dose dependent: oral or intravenous doses of 10 mg/kg cause amnesia and hypotonia; doses of 20–30 mg/kg are sleep inducing and doses of 50 mg/kg or higher produce anesthesia.

It is indicated for the treatment of excessive daytime sleepiness in patients with narcolepsy. It is effective for inducing or maintaining general anesthesia in surgical procedures in combination with barbiturates and opiates. It is also indicated in order to ease alcohol withdrawal.[12]

The most frequently reported adverse effect is transient vertigo. Short-term amnesia has been associated with ingestion of sodium oxybate, which makes this compound interesting for use in DFC. Confusion was reported in 3% of patients receiving sodium oxybate for narcolepsy, dizziness in 9%, somnolence in 1% and tremor in 2%.

Agitation, anxiety, paranoia, hallucinations, panic attack, psychosis and sleepwalking have already been reported in patients receiving sodium oxybate. In large doses it can cause disorientation, nausea and vomiting, and muscle spasms.

It is also used as a party drug, since it causes alcohol-like effects and aroused sexuality. It has been marketed illicitly at gymnasiums and health food stores, where it was promoted as a steroid alternative for bodybuilding and as a tryptophan replacement for weight control and sedation. Several biological precursors to GHB such as gamma-butyrolactone (GBL) and 1,4-butanediol have also been employed as substances of abuse.

It is important to note for the toxicologist that several fermented products such as beer, wine and vinegar often contain trace amounts of sodium oxybate, which may account for 1 to 20 mg/L of GHB.

2.2 Pharmacokinetics (PK) Aspects

Absorption: GHB is readily absorbed after oral administration with an oral bioavailability around 27%.[13] The time to peak concentration after oral administration is 25 minutes to 2 hours. It is rapidly metabolized in the liver by gamma-hydroxybutyrate dehydrogenase to succinic acid in a capacity-limited process or by beta-oxidation with subsequent metabolism to carbon dioxide in the Krebs cycle eliminated by expiration.[15] Less than 5% of an oral dose is eliminated unchanged in urine in 6 to 8 hours, with no drug detectable after 12 hours. Endogenous urine GHB concentrations in healthy adults have been shown to range from 0.1 to 6.6 mg/L,[14] and 4 mg/L in ante-mortem plasma. The terminal half-life of GHB is 20 minutes to 1 hour.

After a single 25 mg/kg (1.75 g/70 kg) oral dose in eight adult subjects the average peak plasma concentration was 80 mg/L at 0.5 hour.[15] A single 75 mg/kg (5.25 g/70 kg) oral dose to four adults produced a peak plasma concentration of 90 mg/L at 2 hours, decreasing to 6 mg/L after 6 hours.[16]

An intravenous dose of 50 mg/kg (3.5 g/70 kg) in one adult produced a peak plasma concentration of 170 mg/L within 15 minutes.[17]

There is a good correlation of blood levels of GHB with the state of consciousness of the patient since a blood concentration under 52 mg/L is associated with wakefulness, a concentration between 52 and 156 mg/L with light sleep, a concentration between 156 and 260 mg/L with moderate sleep, and a concentration more than 260 mg/L with deep sleep.[17]

After a single 25 mg/kg (1.75 g/70 kg) oral dose of 1,4-butanediol in eight healthy adults, peak plasma concentrations of 1,4-butanediol and GHB were 3.8 mg/L and 46 mg/L, achieved after 24 and 42 minutes, with elimination half-lives of 42 and 30 minutes, respectively.[18]

3. BARBITURATES[19–33]

Until the 1960 s, barbiturates formed the largest group of hypnotics and sedatives in clinical use. They can produce all degrees of depression of the CNS from reduction of anxiety at low doses, sedation, unconsciousness and general anesthesia (high doses) to death by respiratory and cardiovascular failure (overdose). They are actually used in anesthesia and treatment of epilepsy. They are extensively used as sedative and hypnotics drugs but it is no longer recommended because they are less safe than benzodiazepines.[19]

However, several compounds are still commercialized worldwide (Table 3.3).

3.1 Pharmacological Properties

Barbiturates reversibly depress activities of excitable tissues: CNS, cardio-vascular system and respiration:

- **Actions on the CNS** (depending on the doses used): non-anesthetic doses preferentially suppress synaptic transmission. The site of inhibition is

TABLE 3.3 Main Indications of Barbiturates

Compound	Trade Name	Forms	Use in Insomnia	Use in Anesthesia	Use in Pre-op Sedation	Use in Seizures
Amobarbital	Amytal Amylobarbitone	VO IM-IV	X		X X	X X
Butabarbital	Butisol Secbutabarbitone	VO	X		X	
Butalbital	Allylbarbital Allylbarbitone Itobarbital Sandoptal Fiorinal	VO			X (analgesic-sedative mixture with aspirin, acetaminophen)	
Mephobarbital	Mebara N-methyl-phenobarbital	VO	X			X
Methohexital	Brevital Methohexitone	IV		X		
Pentobarbital	Nembutal Pentobarbitone	VO-Rectal-IM-IV	X		X	X
Phenobarbital	Luminal Gardenal Phenobarbitone	VO-IM-IV	X			X
Secobarbital	Seconal Quinalbarbitone	VO	X			
Thiopental	Pentothal Thiopentone	IV	X	X	X	X

either pre-synaptic in the spinal cord or post-synaptic in cortical and cere-bellar pyramidal cells, in thalamic relay neurons, cuneate nucleus and substantia nigra. They act partly by enhancing action of the inhibitory neurotransmitter GABA, but they are less specific than benzodiazepines. They bind a different site on the GABA-a chloride receptor. The barbitu-rates may have euphoriant effects. Like other CNS drugs, they are abused and some people can develop dependence and tolerance.

- **Actions on the cardiovascular system:** significant cardiovascular effects occur during overdose. Blood pressure falls because of the action on medullar vasomotor centers. Depression of cardiac contractility and sym-pathetic ganglia also contributes.

- **Actions on respiration:** barbiturates depress both respiratory drive and the mechanisms responsible for the rhythmic character of respiration.

3.2 Pharmacokinetics (PK) Aspects

Absorption: Like benzodiazepines, the selection of a particular barbiturate in therapeutic use is based on pharmacokinetics properties and on dosage form.

For sedative and hypnotic use, barbiturates usually are administered orally. Barbiturates are highly lipid soluble and permit a rapid and complete absorption. Delay for action depends on formulations and is delayed by the presence of food in the stomach.

The intravenous route usually is reserved for the management of status epilepticus and for induction and maintenance of general anesthesia.

Distribution: Redistribution after intravenous injection is important. Uptake into less vascular tissues, especially muscle and fat, leads to a decline in the concentration of barbiturate in the plasma and brain.

Barbiturates cross the placenta.

Metabolism: Complete metabolism and/or conjugation of barbiturates occur in the liver. This phenomenon is reduced for less lipid soluble drugs like aprobarbital and phenobarbital.

Barbiturates strongly induce the synthesis of hepatic cytochrome P-450 (1A2-2C9-2C19-3A4) and conjugating enzymes, thus increasing the rate of metabolic degradation of many drugs and giving rise to a number of poten-tially harmful drug interactions. These effects vary with the duration of expo-sure to the barbiturate, thus facilitating their own metabolism.

The plasma half-life is described for each drug in Table 3.4.

The metabolism of barbiturates is more rapid in young people than in infants and the elderly. Chronic liver disease like cirrhosis often increases the $T_{1/2}$ of the biotransformable barbiturates.

Because of enzyme induction, barbiturates are potentially dangerous for persons suffering from porphyria.

TABLE 3.4 Main Pharmacokinetic Parameters of Barbiturates Helpful in Drug-Facilitated Crimes 9–11

Compound	Bioavailability	Urinary Excretion %	Peak Time	Half-Life T$_{1/2}$	Mean Peak Blood Concentration (after single dose)
Amobarbital	94%	92% excreted in urine in 6 days as 3-hydroxyamobarbital, active (30–50%) and N-glucosylamobarbital (29%); unchanged drug: 1–3%	2 h	8–42 h, dose dependent	1.8 mg/L (120 mg) 3-hydroxyamobarbital < 0.5 mg/L
Butabarbital	–	50% excreted in urine in 9 days as 2-carboxy-butabarbital (24–34%), 2-hydroxybutabarbital (2–3%); unchanged drug (5–9%)	0.5–2 h	34–42 h	2 mg/L (600 mg in 3 h)
Butalbital	–	92% excreted in urine in several metabolites; unchanged drugs: 3.6%	2 h	35–88 h (mean 61 h)	2.1 mg/L (100 mg)
Mephobarbital	About 75% of a single oral dose of mephobarbital is converted to phenobarbital in 24 hours	Excreted in urine as phenobarbital (15%); conjugated p-hydroxy-mephobarbital (35%); conjugated p-hydroxy-phenobarbital (1%); unchanged drug: <1%	2–8 h; Phenobarbital, 144 h	48–52 h; Phenobarbital, 80–120 h	2.5–3.5 mg/L (800 mg) phenobarbital 1.5–3.0 mg/L
Methohexital	IV administration Rectal: 1%	Less than 1% excreted unchanged in the urine in 24 h	IV: 3 min min	1.2–2.1 h	Anesthesia, IV: 3.9–8.6 mg/L (1.5–2.0 mg/kg)

(Continued)

TABLE 3.4 (Continued)

Compound	Bioavailability	Urinary Excretion %	Peak Time	Half-Life $T_{1/2}$	Mean Peak Blood Concentration (after single dose)
Pentobarbital	IV administration Oral: 100%	86% excreted in urine in 6 days as 3-hydroxy-pentobarbital (73%), N-hydroxy-pentobarbital (3%); unchanged drug: 1%	IV: 5 min VO: 0.5–2 h	15–48 h (mean: 20–30 h)	3 mg/L (100 mg IV) 1.2–3.1 mg/L (100 mg VO) 3.0 mg/L (600 mg in 3 h VO)
Phenobarbital	83%	78–87% excreted in urine in 16 days as N-glucosyl-phenobarbital (24–30%), p-hydroxyphenobarbital free and conjugated (18–19%); unchanged drug: 25–33%	2–4 h	50–140 h for adult 40–70 h for child	0.7 mg/L (30 mg) 3.1 mg/L (100 mg) 5.5 mg/L (3 mg/kg, 210 mg) 18 mg/L (600 mg) 6.2 mg/L (3 mg/kg, 30 min IV)
Secobarbital	Sodium secobarbital is well absorbed The free acid is absorbed less readily	50% excreted in urine in 2 days as secodiol and 3-hydroxy-secobarbital (50%); unchanged drug: 5%	3 h	22–29 h	2.0 mg/L (3.3 mg/kg, 231 mg) 4.3 mg/L (600 mg in 3 h VO)
Thiopental	IV administration Rectal absorption of thiopental is variable and not routinely administered via this route	Not well investigated Excreted in urine as a carboxylic acid compound (10–25%) Lesser amount transformed in pentobarbital; unchanged drug: 0.3%	—	3–18 h for adult; in neonates, proximately 15 h, which is twice as long as that in mothers	28 mg/L (400 mg IV in 2 min)

Elimination: Renal excretion is preceded by metabolism and/or conjugation for most drugs. About 25% of phenobarbital and nearly 100% of aprobarbital are excreted unchanged in the urine. The renal excretion can be increased by osmotic diuresis and urine alkalinization.

Table 3.4 summarizes specific PK parameters.

3.3 PK/PD Relationship

None of the barbiturates used for hypnosis appears to have a $T_{1/2}$ that is short enough for elimination to be virtually complete in 24 hours. For this reason, they are easy to detect in serum and urine.

Pharmacodynamic and pharmacokinetic tolerance to barbiturates can occur.

4. H1 ANTAGONISTS[34−41]

In this paragraph, we only expose the first generation H1 antagonists, which can depress CNS and be used in DFC.

4.1 Pharmacological Properties

The antihistamine, sedative and antiemetic effects of H1 antagonists come from their H1-receptor blocking properties, which make their effects easy to predict (Table 3.5).

H1-receptor antagonists inhibit most of the effects of histamine on smooth muscles, especially the constriction of respiratory smooth muscle.

H1-receptor antagonists affect various inflammatory and allergic mechanisms. They are indicated for various types of allergic reactions, and as an adjunctive therapy for anaphylactic reactions.

They are also used to relieve preoperative anxiety and tension, facilitate sleep, and reduce postoperative nausea and vomiting.

Some drugs are fairly strong sedatives and may be used for this action in the short-term treatment of insomnia.

Many of the first generation H1 antagonists tend to inhibit response to acetylcholine that is mediated by muscarinic receptors. Therefore they also can be indicated for the active and prophylactic treatment of motion sickness.

Central depression usually occurs with therapeutic doses of older drugs, which diminish alertness, slow reaction times and induce somnolence. The ethanolamines (diphenhydramine) are especially prone to induce sedation.

Poisoning is common but rarely severe and may occur via oral, parenteral or dermal (patches or cream) routes.

TABLE 3.5 Main Indications of H1 Antagonists

Compound	Trade Name	Chemical Class	Forms	Insomnia	Pain, Adjunction in Anesthesia, Pre-Op Sedation, Post-Operative Nausea and Vomiting	Inflammation Allergy	Motion Sickness
Alimemazine or trimeprazine	Methyl-promazine Temaril Theralene Vallergan	Phenothiazines	VO: solid and liquid	X		X	
Brompheniramine	Bromphed Dimetane Puretane	Alkylamines	VO: solid and liquid IV			X	
Carbinoxamine	Rondex Ciberon Polistin Tussafed	Ethanolamines	VO: solid and liquid			X	
Chlorpheniramine	Chlor-trimeton Chlorphenamine Piriton	Alkylamines	VO: solid and liquid IV			X	
Clemastine	Tavist Meclastine Clastinol	Ethanolamines	VO: solid and liquid			X	

Drug	Brand names	Class	Route/Form			
Cyclizine	Marezine, Valoid, Diconal, Migril	Piperazines	VO: solid, IV	X		X
Cyproheptadine	Periactin	Piperidines	VO: solid and liquid		X	
Dimenhydrinate	Dramamine	Ethanolamines	VO: solid and liquid, IV	X		X
Diphenhydramine	Benadryl, Nytol, Unisom, Panadol	Ethanolamines	VO: solid and liquid, IV		X	X
Doxylamine	Donormyl, Bencectin, Diclectin, Unisom	Ethanolamines	VO solid		X	X
Hydroxyzine	Atarax, Vistaril	Piperazines	VO: solid and liquid, IV		X	X

(Continued)

TABLE 3.5 (Continued)

Compound	Trade Name	Chemical Class	Forms	Insomnia	Pain, Adjunction in Anesthesia, Pre-Op Sedation, Post-Operative Nausea and Vomiting	Inflammation Allergy	Motion Sickness
Meclizine	Antivert Meclozine Bonamine Bonine	Piperazines	VO: solid		X		X
Niaprazine	Nopron	Piperazines		X in child			
Promethazine	Phenergan Remsed Zipan	Phenothiazines	VO: solid and liquid IV and rectal	X	X	X	X
Pyrilamine	Mepyramine Ryna 12	Ethylene-diamines	VO: solid and liquid	X	X	X	
Tripelennamine	PBZ Pyri-benzamine	Ethylene-diamines	VO: liquid		X	X	

4.2 Pharmacokinetics Aspects

Absorption: The H1 antagonists are well absorbed. Following oral administration, peak plasma concentrations are achieved in 2−3 hours and major effects usually last 4−6 hours. However, some drugs are much longer acting.

Distribution: The drugs are distributed widely throughout the body, including the CNS. The volume of distribution tends to be large. Most are highly protein bound.

Metabolism: H1-receptor antagonists also induce hepatic CYPs and thus facilitate their own metabolism.

Like other metabolized drugs, H1 antagonists are eliminated more rapidly by children than by adults and more slowly in those with severe renal disease.

Hydroxyzin is metabolized to an active drug, cetirizine.

Elimination: H1-receptor antagonists are excreted unchanged in the urine. Some drugs are excreted in the urine as inactive metabolites.

Table 3.6 summarizes specific PK parameters.

4.3 PK/PD Relationship

Some H1 antagonist drugs can be used in DFC. Indeed, they reduce alertness and induce somnolence. The ethanolamines are especially prone to induce sedation. They are available in liquid form and peak plasma concentrations are achieved in 2−3 hours.

5. ANTIPSYCHOTIC DRUGS[42−49]

Many antipsychotic drugs are available for clinical use, but with some exceptions, and differences between them are minor. They are effective in controlling symptoms of acute schizophrenia (large doses are necessary). Long-term antipsychotic treatment is also necessary in schizophrenia maintenance and the same drugs are used (depot preparations).

A distinction is drawn between the drugs that were originally developed (haloperidol, chlorpromazine), called *classical* or *typical* antipsychotic drugs, and more recently developed drugs like risperidone and clozapine, called *atypical* (Table 3.7).

5.1 Pharmacological Properties

All antipsychotic drugs are antagonists at dopamine D2 receptors but most also block other receptors like 5-HT2, histamine H1, muscarinic receptors and alpha-adrenoceptors. Clozapine also blocks dopaminergic D4 receptors. Activities on D2 receptors determine antipsychotic activity. Extrapyramidal

TABLE 3.6 Main Pharmacokinetic Parameters of H1 Antagonists Helpful in Drug-Facilitated Crimes[9–11]

Compound	Bioavailability	Urinary Excretion %	Peak Time	Half-Life T$_{1/2}$	Mean Peak Blood Concentration (After Single Dose)
Alimemazine (trimeprazine)	70%	70% excreted in urine in 5 days mostly as sulfoxide metabolites and glucuronides	Oral tablets: 4.5–6.0 h Oral syrup: 3.5 h	6–18 h	1.0 μg/L (5 mg) 2.0 μg/L (10 mg)
Brompheniramine	Absorption is rapid Bioavailability has not been determined	53% excreted in urine in 5 days as norbrompheniramine (11.5%), unchanged drug (10.5%), dinorbrompheniramine (9.9%)	2–5 h 3.2 in 14 pediatric patients after a single 4 mg dose of oral elixir	25 h; mean of 12.4 h in 14 pediatric patients	15 μg/L (8 mg)
Carbinoxamine	Oral: good	Carbinoxamine is excreted in the urine as inactive metabolites; unchanged drug not found	Oral: 1.5–2 h Extended-release suspension: 6.7 h	10–15 h	8.0 μg/L (4 mg)
Chlorpheniramine	41 ± 16%	34% excreted in urine in 48 h as norchlorpheniramine (2%), dinorchlorpheniramine (1%); unchanged drug (3%)	Oral: 2–3 h	12–43 h	3.0 μg/L (2 mg) 9.9 μg/L (8 mg) 17 μg/L (12 mg)
Clemastine	39%	42% excreted in urine in 72 h as inactive metabolites; unchanged drug not found or very low	4.8 h	10–32 h (mean 21 h)	0.6 μg/L (1 mg) 2.3 μg/L (4 mg)
Cyclizine	—	Norcyclizine, inactive; unchanged drug 0.5%	2 h	7–24 h (mean 14 h)	69–77 μg/L (50 mg)

Drug	Absorption	Metabolism/Excretion	Peak time	Half-life	Plasma concentration
Cyproheptadine	—	72% excreted in urine in 6 days. In the first 24 h, free unchanged drug 1% and conjugated 10%	4 h	8–9 h	30 µg/L after glucuronidase hydrolysis (8 mg)
Dimenhydrinate	Well absorbed	In fact, precursor of diphenhydramine		Unknown	—
Diphenhydramine	55%	Nordiphenhydramine and dinordiphenhydramine; 64% excreted in urine in 96 h, unchanged drug 1%, glucuronide 11%	Oral: 2–3 h Nordiphenhydramine: 3.9 h	4–8 h Elderly subject: 14 h	15 µg/L (12.7 mg) 66 µg/L and nordiphenhydramine: 17 µg/L (50 mg) 112 µg/L (100 mg)
Doxylamine	Oral: good	Little studied Excreted in urine as unchanged drug, nordoxylamine and dinordoxylamine	1–4 h	7–13 h Mean: 10.1 h	99 µg/L (25 mg)
Hydroxyzine	—	Cetirizine with antihistaminic activity but devoid of sedative properties Excretion not studied in humans; unchanged drug not found in urine	2–4 h Cetirizine: 4 h	13–27 h (mean 20 h) Cetirizine: 11 h Children: 1–3 h Elimination half-life increased with increasing age in children	43 µg/L (25 mg) 70 µg/L (0.7 mg/kg, 49 mg/70 kg) 78 µg/L (100 mg) Cetirizine: 5 times those of the parent drug
Meclizine	—	Not studied in humans	3 h	4–6 h	80 µg/L (25 mg)
Niaprazine	Oral: good and rapid	62% excreted in urine in 4 days mostly as metabolites and unchanged drug	1 h	—	—

(Continued)

TABLE 3.6 (Continued)

Compound	Bioavailability	Urinary Excretion %	Peak Time	Half-Life $T_{1/2}$	Mean Peak Blood Concentration (After Single Dose)
Promethazine	25% (extensive first-pass hepatic metabolism)	Excreted in the urine as metabolites: promethazine sulfoxide (10.3% in the first 24 h); unchanged drug: 0.6%	2–3 h; 3–16 h, mean 8.6 h rectal form; 2 h IM	16 h VO 18 h IM	11 µg/L (30 mg) 29 µg/L (50 mg) 20 µg/L (12 .5 mg, IV, 15 min post-injection)
Pyrilamine	Not established	Excreted in the urine as conjugated O-desmethylpyrilamine (48%); free 2%; unchanged drug not found	4 h	Not established	Not established
Trimeprazine (see alimemazine)					
Tripelennamine	–	Excreted in urine: tripelennamine-N-glucuronide (4.4%), conjugated hydroxy-tripelennamine (23%); unchanged drug: 1.2%	2–3 h; 0.25–0.5 h IM	2.9–5.3 h	60 µg/L (100 mg) 105 µg/L (50 mg IM) 199 µg/L (100 mg IM)

(according to 9–11)

TABLE 3.7 Indications of Antipsychotic Drugs

Compound	Trade Name	Chemical Class	Forms	Use	Sedation
Chlorpromazine *typical*	Largactil Thorazine	Phenothiazines	VO: solid and liquid IM	Acute psychosis Schizophrenia maintenance	++
Clozapine *atypical*	Leponex Cozaril	Dibenzodiazepines	VO	Psychosis	++
Cyamemazine	Cyamepromazine Tercian	Phenothiazines	VO: solid and liquid IM	Acute psychosis	++
Droperidol	Inapsine Droleptan	Butyrophenones	IM; IV	Neuroleptic, adjunct to general anesthesia	++
Flupenthixol	Fluanxol Depixol Emergil Metamin Viscoleo	Thioxanthenes	VO IM	Schizophrenia maintenance	+
Fluphenazine *typical*	Stelazine Permitil Prolixin	Phenothiazines	VO: solid and liquid IM	Acute psychosis Schizophrenia maintenance	++
Haloperidol *typical*	Prolixin Haldol Dozic	Butyrophenones	VO: solid and liquid IM	Acute psychosis Schizophrenia maintenance	+

(*Continued*)

TABLE 3.7 (Continued)

Compound	Trade Name	Chemical Class	Forms	Use	Sedation
Loxapine *typical*	Daxoline Loxitane Loxapac	Dibenzo-oxazepines	VO: solid and liquid IM	Acute psychosis Schizophrenia maintenance	+
Molindone *typical*	Moban Lidone	Phenothiazines	VO: solid and liquid	Acute psychosis Schizophrenia maintenance	+
Perphenazine *typical*	Trilafon Triavil	Phenothiazines	VO: solid and liquid IM	Acute psychosis Schizophrenia maintenance	+
Quetiapine *atypical*	Xeroquel Ketipinor Quepin Seroquel	Dibenzothiazepines	VO	Acute psychosis Schizophrenia maintenance	+ +
Risperidone *atypical*	Risperdal	Benzisoxazoles	IM VO	Acute psychosis Schizophrenia maintenance	+ +
Thioridazine *typical*	Mellaril Melleril	Piperidines	VO	Acute psychosis Schizophrenia maintenance	+ +
Trifluoperazine *typical*	Stelazine	Phenothiazines	VO: solid and liquid IM	Acute psychosis Schizophrenia maintenance	+

motor disturbances and endocrine perturbations (prolactin release) are due to dopamine D2 receptor block.

Other activities run parallel to the side-effect profile.

Sedation, which tends to decrease with continued use, occurs with many antipsychotic drugs. Antihistaminic H1 activity is a property of phenothiazines and contributes to their sedative and antiemetic profile. The sedation profile is described in Table 3.7.

Blocking muscarinic receptors produces a number of peripheral effects: dry mouth and dry eyes, blurring of vision, increased intraocular pressure, constipation and urinary retention.

Blocking alpha-adrenoceptors produces orthostatic hypotension.

Weight gain and troublesome side-effects are particularly associated with atypical drugs and are probably related to their action on HT antagonism.

5.2 Pharmacokinetics Aspects

Absorption: Most antipsychotic drugs are given orally or by intramuscular injection, once or twice a day. Depot preparations are also available; this allows less frequent administration (monthly) and optimizes compliance.

Chlorpromazine, a large representative of antipsychotic drugs, is well absorbed in the bloodstream after oral administration. Others drugs have a lower bioavailability (Table 3.8).

Distribution: The relationship between plasma concentration and clinical effects of antipsychotic drugs is highly variable.

Metabolism: The plasma half-life of most antipsychotic drugs is 15–30 hours. Clearance depends entirely on hepatic transformation by a combination of oxidative and conjugative reactions.

Elimination: Metabolites are eliminated in the urine.

Table 3.8 summarizes specific PK parameters.

5.3 PK/PD Relationship

Drowsiness and dizziness often appear with high doses of antipsychotic drugs and at the beginning of the treatment. For naïve patients, these side-effects may be increased. This effect can be sought in DFC. Long half-lives permit the detection of drugs for a long time in biological samples.

6. OTHER DRUGS

6.1 Atropine[50–53]

The main effect of atropine occurs on the heart. Atropine can alter heart rate. Although the dominant response is tachycardia, the heart rate often decreases transiently with average clinical doses (0.4 to 0.6 mg).

TABLE 3.8 Main Pharmacokinetic Parameters of Antipsychotic Drugs Helpful in Drug-facilitated Crimes[9–11]

Compound	Bio Availability	Urinary Excretion %	Peak Time	Half-Life $T_{1/2}$	Mean Peak Blood Concentration (After Single Dose)
Chlorpromazine	Oral: 32%	23% excreted in urine as metabolites (more than 168); unchanged drug: 1%	Oral: 2–3 h IM: 4 h IV: 2–4 h	18 h A half-life of 7–119 h has been reported	1 µg/L (25 mg) 18 µg/L (150 mg) 17–140 µg/L (50 mg, IM)
Clozapine	Oral tablet: 50% to 60%	80% excreted in urine; two active metabolites: norclozapine and clozapine-N-oxide; unchanged drug: trace amount	1–2 h	8–12 h N-desmethylclozapine: 13.2 h	57 µg/L (25 mg in Chinese) 140 µg/L (70–340 µg/L, 100 mg)
Cyamemazine	–	Little studied. Excreted in urine as sulfoxide and desmethyl cyamemazine in 72 h	–	10 h	–
Droperidol	–	74% excreted in urine in 4 days as unidentified metabolite; unchanged drug: 0.3%	IM: 1 h	1.3–2.7 h	60 µg/L (5 mg IM) 3.5 mg/70 kg IV: 300 µg/L at 2 min, 50 µg/L at 1 h, 30 µg/L at 2 h

Flupenthixol	Oral: 40% to 50%	Renal excretion is negligible; major: flupentixol sulfoxide; unchanged drug: trace amount	Oral: 3–8 h	19–39 h	3–9 µg/L (1 mg) 38 µg/L (12 mg)
Fluphenazine	Oral: immediate release: 2.7%	Renal excretion is less than 20%; active metabolite: fluphenazine- sulfoxide, 7-hydroxy-fluphenazine; unchanged drug: trace amount	Oral: 2–3 h; IM: 1.5–2 h	13–58 h, mean 33 h	0.26–1.1 µg/L (5 mg) 1.7 µg/L (25 mg) 13–23 µg/L (25 mg IM)
Haloperidol	Oral: 60%	33% to 40% excreted in urine as metabolite; unchanged drug: 1%	Oral: 2–6 h; IM: 20 min	14–41 h Reduced in children	2.0 (5 mg) 3.0 µg/M (10 mg) 5 µg/L (2 mg IM, 20 min post-injection)
Loxapine	Complete but extensive metabolism in 7- and 8-OH-loxapine and 7- and 8-OH-amoxapine	70% excreted in urine as conjugated metabolites, major being 8-OH-loxapine; unchanged drug: 1%	IM: 2 h; VO: 1 h, 8-OH-loxapine: 2 h, 8-OH-amoxapine: 6 h	3–8 h	17 µg/L (29.5 mg IM) 257 µg/L (10 mg inhalation) 17 µg/L (29.5 mg VO) with 30 µg/L 8-OH-loxapine and 5 µg/L 8-OH-amoxapine

(Continued)

TABLE 3.8 (Continued)

Compound	Bio Availability	Urinary Excretion %	Peak Time	Half-Life T$_{1/2}$	Mean Peak Blood Concentration (After Single Dose)
Molindone	–	At least 36 metabolites; unchanged drug excreted in urine: 2–3%	Oral: 0.5–1.5 h	1.2–2.8 h Existence of active metabolite with long half-time is hypothesized	5.0 µg/L (50 mg)
Perphenazine	Oral: 20%	Excreted in urine as sulfoxide metabolite (13%), glucuronide conjugates (30%); unchanged drug: 1%	Oral: 3–8 h	8–12 h (mean 9.4 h)	16 µg/L (6 mg)
Quetiapine	9% enhanced by food	73% excreted in urine in 4 days as 20 metabolite, one active: 7-hydroxy-quetiapine; unchanged drug <1%	Oral: 1–1.5 h	2.6–9 h 7-hydroxy-quetiapine: 6.2 h	45 µg/L (25 mg)
Risperidone	Oral: 70%	70% eliminated in urine in 1 week; unchanged drug: 4% in EM with 32% of 9-hydroxy-risperidone; to 30% in PM with 8% of 9-hydroxy-risperidone	1–2 h 9-hydroxy-risperidone: 3–4 h	Oral: 3 (extensive metabolizers, EM) to 20 (poor metabolizers PM) h IM: 2.9–6 days	7.9 µg/L and 6.5 µg/L 9-hydroxyrisperidone (EM, 1 mg) 16 µg/L and 19 µg/L

			t_{max}	$t_{1/2}$	Concentration
				9-hydroxyrisperidone: 21 (EM) to 30 (PM) h	9-hydroxyrisperidone (Chinese, 2 mg) 27 µg/L and 38 µg/L 9-hydroxyrisperidone (EM, 4 mg)
Thioridazine	—	2.5–17% excreted in urine, mesoridazine, and sulforidazine, both actives; unchanged drug: 0.5%	1–2 h Mesoridazine: 4 h Sulforidazine 6.9 h	21–24 h	50 µg/L, mesoridazine: 170 µg/L, sulforidazine: 50 µg/L (25 mg); 240 µg/L, mesoridazine: 320 µg/L, sulforidazine: 80 µg/L (100 mg)
Trifluoperazine	Oral: readily absorbed	Low excretion in urine, 1.3–6% as sulfoxide; unchanged drug: 0.3–1.0%	Oral: 1.5–4 h	7–18 h (mean 11 h) 7-hydroxy-trifluoperazine: 11 h	1.4 µg/L (0.5–3.1 µg/L) (5 mg) 0.9–4.0 µg/L (20 mg)

(according to 9–11)

6.1.1 Pharmacological Properties

Atropine is a competitive antagonist of the actions of acetylcholine and other muscarinic agonists. Atropine competes for a common binding site on all muscarinic receptor. Cardiac muscle muscarinic receptors are blocked. Muscarinic receptors in exocrine glands, smooth and ganglia and intramural neurons are also blocked by atropine.

Atropine is indicated for the management of poisoning by organophosphorous nerve agents with cholinesterase activity as well as organophosphorous or carbamate insecticides.

Atropine is also used in cardiac dysrhythmia, asthma, heart block, general anesthesia, carotid sinus massage, etc.

Sedation is a side-effect of atropine. Some patients who received atropine as a preanesthetic medication and also during surgery for several episodes of bradycardia remained somnolent several hours postoperatively.

6.1.2 Pharmacokinetics Aspects

Absorption: After oral administration, bioavailability is high. It is variable after inhalation.

After sublingual administration, absorption is significantly slow and incomplete compared with that of intramuscular or subcutaneous administration.

Time to peak concentration is 30 minutes after intramuscular administration.

Distribution: Atropine was widely distributed in tissues following intravenous injection in healthy adults. The estimated value of 230.79 L (3.297 L/kg) exceeds total body water.

Metabolism: Atropine is metabolized in noratropine and N-oxide-atropine.

Elimination: Half-life is 2 to 4 hours for adults and 6.5 hours for children.

After intravenous administration, serum levels drop rapidly within 10 minutes, and decrease more gradually thereafter.

Up to 93% of a single dose is eliminated in the urine in 24 hours as unchanged drug for 50% after IV administration, 30% after IM administration and 13% after oral administration. Twenty-four percent is present as noratropine.

6.1.3 PK/PD Relationship

Therapeutic drug concentration in bronchitis after inhalation is 1.3 to 5.8 ng/L.

Unpredictable serum levels may be high enough to lead to systemic anticholinergic effects.

Sedation, a side-effect of atropine, can be sought in DFC. Bioavailability is high after oral administration and this form can be used in DFC. It is not easy to identify the drug in biological fluids since the half-life is short and circulating blood levels are very low.

A single oral 0.3 mg/kg (2.1 mg/70 kg) dose in children (average age: 4.8 years) leads to an average blood concentration of 1.9 µg/L at 2 hours.

6.2 Scopolamine[54–56]

6.2.1 Pharmacological Properties

This drug is used by transdermal patch.

Transdermal scopolamine is indicated for treating motion sickness. This drug is effective in preventing seasickness when applied behind the ear 5 hours prior to sailing. It is also indicated for reducing postoperative nausea and vomiting.

Confusion and memory loss are side-effects of transdermal scopolamine. Restlessness has been also reported.

During clinical trials of transdermal scopolamine for motion sickness, drowsiness was reported to occur in less than one-sixth of patients.

Deep coma and meningism were described in a 52-year-old woman following premedication with scopolamine 0.4 mg IM, hydroxyzine 50 mg IM and meperidine 100 mg IM for a pancreatoduodenectomy.

6.2.2 Pharmacokinetics Aspects

Absorption: Scopolamine is well absorbed following application of a scopolamine transdermal patch. The oral bioavailability is 27%.

Scopolamine hydrobromide 0.25% ophthalmic solution is rapidly absorbed after ocular administration.

Distribution: The distribution of scopolamine is not well characterized, but may be reversibly bound to plasma proteins and is known to cross the placenta and blood−brain barrier.

Time to peak concentration after transdermal administration is 24 hours.

Metabolism: Scopolamine is extensively metabolized and conjugated.

Elimination: Renal excretion is less than 10%, and less than 5% is unchanged.

Following removal of a transdermal scopolamine patch, plasma levels decrease with a half-life of 9.5 hours.

6.2.3 PK/PD Relationship

Therapeutic drug concentration in motion sickness after transdermal administration is 87 ng/L. A single oral 0.4 mg dose given to healthy men yielded an average plasma concentration of 0.5 µg/L at 0.8 hours. In a subject with a 0.9 mg dose, a concentration of 1.1 µg/L was measured after 1 hour.

Circulating blood levels are very low. It is difficult to identify the drug in biological fluids.

6.3 Meprobamate[57–58]

6.3.1 Pharmacological Properties

Meprobamate (oral and IM) is indicated for the treatment of anxiety disorders. The usual dose is 400 milligrams three or four times daily.

Dizziness, vertigo, drowsiness, feelings of hangover, ataxia, slurred speech, headache, weakness, overstimulation, seizures, fast electroencephalogram (EEG) activity and paradoxical excitement may occur with meprobamate therapy. Euphoria, paranoia and hallucinations have also been reported with meprobamate therapy. Few studies have described depression as a side-effect of meprobamate therapy.

6.3.2 Pharmacokinetics Aspects

Absorption: Meprobamate is well absorbed after oral administration.

Distribution: Protein binding is 0% to 30%. Volume of distribution is 0.5 to 0.8 L/kg.

Meprobamate can cross the placenta barrier. Time to peak concentration after oral administration is 2 to 3 hours.

Metabolism: Meprobamate is metabolized by liver to hydroxymeprobamate, a non-active metabolite.

Elimination: Renal excretion is 10% to 20%. Elimination half-life is 9 to 11 hours.

6.3.3 PK/PD Relationship

Therapeutic drug concentrations in anxiety are 5 to 30 µg/mL after recommended doses (400–600 mg). A single 400 mg oral dose to healthy men produced average plasma concentrations of 7.7 mg/L at 2 hours, 4.4 mg/L at 4 hours and 1.6 mg/L at 24 hours. After 800 mg, a plasma concentration of 16 mg/L was achieved 2 hours after ingestion.

Meprobamate is especially prone to induce sedation. This effect can be sought in DFC. A long half-life permits the drug to be detected for a long time in biological samples.

6.4 Imidazoline Decongestants: Tetrahydrozoline, Naphazoline, Oxymetazoline and Xylometazoline

6.4.1 Pharmacological Properties

These drugs are decongestant compounds used in rhinitis (nasal sprays or drops) or in conjunctivitis (ophthalmic solution). Intranasal administration constricts dilated blood vessels in the nasal mucosa, reducing blood flow to engorged, edematous tissue.

Imidazoline decongestants can depress rather than stimulate the CNS. Presumably this is related to preferential effects of the drug on alpha-2 receptors, which effect is similar to that of clonidine.

Drowsiness may occur following topical administration (intranasal) in adults and children, especially with administration of larger than recommended doses. Coma and hypothermia may occur in children following administration of larger than recommended doses.

6.4.2 Pharmacokinetics Aspects

Mucosal and nasal solution absorption is good.

The distribution, metabolism and elimination are not well characterized.

6.4.3 PK/PD Relationship

Systemic reactions appear to be most prevalent in infants, young children and the elderly.

Drowsiness is a side-effect and can be sought in DFC, especially in infants, young children and the elderly.

6.5 Ketamine [59-63]

6.5.1 Pharmacological Properties

This drug is an anesthetic and analgesic agent structurally related to phencyclidine and cyclohexamine.

Ketamine is the only single-agent anesthetic capable of producing a "dissociative" anesthesia. This agent also produces analgesia at lower therapeutic concentrations.

Mechanism is not well known. Several theories have been proposed to explain these effects, including binding to N-methyl-aspartate (NMA) receptors in the CNS, interactions with opiate receptors at central and spinal sites, and interaction with norepinephrine, serotonin and muscarinic cholinergic receptors.

Psychiatric disorders can often occur (12% to 50%). The reactions are characterized by vivid dreams, dissociative or extracorporeal (out-of-body) experiences, floating sensations, hallucinations, delirium, confusion or "weird trips." Increases in cerebrospinal fluid pressure and intracranial blood flow have also been reported with ketamine administration.

6.5.2 Pharmacokinetics Aspects

Absorption: Bioavailability after oral administration is 16%. Bioavailability after IM administration is above 90%. Absorption after IM administration appears to be more rapid in children than in adults. Systemic bioavailability after epidural doses is 77%, with rapid increases in plasma levels. Time to peak concentration after IM administration is 15 to 30 minutes. Time to peak concentration after oral administration is 20 to 45 minutes (mean 30 minutes).

Distribution: Protein binding is 47%.

The drug is initially distributed to highly perfused tissues (brain, heart, lungs) with levels achieved being four to five times higher than corresponding plasma concentrations. Ketamine is then redistributed to muscle and peripheral tissues, and eventually fat tissue.

Volume of distribution is 2 to 3 L/kg.

Metabolism: The primary metabolic pathway involves hepatic N-demethylation via the cytochrome P450 system; norketamine, an active metabolite is subsequently hydroxylated and conjugated to water-soluble compounds. Other hydroxylated metabolites have also been reported.

Children metabolize ketamine more rapidly than adults.

Elimination: Most of a dose appears in the urine as hydroxylated and conjugated metabolites; 4% is excreted unchanged or as norketamine.

Less than 5% is excreted in the feces.

Elimination half-life is 2 to 3 hours.

6.5.3 PK/PD Relationship

Anesthesia usually requires serum levels over 1000 μg/L. Norketamine (its active metabolite) serum levels are higher in children.

Analgesic effects were observed with plasma levels of 100 to 200 μg/L following IM or IV administration.

A single 50 mg oral dose achieved plasma concentrations of 80 μg/L after 0.5 hour for ketamine and 360 μg/L at 0.8 hour for norketamine.

Ketamine is especially prone to induce sedation. This effect can be sought in DFC.

REFERENCES

1. Schallek W, Horst WD, Schlosser W. Mechanisms of action of benzodiazepines. *Adv Pharmacol Chemother* 1979;**16**:45–87.
2. Study RE, Barker JL. Cellular mechanism of benzodiazepines action. *JAMA* 1982;**247**:2147–51.
3. Richter JJ. Current theories about mechanism of benzodiazepines in neuroleptic drugs. *Anesthesiology* 1981;**54**:66–72.
4. Squires RF, Braestrup C. Benzodiazepine receptors in rat brain. *Nature* 1977;**266**:732–4.
5. Wagner J, Wagner ML, Hening WA. Beyond benzodiazepines: alternative pharmacologic agents for the treatment of insomnia. *Ann Pharmacother* 1998;**32**:680–91.
6. Shimizu K, Matsubara K, Uezono T, Kimura K, Shiono H. Reduced dorsal hippocampal glutamate release significantly correlates with the spatial memory deficits produced by benzodiazepines and ethanol. *Neuroscience* 1998;**83**:701–6.
7. Lader M. Psychiatric disorders. In: Speight T, Holford N, editors. *Avery's drug treatment*. 4th ed. Auckland: ADIS Internation Press; 1997. p. 1437.

8. Michel L, Lang JP. Benzodiazepines et passage à l'acte criminel (benzodiazepine and forensic aspects). *Encephale* 2003;**29**:479−85.

9. Database Thomson Reuters Micromedex 2.0, New York.

10. Baselt RC, editor. 9th ed. New York: Biomedical Publications; 2011.

11. Moffat AC, Osselton MD, Widdop B, editors. *Clarke's analysis of drugs and poisons.* 3rd ed. London: Pharmaceutical Press; 2004.

12. 15th ed. Aronson JK, editor. *Meyler's side effects of drugs. The international encyclopedia of adverse drug reactions and interactions,* vol. 3. Oxford: Elsevier; 2006.

13. Vree TB, Damsma J, Van den Bogert AG, Van der Kleijn. Pharmacokinetics of 4-hydroxybutyric acid in man, rhesus monkey and dog. *Anaesth Intensivemed Praxis* 1978;**110**:21−39.

14. Lebeau MA, Christenson RH, Levine B, et al. Intra- and interindividual variations in urinary concentration of endogenous gamma-hydroxy-butyrate. *J Anal Tox* 2002;**26**: 340−6.

15. Palatini P, Tedeschi L, Frison G, et al. Dose-dependent absorption and elimination of gamma-hydroxybutyric acid in healthy volunteers. *Eur J Clin Pharmacol* 1993;**45**:353−6.

16. Hoes MJAJM, Vree TB, Guelen PJM. Gamma-hydroxybutyric acid as a hypnotic. *L'encephale* 1980;**6**:93−9.

17. Helrich M, McAslan TC, Sholnick S, Bessman SP. Correlation of blood levels of 4-hydroxybutyrate with state of consciousness. *Anesthesiology* 1964;**25**:771−5.

18. Thai D, Dyer JE, Jacob P, Haller CA. Clinical pharmacology of 1,4-butanediol and GHB after oral 1,4-butanediol administration to healthy volunteers. *Clin Pharmacol Ther* 2007;**81**:178−84.

19. Gilman AG, Rall TW, Nies AS, editors. *Goodman and Gilman's the pharmacological basis of therapeutics.* 8th ed. New York, NY: Pergamon Press; 1990.

20. Tang BK, Kalow W, Inaba T, et al. Variation in amobarbital metabolism: evaluation of a simplified population study. *Clin Pharmacol Ther* 1983;**34**:202−6.

21. Saunders PA, Ito Y, Baker ML, Hume AS, Ho IK. Pentobarbital tolerance and withdrawal: correlation with effects on the GABAA receptor. *Pharmacol Biochem Behav* 1990;**37**:343−8.

22. Saunders PA, Ho IK. Barbiturates and the GABAA receptor complex. *Prog Drug Res* 1990;**34**:261−86.

23. Mather LE, Ladd LA, Copeland SE, Chang DH. Effects of imposed acid−base derangement on the cardiovascular effects and pharmacokinetics of bupivacaine and thiopental. *Anesthesiology* 2004;**100**:1457−68.

24. Perucca E. The clinical pharmacokinetics of the new antiepileptic drugs. *Epilepsia* 1999;**40**:S7−13.

25. Blakey GE, Nestorov IA, Arundel PA, Aarons LJ, Rowland M. Quantitative structure−pharmacokinetics relationship: I. Development of a whole-body physiologically based model to characterize changes in pharmacokinetics across a homologous series of barbiturates in the rat. *J Pharmacokinet Biopharm* 1997;**25**:277−312. Erratum in: J Pharmacokinet Biopharm 1998; 26:131.

26. Eriksson K, Baer M, Kilpinen P, Koivikko M. Effects of long barbiturate anaesthesia on eight children with severe epilepsy. *Neuropediatrics* 1993;**24**:281−5.

27. Browne TR. The pharmacokinetics of agents used to treat status epilepticus. *Neurology* 1990;**40**:28−32.

28. Beard WJ, Free SM. Two double-blind, controlled studies compared chlorethate, a new sedative-tranquilizer, with phenobarbital. *J Clin Pharmacol* 1967;**7**:41−5.

29. Homer TD, Stanski DR. The effect of increasing age on thiopental disposition and anesthetic requirement. *Anesthesiology* 1985;**62**(6):714–24.

30. Quaynor H, Corbey M, Bjorkman S. Rectal induction of anaesthesia in children with methohexitone. *Br J Anaesth* 1985;**57**:573–7.

31. Hudson RJ, Stanski DR, Burch PG. Pharmacokinetics of methohexital and thiopental in surgical patients. *Anesthesiology* 1983;**59**:215–9.

32. Lauven PM, Schwilden H, Stoeckel H. Threshold hypnotic concentration of methohexitone. *Eur J Clin Pharmacol* 1987;**33**:261–5.

33. Breimer DD. Clinical pharmacokinetics of hypnotics. *Clin Pharmacokinet* 1977;**2**:93–109.

34. Simons FER, Roberts JR, Gu X, et al. The clinical pharmacology of brompheniramine in children. *J Allergy Clin Immunol* 1999;**103**:223–6.

35. Simons FER, Simons KJ. H1 receptor antagonists: clinical pharmacology and use in allergic disease. *Ped Clin North Am* 1983;**30**:899–914.

36. Peets EA, Jackson M, Symchowicz S. Metabolism of chlorpheniramine maleate in man. *J Pharmacol Exp Ther* 1972;**180**:364–74.

37. Glazko AJ, Dill WA, Young RM, et al. Metabolic disposition of diphenhydramine. *Clin Pharmacol Ther* 1974;**16**:1066–76.

38. Albert KS, Hallmark MR, Sakmar E, et al. Pharmacokinetics of diphenhydramine in man. *J Pharmcokinet Biopharm* 1975;**5**:159–70.

39. Friedman H, Greenblatt DJ, Scavone JM, et al. Clearance of the antihistamine doxylamine reduced in elderly men but not in elderly women. *Clin Pharmacokinet* 1989;**16**: 312–6.

40. Fouda HG, Hobbs DC, Stambaugh JE. Sensitive assay for determination of hydroxyzine in plasma and its human pharmacokinetics. *J Pharm Sci* 1979;**68**:1456.

41. Simons FER, Simmons KJ, Frith EM. The pharmacokinetics and antihistaminic of the H1 receptor antagonist hydroxyzine. *J Allergy Clin Immunol* 1984;**73**:69–75.

42. Rivera-Calimlim L, Castaneda L, Lasagna L. Effects of mode of management on plasma chlorpromazine in psychiatric patients. *Clin Pharmacol Ther* 1973;**14**:978–86.

43. Hollister LE, Curry SH. Urinary excretion of chlorpromazine metabolites following single doses and in steady-state conditions. *Res Commun Chem Pathol Pharmacol* 1971;**2**:330–8.

44. Olesen OV. Therapeutic drug monitoring of clozapine treatment: therapeutic threshold value for serum clozapine concentrations. *Clin Pharmacokinet* 1998;**34**:497–502.

45. Koytchev R, Alken R-G, McKay G, et al. Absolute bioavailability of oral immediate and slow release fluphenazine in healthy volunteers. *Eur J Clin Pharmacol* 1996;**51**:183–7.

46. Omerov M, Wistedt B, Bolvig-Hansen L, et al. The relationship between perphenazine plasma levels and clinical response in acute schizophrenia. *Prog Neuropsychopharmacol Biol Psychiatry* 1989;**13**:159–68.

47. Ulrich S, Wurthmann C, Brosz M, et al. The relationship between serum concentration and therapeutic effect of haloperidol in patients with acute schizophrenia. *Clin Pharmacokinet* 1998;**34**:227–63.

48. Fabre Jr LF, Arvanitis L, Pultz J, et al. ICI 204,636, a novel, atypical antipsychotic: early indication of safety and efficacy in patients with chronic and subchronic schizophrenia. *Clin Ther* 1995;**17**:366–78.

49. Huang M, Peer A, Woestenborghs R, et al. Pharmacokinetics of the novel antipsychotic agent risperidone and the prolactin response in healthy subjects. *Clin Pharmacol Ther* 1993;**54**:257–68.

50.   Berghem L, Bergman U, Schildt B, et al. Plasma atropine concentrations determined by radioimmunoassay after single-dose IV and IM administration. *Br J Anaesth* 1980;**52**:597−601.

51.   Kalser SC, McLain PL. Atropine metabolism in man. *Clin Pharmacol Ther* 1970;**11**: 214−27.

52.   Smith DS, Orkin FK, Gardner SM, et al. Prolonged sedation in the elderly after intraoperative atropine administration. *Anesthesiology* 1979;**51**:348−9.

53.   Adams RG, Verma P, Jackson AJ, et al. Plasma pharmacokinetics of intravenously administered atropine in normal human subjects. *J Clin Pharmacol* 1982;**22**:477−81.

54.   Honkavaara P. Effect of transdermal hyoscine on nausea and vomiting during and after middle ear surgery under local anaesthesia. *Br J Anaesth* 1996;**76**:49−53.

55.   Attias J, Gordon C, Ribak J, et al. Efficacy of transdermal scopolamine against seasickness: a 3-day study at sea. *Aviat Space Environ Med* 1987;**58**:60−2.

56.   Samuels SI, Washington E. Coma and abnormal neurologic signs following premedication. *Anesth Analg* 1980;**59**:79−80.

57.   Haizlip TM, Ewing JA. Meprobamate habituation: a controlled clinical study. *N Engl J Med* 1958;**258**:1182−6.

58.   Thompson RE. Nose-drop intoxication in an infant (letter). *JAMA* 1970;**211**:123−4.

59.   Reich DL, Silvay G. Ketamine: an update on the first twenty-five years of clinical experience. *Can J Anaesth* 1989;**36**:186−97.

60.   Green SM, Johnson NE. Ketamine sedation for pediatric procedures: part 2, review and implications. *Ann Emerg Med* 1990;**19**:1033−46.

61.   White PF, Dworsky WA, Horai Y, et al. Comparison of continuous infusion fentanyl or ketamine versus thiopental—determining the mean effective serum concentrations for outpatient surgery. *Anesthesiology* 1983;**59**:564−9.

62.   Grant IS, Nimmo WS, Clements JA. Pharmacokinetics and analgesic effects of IM and oral ketamine. *Br J Anaesth* 1981;**53**:805−10.

63.   White PF, Way WL, Trevor AJ. Ketamine—its pharmacology and therapeutic uses. *Anesthesiology* 1982;**56**:119−36.

Chapter 4

Ethanol- and Drug-Facilitated Crime

Christian Staub and Aline Staub Spörri

1. INTRODUCTION

As mentioned in the preceding chapters, the term drug-facilitated crime (DFC) is used when a person is subjected to a criminal act through the incapacitating effects of drugs. Under this name, we generally find rape, sexual assault, robbery or the sedation of elderly persons, but the most prevalent DFCs are drug-facilitated sexual assault (DFSA). It has been suggested that DFSAs should be divided into proactive DFSA, i.e. "the covert or forcible administration to a victim of an incapacitating or disinhibiting substance by an assailant for the purpose of sexual assault," and opportunistic DFSA, i.e. "sexual activity by an assailant with a victim who is profoundly intoxicated by his or her own actions to the point of near or actual unconsciousness".[1,2]

Some data show that humans have been making and consuming alcohol (or ethanol, its chemical name) for at least 7000 years. Furthermore, alcohol is extensively used in western society, especially among young people. Therefore, it is not surprising that it is the most common substance involved in DFCs, either alone or in combination with other drugs. A literature review of studies based in the following seven countries: France (1752 DFC cases), United Kingdom (1428), United States (6835), Canada (1128), Australia (434), Sweden (1806) and Poland (168) has shown that ethanol is the most prevalent drug in five of these seven countries.[3]

In DFC cases, the excessive consumption of alcohol is often more dangerous than the intake of any other psychotropic drug. In many cases, the perpetrators take advantage of the fact that an individual has been drinking heavily and is thus less able to resist. In other instances, the perpetrator has been closely involved in ensuring that the future victim gets drunk by ordering drinks and by encouraging her or him to drink more than usual.[4]

Toxicological Aspects of Drug-Facilitated Crimes. DOI: http://dx.doi.org/10.1016/B978-0-12-416748-3.00004-9

In the particular context of DFSAs, women under the influence of ethanol are more often victims of rape. It seems that intoxicated women seem to be less capable of evaluating the risks and effectively resisting. Women who were drinking before being sexually assaulted have reported that their intoxication made them more likely to take risks that they normally would avoid. For example, "the women felt comfortable accepting a ride home from a party with a man they did not know well or letting an intoxicated man enter their apartment".[5] Furthermore, some studies indicate that completed rapes (as opposed to attempted rapes) are more common among intoxicated victims than among sober victims, suggesting again that intoxicated women are less able than sober women to effectively resist an assault.

Unlike other drugs, alcohol consumption is frequent among perpetrators. Men are usually socialized to be the initiators of sexual interactions and they feel that they must make the first move. An intoxicated man may misinterpret a woman's friendly attitude as a sexual message that pushes him to act sexually. Date rapists may also intentionally get drunk to decrease their inhibitions when they want to act in a sexually aggressive fashion. Finally, the co-occurrence of alcohol consumption by both the perpetrator and victim is frequent because when one of them is drinking, the other one is generally drinking as well.

Another reason for the high prevalence of alcohol in DFCs is that it is common to administer alcohol along with psychoactive drugs such as sedatives, hypnotics, anticonvulsants, tranquilizers or analgesics. Thus, the effects of these drugs are enhanced by the presence of ethanol, even at low levels. Therefore, it is not surprising that DFCs often occur when the victim is under the influence of both alcohol and another drug(s).

Due to the high prevalence of alcohol (ethanol) and to its dual role (active and passive) in DFCs, it is important to devote a whole chapter to this old but potent drug.

2. ETHANOL

Ethanol is also called *ethyl alcohol*, *pure alcohol*, *grain alcohol* or *drinking alcohol*. It is the vector of alcoholism and its presence is the first direct marker used for the detection of alcohol consumption.

2.1 Physical Properties of Ethanol

Ethanol (CH_3CH_2OH) is a volatile, flammable, colorless liquid. It is a psychoactive drug and one of the oldest known recreational drugs. Unlike THC or delta-9-tetrahydrocannabinol, which is fat soluble and has a high molecular weight, ethanol is an aliphatic compound of low molecular weight (46.05 grams) that is only slightly soluble in lipids but is fully miscible in water.

Ethanol is generally consumed as an alcoholic beverage. Two types of alcoholic beverages are usually consumed, depending on their use in the country in question. The first type includes fermented beverages (e.g. wines and beers) and distilled beverages (e.g. cognac and whiskey), which naturally contain alcohol. The second type includes drinks to which ethanol has been added (e.g. orange juice and vodka or whiskey and cola).

The centesimal degree of a beverage is the volume of pure alcohol contained in 100 volumes of beverage. By using a density of 0.8 for ethanol and by considering standard glasses, each glass consumed includes close to 10 grams of ethanol.[6]

2.2 Classification of Alcohol Consumers

Chronic and excessive alcohol consumption is recognized as a major public health concern. In Western Europe, it is generally acknowledged that approximately 20% of the population engages in chronic and excessive alcohol consumption. According to WHO recommendations, alcohol consumers are classified into four categories[7]:

Teetotalers: subjects who declared total abstinence from alcohol consumption (0 g/day), generally over a period of 12 months.
Low-risk drinkers: subjects who consumed ≤20 g/day for women and ≤30 g/day for men.
At risk drinkers: subjects who consumed >20 g/day for women and >30 g/day for men.
Heavy drinkers: subjects with an alcohol consumption of >40 g/day for women and >60 g/day for men.

The possibility that the victim and/or perpetrator of a DFC belongs to one of these four categories of consumers introduces a new parameter to the interpretation of DFC cases. Therefore, experts should try to collect these data before making a final conclusion.

Later in this chapter, the categorization of drinkers and their biomarkers will be introduced.

2.3 Metabolism and Pharmacokinetics

Ethanol differs from most other drugs by the way it is absorbed into the blood, metabolized in the liver and enters the brain. Because of its chemical and physical properties, ethanol is rapidly distributed throughout the whole organism and can cross important biological membranes, such as the blood–brain barrier, to act on a large number of organs and biological processes.

Because the aim of this book is not to provide exhaustive information about a particular drug, this section will be focused only on the primary aspects of the issue, and the reader is asked to consult specialized literature if needed.

After absorption into the portal blood, ethanol passes through the liver, where dedicated enzymes begin converting the compound into acetaldehyde and acetate. The end products of ethanol metabolism are carbon dioxide and water. Alcohol dehydrogenase is only present in small amounts in children below 5 years of age; this fact explains their comparatively high sensitivity to alcohol. One form of aldehyde dehydrogenase is commonly deficient in a high proportion of people with East Asian genetic backgrounds; individuals with this form do not enjoy alcohol ingestion because of the build-up of acetaldehyde, which causes flushing and nausea. In all cases, the limiting step is the conversion of alcohol to acetaldehyde.[8] This process constitutes the main metabolic pathway, i.e. oxidative metabolism (Figure 4.1).

A second metabolic pathway, which is non-oxidative (see Figure 4.2), produces some direct markers of alcohol consumption, namely, ethyl-glucuronide and ethyl-sulfate, phosphatidylethanol, and fatty acid ethyl esters.

At the beginning of the twentieth century, the Swedish scientist Erik M.P. Widmark (1889–1945) made major contributions to pharmacokinetic understanding of ethanol consumption.[9] Widmark observed that after the peak ethanol concentration has been reached, the elimination phase appears to follow a nearly straight line. He explained this observation by noting that the system for metabolizing alcohol was saturated and fully occupied. The major consequence of this pharmacokinetic profile is that the amount of alcohol metabolized per hour is independent of the blood alcohol concentration (BAC) (Figure 4.3).

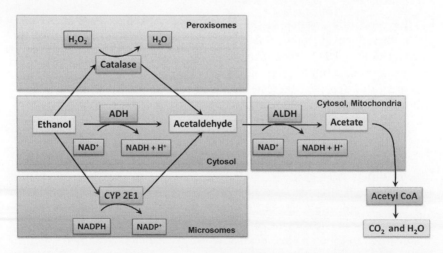

FIGURE 4.1 Oxidative metabolism of ethanol. ALDH: acetaldehyde dehydrogenase; ADH: alcohol dehydrogenase; MEOS: microsomal oxidation system. *Adapted from (6).*

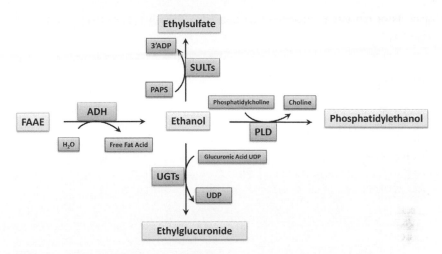

FIGURE   4.2 Non-oxidative   metabolism   of   ethanol.   PAPS: 3′phosphoadenosine 5′phosphosulfate; PLD: phospholipase D; UGTs: UDP-glucuronyl transferases; SULTs: sulfotrans-ferases; ADP: adenosine 5′diphosphate; UDP: uridine 5′diphosphate; *adapted from (6).*

Pharmacokinetic of ethanol

Example: consumption of 60 g of ethanol (about 6 glasses)

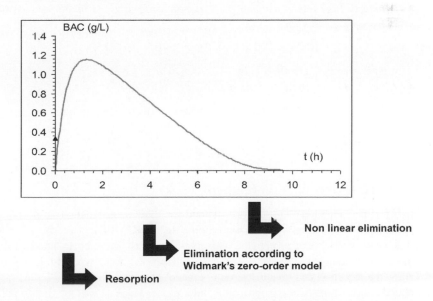

FIGURE 4.3 Elimination kinetic of ethanol. Schematic diagram illustrating the Widmark's zero order model.

2.4 Theoretical Evaluation of Blood Alcohol Concentrations (BACs)

The Widmark equation (4.1) is generally used to estimate the blood alcohol concentration (BAC). Widmark found that the distribution constant r for men was 0.68 (within a range of $0.51-0.85$) but lower for women, at an average of 0.55 (within a range of $0.44-0.66$). These discrepancies between the sexes derive from differences in body-tissue composition; women have a higher percentage of fat and less percentage of water than do men. Accordingly, women reach higher BACs than men at the same proportional dose of ethanol (i.e. per body weight). A similar observation was made in studies of men at different ages, because body water composition decreases with age.

$$C_t = (A/(r \times p)) - \beta t \tag{4.1}$$

where:

A: amount of alcohol consumed (g)
r: Widmark constant (distribution constant, man: 0.68; woman: 0.55)
p: body weight (kg)
C_t: blood alcohol concentration (BAC in g/kg)
β: elimination rate (g/kg/h)
t: time since first drink (h)

Examples:

- *A man (72 kg) has consumed 0.25 liter of wine at 12°C in 2 hours. What is his BAC at this time?*

$$C_0 = (0.25 \times 120 \times 0.8)/(0.68 \times 70(kg)) = 0.50 g/kg$$

after 2 hours: $C_{2h} = 0.30$ g/kg.
- *In the same situation, but for a woman (50 kg)?*

$$C_0 = (0.25 \times 120 \times 0.8)/(0.55 \times 50(kg)) = 0.87 g/kg$$

after 2 hours: $C_{2h} = 0.67$ g/kg.

2.5 BAC Determination Methods

In a forensic situation the reference method for BAC determination is gas chromatography coupled to a flame ionization detector (GC-FID). Because of their lack of sensitivity and selectivity, enzymatic methods must be avoided in the medico-legal context. The GC-FID methods, described in the scientific literature, allow the detection and quantification of ethanol and other aliphatic volatile compounds, such as methanol, isopropanol and acetone. Machata was the first to publish a GC-FID method for analyzing simple volatiles in blood by direct[10] and headspace (HS-GC-FID) injections.[11] The last method is now the most common.

The gas chromatograph is equipped with a special headspace injector (HS) that protects the column from non-volatile blood components, which is necessary because the injected sample corresponds to a gas phase portion. For this purpose, a blood sample (0.1 to 1 ml) with an ionic solution (e.g. H_2SO_4 saturated in sulfates) is used and an internal standard is introduced into a headspace vial. The solution is heated to $50-60°C$, and the upper gas phase is injected into the GC-FID. The choice of internal standard is very important and can include n-propanol, t-butanol, methyl ethyl ketone, acetonitrile and dioxane. However, n-propanol must be used with precaution because of its postmortem formation.

Even if GC-FID is clearly the method of choice for the quantitative analysis of alcohol in the modern forensic laboratory, and although it is sufficiently specific for routine practice, some results of this form of analysis could be misleading. For example, an ethanol-like peak was detected during a routine GC-FID test for alcohol. Subsequent gas chromatography coupled to mass spectrometry (GC-MS) identified the peak as ethyl chloride.[12]

Specificity is the primary concern in forensic situations, so it is recommended that the results be confirmed by GC-MS or even gas chromatography coupled to tandem mass spectrometry (GC-MS-MS).

According to Swiss law, BAC forensic determinations must be carried out in duplicate and analyzed using two independent GC-FID methods. The methods must employ different columns and internal standards, but the same injection technique (e.g. headspace) can be used. The result is presented as the mean (m) of the four determinations and should include the uncertainty measurement (ε) or ($\varepsilon \times m$), depending on the measured blood alcohol concentration (≤ 1 g/kg or > 1 g/kg) (see Table 4.1). The

TABLE 4.1 EtG Concentrations in Different Biological Fluids (mg/l) and Tissues (μg/g) as a Function of BAC

Biological Fluids and Tissues	BAC 0.1−0.6 (g/l)	BAC 1−1.5 (g/l)	BAC >2 (g/l)
Urine	3.8−80	15	33−509
Blood	0.1−4.9	0.5−56	12−40
Bile	1.1−7.0	2.8	6.3−42
Liver	7.9−13	6.7	43−77
Bone marrow	0.5−1.0	0.8	1.0−9.4
Muscle	0.1−0.6	0.3	0.6−1.8
Adipose tissue	0.0−0.4	0.2	0.4−1.2

Adapted from (18).

following equations show BAC forensic measurements with uncertainty, according to Swiss law:

$$m[m - \varepsilon; m + \varepsilon] \tag{4.2}$$

where:

$\varepsilon = 0.05$ g/kg if $m \leq 1$ g/kg, e.g. 0.8‰ 0.75−0.85‰ or g/kg.

$$m[m - (\varepsilon \times m); m + (\varepsilon \times m)] \tag{4.3}$$

where:

$\varepsilon = 0.05$ if $m > 1$ g/kg, e.g. 2.0‰ 1.90−2.10‰ or g/kg.

2.6 Retrospective BAC Calculation at the Moment of the Crime

Blood sampling generally takes place a few hours after a crime. Therefore, the measured ethanol concentration does not represent the BAC at the moment of the crime. According to the Swiss Society of Legal Medicine and the Federal Roads Office,[13a,13b] it is possible to estimate the BAC of either the victim or the perpetrator at the moment of the crime. This calculation is based on the following important phases: resorption and elimination (see Figure 4.4a).

2.6.1 The Resorption Phase

The resorption of ingested alcohol begins at the onset of consumption. The resorption phase corresponds to the non-linear portions of the blood alcohol curve, from the beginning of consumption to the beginning of linear alcohol elimination. After this time, resorption is considered to be essentially finished. The resorption time corresponds to the elapsed time during this phase. The minimum and maximum resorption times are 20 and 120 minutes, respectively, depending on different factors, including food and digestion.

2.6.2 The Elimination Phase

This phase is represented by the linear decrease of the blood alcohol curve. It directly follows the resorption phase and finishes when the measured alcohol concentration reaches 0.15 g/kg. The elimination phase should not be confused with the elimination of alcohol, which begins immediately after the onset of alcohol consumption. The elimination rate β_{60} is defined as the diminution of alcohol within 1 hour. Individual differences are expressed by the following two parameters:

β_{60} minimum: 0.1 (‰ or g/kg) per hour
β_{60} maximum: 0.2 (‰ or g/kg) per hour

plus one unique addition of 0.2 (‰ or g/kg) for the accelerated decrease during the first hour after the end of resorption.

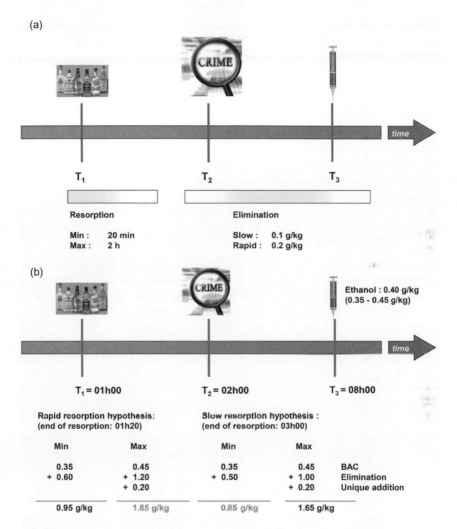

FIGURE 4.4 (a) General principles of retrospective BAC calculation. (b) Example of retrospective BAC calculation. *Adapted from (13b).*

2.6.3 Example of a Retrospective BAC Calculation

A victim of an alleged crime came to the urgent service clinic at 8 a.m. A blood sample was collected, and one BAC analysis was ordered. The victim admitted to having spent the preceding evening drinking in a bar until 1 a.m. and claimed that the time of the alleged crime, of which he was the victim, was 2 a.m. Considering that the result of the BAC analysis is 0.40 ± 0.05 g/kg, what were the minimum and maximum BACs at 2 a.m.?

The details of the calculation are given in Figure 4.4b. As shown, the minimum and maximum BACs at the moment of the alleged crime were estimated at 0.85 and 1.85 g/kg, respectively. It is clear that the first or second value could change the interpretation of the degree of intoxication.

2.6.4 Alcohol Consumption after the Crime

BAC estimation is sometimes necessary in a situation during which alcohol consumption occurred after the crime and before blood sampling. When the quantities of alcohol and the period of consumption are precisely known, as previously mentioned (see 2.4), it is possible to calculate the BAC at the moment of the crime.

2.7 Determination of Urine Alcohol Concentration (UAC)

The methods used for blood alcohol analysis can also be used to determine the amount of ethanol in urine samples. The quantitative relationship between the urine alcohol concentration (UAC) and the BAC has been extensively studied by Jones.[14,15] In addition to the higher water content in urine ($\approx$99%) compared to whole blood ($\approx$80%), the concentration−time curves are shifted in time. In an interesting study from the same group,[16] the UAC/BAC ratio was determined after volunteer subjects drank a standard dose of ethanol (0.85 g/kg body weight) in the form of neat whiskey over 25 min on an empty stomach. The subjects emptied their bladders of any residual urine before starting to drink, and further voids were collected every 60 minutes for up to 8 hours. Temporal variations in the UAC/BAC ratio were measured, and the mean ratio was less than unity for the 60 minute void, whereas at 120 minutes (the post-resorption phase) and all later times, the UAC/BAC ratio was 1.25 or more (a ratio equal to 3.6 after 8 hours). After 360 minute post-drinking, as the BAC decreased below 0.5 g/kg, the mean UAC/BAC increased significantly and continued to increase as the BAC approached zero. Therefore, when the time between the alleged crime and the blood sampling is more than 8 hours or when the BAC is close to 0 g/kg, it is recommended to collect one urine sample and to determine the urine alcohol (ethanol).

3. BIOMARKERS

3.1 Classification of Biomarkers

The exploration of markers linked to alcohol consumption and abuse has attracted a great deal of attention over the past three decades. Alcohol consumption leads to the formation of direct metabolites, such as ethyl glucuronide (EtG), ethyl sulfate (EtS), fatty acid ethyl esters (FAEEs) and

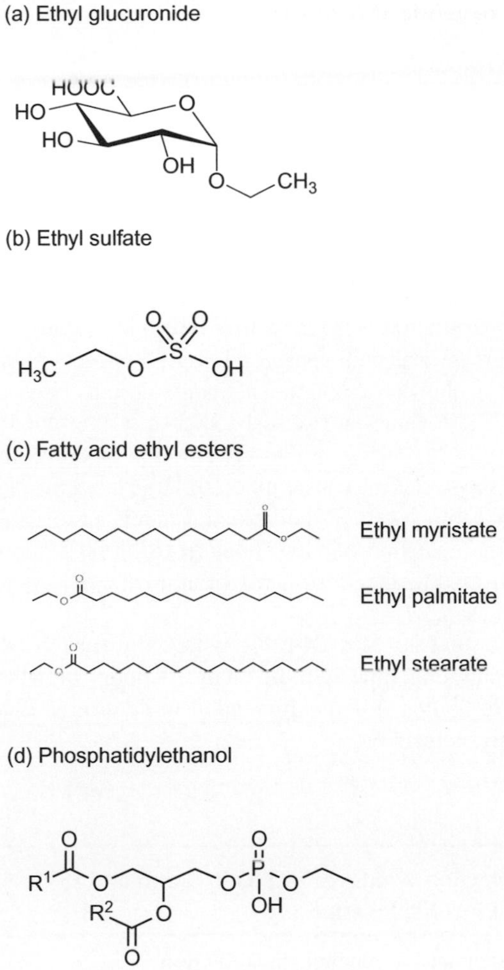
(a) Ethyl glucuronide
HOOC
HO
HO
OH
O
CH3
(b) Ethyl sulfate
H3C
O
S
OH
(c) Fatty acid ethyl esters
Ethyl myristate
Ethyl palmitate
Ethyl stearate
(d) Phosphatidylethanol
R1
R2
P
OH

FIGURE 4.5 Structures of the direct biomarkers: (a) EtG, (b), EtS (c), FAEEs, (d) PEth.

phophatidylethanol (PEth) (Figure 4.5). These biomarkers are recognized as direct and specific markers of ethanol. On the other hand, alcohol congeners (CAs) are indirect biomarkers because they are ingredients in alcoholic beverages. Alcohol abuse also induces changes in endogenous compound levels including liver enzymes, carbohydrate-deficient transferrin (CDT), the urinary ratio of 5-hydroxytryptophol and 5-hydroxyindolacetic acid and cytokines. These types of biomarkers are less specific to alcohol consumption and less relevant to the problem of DFCs. Therefore, they will not be discussed here.

3.2 Ethylglucuronide (EtG)

3.2.1 EtG in Biological Fluids and Tissues

As discussed earlier, EtG is produced through non-oxidative metabolism (see Figure 4.2) in the liver and through a reaction that is catalyzed by isoenzymes, namely, UDP-glucuronyl transferases (UGTs), the most active forms of which are UGT 1A1 and 2B7.[17] Hydrophilic EtG is mainly found in the urine, liver, bile and blood. However, it is also present in much smaller quantities in hair, where it is incorporated by sweat.

EtG appears in the blood less than 45 minutes after alcohol consumption, and its maximum concentration is reached after 3.5 to 5.5 hours. EtG is detected in the blood 17 hours after alcohol consumption. EtG appears in the urine less than 60 minutes after alcohol consumption, and its maximum concentration is reached after 5.5 hours. These values are similar to those in the blood, but EtG can be detected in the urine 24 hours after the consumption of small amounts of ethanol and more than 5 days after the consumption of large amounts of ethanol.

As shown in Table 4.2, EtG is eliminated much more slowly than ethanol, which extends the detection window relative to blood ethanol measurements and, in comparison to other long-term biomarkers, allows the detection of lower alcohol intakes.

Therefore, in the case of a DFC, in which the time between the alleged crime and the sampling time is more than 20 hours or when the BAC and UAC are close to 0 g/kg, it is recommended to determine the EtG and to use urine as the analysis matrix.

TABLE 4.2 Detection Windows for EtG in Blood and Urine According to the Amount of Alcohol Ingested

References	Samples	Alcohol Ingested (g/kg)	Detection Window in Blood (hours)	Detection Window in Urine (hours)
19	urine	0.1	–	≤6
20	urine	0.25	–	<24
21	urine	0.5	–	22–32
22	urine/ blood	0.5	10–14	25–35
23	blood	1.7	≤17	–
24	urine	high	–	40–130

3.2.2 EtG Analysis in Urine

The determination of EtG in urine has become a routine analysis. Because it is possible to find EtG in urine without the consumption of alcoholic beverages,[25,26] the use of a cut-off limit is recommended to avoid false-positive results. No well-accepted cut-off is fixed by international guidelines. However, the most accepted value is generally 0.1 μg/ml, because this limit seems to be appropriate for determining the repeated consumption of alcohol, and urine analysis from teetotalers shows no EtG above 0.1 μg/ml.[27,28]

The most common technique for EtG quantification in the urine is liquid chromatography coupled to mass spectrometry (LC-MS)[21,24] or tandem mass spectrometry (LC-MS/MS)[29–31] in combination with simple dilution (generally 1/10) or with protein precipitation as the sample preparation. An interesting study[32] presented the comparison of five analytical strategies for determining urinary EtG based on LC-MS or LC-MS/MS with or without prior SPE sample cleanup. Based on the concept of "identification points" (IPs), the authors showed that for urinary EtG, single MS procedures were demonstrated to perform well at a reporting limit ≥ 0.3 mg/l, whereas SPE-LC/MS/MS was indicated as the most reliable method with the lowest cut-off = 0.1 mg/l. Two fully validated UPLC-MS-MS methods have been published with regards to improving chromatographic separation.[33,34] The authors proposed the normalization of EtG concentrations to 1000 mg/l creatinine and to use a consensual cut-off of 0.1 mg/l.

A few methods have been published on GC-MS[35] or capillary zone electrophoresis (CZE)[36] for EtG analysis in urine or serum. Recently, the use of LC-ESI-MS/MS to analyze dried urine spots (DUS), an innovative method for sampling, was published.[37] The method proved to be interesting not only because it allows the determination of EtG and creatinine in urine but also because it inhibits the degradation of EtG by *Escherichia coli* or other pathogens observed in classical urine samples.

3.2.3 EtG Analysis in Hair

As mentioned before, EtG also accumulates in the hair allowing for a larger retrospective window of time for alcohol consumption detection. Therefore, EtG could be used as a long-term alcohol marker. The analysis of EtG in this matrix requires highly sensitive analytical methods, because EtG concentrations in hair are generally in the pg/mg range. In contrast to the methods used for urine, the most frequently used analytical methods to measure EtG in hair are based on GC-MS.[38,39] However, the first fully validated method to combine GC-MS/MS with negative chemical ionization (NCI) was published in 2009.[40] The limit of detection (LOD) and the limit of quantification (LOQ) were 3 and 8.4 pg/mg, respectively. Some years later, the same authors published a study[41] in which they evaluated the diagnostic performance of EtG in hair for the investigation of alcohol drinking behavior. Diagnostic performances for EtG (sensitivity,

TABLE 4.3 Diagnostic Performances of EtG in Hair

Classification Alcohol Consumption (g/day)	Teetotalers 0	At-risk Drinkers >20/30	Heavy Drinkers >60
Cut-off (pg/mg)	0	>9	>25 >30
AUC	0.95	0.95	0.99 –
Sensitivity	0.93	0.82	0.95 0.81
Specificity	0.94	0.93	0.97 0.97

AUC area under the ROC curve; a test with $0.9 < AUC < 1.0$ is highly accurate. Adapted from (41).

specificity) were calculated for the optimal cut-off values selected from the receiver operating characteristic (ROC) curves (see Table 4.3).

This study showed that EtG provides a better diagnostic performance in detecting heavy drinkers than at-risk drinkers, with a false-negative rate of 5% and a false-positive rate of 3%. Using the 30 pg/mg cut-off recommended by the Society of Hair Testing (SOHT), the authors would have obtained the same specificity (0.97); however, the sensitivity would have decreased to a small degree (0.81). Interestingly, the same study demonstrated that EtG was not influenced by gender, age or BMI.

In May 2012, a systematic multi-database search retrieved 366 records related to hair EtG concentrations and further screened for relevant publications in the field. Fifteen (4.1%) records matched the selection criteria and were included in a meta-analysis.[42] Although larger and well-designed population studies are required to draw any definitive conclusion, these data show that a cut-off of 30 pg/mg limits the false-negative effects in differentiating heavy from social drinkers, whereas the recently proposed 7 pg/mg cut-off value might only be used for suspected active alcohol use and not for demonstrating complete abstinence.

A fully validated method based on UPLC-ESI-MS/MS with an LOQ of 10 pg/mg was recently presented.[43] To the best of our knowledge, it is the first LC-MS/MS with LOQ values close to those found by GC-MS/MS methods.

3.3 Ethylsulfate (EtS)

EtG was first detected in human urine in 1995 by Schmitt,[35] but it was not until 2004 that Helander[44] showed that EtS was also present in humans after alcohol ingestion. The properties and detection times of EtS are very similar to those of EtG. Therefore, many of the urinanalysis methods presented in this chapter can be used for both compounds.[28,29,32−34,36]

However, EtS has been detected in classical biological fluids (urine, blood) but not in hair.[45] For urine, as with EtG, a well-accepted cut-off is not fixed in international guidelines. However, the most accepted value is generally 0.1 µg/ml as it is for EtG.[33]

3.4 Fatty Acid Ethyl Esters (FAEEs)

FAEEs are formed during the non-oxidative metabolism of ethanol by the conjugation of ethanol to endogenous free fatty acids and fatty acyl-CoA. FAEE formation can be spontaneous but is often catalyzed by microsomal acyl-CoA: ethanol O-acetyltransferase or cytosolic FAEE synthase found throughout the body (see Figure 4.2). Some studies[46,47] have shown that FAEEs are also involved in ethanol-induced organ damage. Finally, FAEE concentrations should be recognized as short-term markers in serum[48] and as long-term markers in hair.[49]

3.4.1 Determination of Serum FAEEs

Serum FAEE concentrations are measured by GC-MS and the measured FAEE values shown here are the sum of E16:0 and E18:0 ester concentrations.[48] The LOQ estimated using this technique is approximately 0.02 µmol/l. In this study, FAEEs have been reported to be measurable after alcohol consumption for up to 24 hours and in heavy drinkers for about two days.

3.4.2 Determination of Hair FAEEs

FAEEs are incorporated into the hair through sebum. Hair FAEE concentrations are most often measured by headspace solid phase microextraction (HS-SPME) and GC-MS.[49–51] A fully validated HS-SPME-GC-MS method[52] was recently proposed for the four primary FAEEs, namely, ethyl myristate, ethyl palmitate, ethyl oleate and ethyl stearate. The resulting LOQs were 0.027, 0.074, 0.087 and 0.032 ng/mg, respectively. Six hundred and forty-four hair samples were analyzed, and their FAEE concentrations ranged from 0.11 to 31 ng/mg (mean 1.77 ng/mg, median 0.82 ng/mg).

For interpretation, the SOHT consensus[53] recommend the sum of the four FAEEs with a cut-off of 0.5 ng/mg for the proximal scalp hair segment at 0−3 cm or less and 1.0 ng/mg for scalp hair samples with a length between 3 and 6 cm and for body hair.

According to this consensus, the diagnostic performance for detecting heavy drinkers (with a cut-off of 1 ng/mg in the proximal 6 cm hair segment) was evaluated in 229 hair samples.[54] The AUC, specificity and sensitivity were 0.955, 0.96 and 0.77, respectively, for the hair FAEE test. A sensitivity of 0.77 indicates that 23% of samples are interpreted as "false negatives." In comparison, the specificity and sensitivity for EtG were 0.97 and 0.81, respectively, using an EtG cut-off of 30 pg/mg.[41]

3.5 Phosphatidylethanol (PEth)

3.5.1 Definition and Formation

Phosphatidylethanol (PEth) is an abnormal cellular membrane phospholipid that was discovered for the first time in 1983 in rats.[55] The formation of PEth is catalyzed by phospholipase D (PLD), an enzyme[56] normally responsible for the hydrolysis of phosphatidylcholine (PC) into phosphatidic acid (PA). In the presence of ethanol, PLD promotes a transphosphatidylation reaction, resulting in the production of PEth.[57] During preliminary studies of rat exposure to ethanol, it was observed that PEth is not a single molecule but rather a group of glycerophospholipid homologs with a common head group onto which two long carboxylic acid side chains are attached. These homologs are commonly named "PEth A:B/C:D," where A and C indicate the number of carbons in the carboxylic side chains, and B and D indicate the number of double bonds in each side chain.[58]

3.5.2 PEth Degradation in Human Blood

Several studies[59–61] have shown that the kinetics of elimination are well approximated by a one-compartment model. PEth was found to decrease over time with a half-life of approximately 3−5 days, and it was detectable in blood up to 28 days after the start of sobriety. In a recent study, 11 test persons drank sufficient EtOH to lead to an estimated blood ethanol concentration of 1 g/kg on each of 5 successive days after 3 weeks of alcohol abstinence. After the drinking episode, subjects remained abstinent for 16 days and were subjected to regular blood sampling. The mean half-life of PEth (measured as PEth 16:0/18:1) ranged from 4.5 to 10.1 days during the first week and from 5.0 to 12.0 during the second week.[62] Although 48 PEth species homologs have been identified in postmortem human blood,[63] the preliminary available data suggest that five molecular species (16:0/18:1, 16:0/18:2, 16:0/20:4, 18:1/18:1 and 18:1/18:2) could constitute more than 80% of the total PEth.

3.5.3 Analytical Techniques for PEth Determination in Blood

For the PEth determination, venous blood should be collected in tubes containing EDTA, and the sample should not be centrifuged. Blood samples for PEth analysis are stable for 24 hours at room temperature and for 3 weeks at +4°C.[58] Work carried out in 2013[64] has shown that differences in temperature storage appear not to have a significant influence for the stability of PEth homologs when blood is spotted into dried blood spots (DBS). The PEth concentrations diminished only up to 20% during 3 weeks of storage at room temperature in DBS form. The decrease was lower when fluorinated blood was spotted.

Several analytical techniques have been proposed for the quantification of PEth. Examples of each type of analytical techniques are indicated below, as follows:

- Thin layer chromatography (TLC)[65]
- Capillary electrophoresis (CE)[66]
- GC-MS[67]
- Immunoassay[68]
- HPLC coupled to an evaporative light-scattering detector (ELSD)[58]
- HPLC-MS or HPLC-MS/MS[63,64]

TLC, CE, GC-MS and immunoassays have not been used in clinical or forensic toxicology, and the HPLC-ELSD method remains the most commonly used analysis method in clinical toxicology. However, multiple mass spectrometry methods (LC-MS/MS) are being developed for the identification of PEth homologs in blood, and the majority of these novel methods employ electrospray ionization (ESI) for MS coupling.

3.5.4 PEth as a Marker of Chronic Alcohol Use

In March 2012, a systematic multi-database search retrieved 444 records related to the formation, distribution and degradation of PEth in human blood. Twelve papers (2.7%) were included in the meta-analysis.[69] The mean (M) and 95% confidence interval (CI) of total PEth concentrations in social drinkers ($M = 0.288\ \mu M$; CI $0.208-0.367\ \mu M$) and heavy drinkers ($M = 3.897\ \mu M$; CI $2.404-5.391\ \mu M$) were calculated. This analysis demonstrated the good clinical efficiency of PEth analysis for detecting chronic heavy drinking, displaying a mean concentration one order of magnitude higher than the remaining group (heavy drinkers $= 3.897\ \mu M$; social drinkers $= 0.288\ \mu M$). Although the international scientific community has not yet established a cut-off value for differentiating acceptable social ethanol intake from at-risk alcohol use and chronic excessive drinking behavior, nine of the 12 mentioned studies that applied HPLC-ELSD for total PEth quantification in blood used the LOQs of the analytical method as cut-offs: $0.22\ \mu M$ (five methods); $0.30\ \mu M$ (three methods); $0.80\ \mu M$ (one method). The sensitivity and the specificity of these cut-offs were $98-100\%$ and $95-100\%$, respectively.

An interesting question remains regarding the quantity of ethanol that must be consumed over a certain period to give a positive blood PEth response. One study,[62] which was conducted in 11 healthy volunteers who drank $50-109\ g$ of ethanol/day, showed that the formation of PEth began immediately after the first consumption of alcohol ($0.5-8$ hours), reaching a concentration of $0.05-0.10\ \mu M$. These observations show novel potential applications for PEth in the diagnosis of excessive drinking episodes and/or "binge drinking" behaviors found frequently in the context of DFCs.

3.6 Alcohol Congeners

Alcohol congeners are minor chemical compounds other than ethanol that are present in alcoholic beverages, and they are classified as the following two types:

- Fermentation by-product congeners
- Ingredient biomarker congeners

3.6.1 Fermentation By-product Congeners

Fermentation by-product congeners are mostly a result of the fermentation and aging process or they are added during production. The quantities of each alcohol congener are dependent on the amount and type of beverage consumed.[70] The most commonly encountered alcohol congeners[71] are listed in order of importance as follows: methanol, isopropanol, 1-propanol, 1-butanol, 2-butanol, isobutanol, 2-methyl-1-butanol and 3-methyl-1-butanol. The number of congeners found in common beverages varies from 28 in rum to approximately 800 in wine (Table 4.4).

After publishing his well-known works on the direct determination of ethanol in blood,[10,11] Machata presented his initial workup and concept of *alcohol congener analysis* (ACA) by correlating congeners detected in blood with the concentrations found in the beverage consumed.[72]

The current analytical method for determining by-product congeners in beverages and blood is HS-GC-FID and can include trapping and/or cryofocusing techniques. Generally $0.1-0.3$ ml of blood is used to achieve the required LODs, with 0.1 mg/l for methanol and 0.01 mg/l for the other alcohol congeners.[73]

However, the fermentation by-product ACA causes some important limitations.[70] First, many fermentation by-product congeners can either be produced endogenously by bacterial putrefaction or obtained from sources other than the claimed alcoholic beverage. Second, blood must be sampled within 3 hours after drinking cessation, and a significant BAC of 0.1‰ must be present.

3.6.2 Ingredient Biomarker Congeners

Congeners are also found in beverages as a result of the ingredients and materials used during production. These materials include aldehydes, esters, histamines,

TABLE 4.4 Number of Congeners in Common Beverages

Alcoholic beverage	Beer	Wine	Brandy	Whiskey	Rum	Vodka
Number of congeners	653	813	120	113	28	31

Data from (71).

additives, coloring agents, tannins, phenols and others. In contrast with by-product congeners, they are often very specific to the beverage ingested.[71]

Analytical strategies for the detection of ingredient biomarker congeners have employed wider techniques than classical ACA by HS-GC-FID, because they have larger molecular weights. For example, aromatic compounds from alcoholic beverages have been determined in blood samples by HS-GC-MS[74] and with SPME pretreatment to detect congeners coming from herbs.[75] LC-MS/MS was also used for analyzing flavonoids in beer.[76]

Although alcohol congeners are not often investigated at present, they will constitute a powerful tool for determining the specific source of alcohol in the future.

3.6.3 DFC Case Applications

The specific analysis of fermentation and ingredient congeners can help to determine what type of beverage has been consumed, which might constitute a helpful tool in the following situations:

- When a higher strength spirit was added to a lower strength beverage, unknowingly increasing the ethanol intake of the victim.
- When the victim claimed to have consumed a drink (usually a strong spirit) after the incident to calm their nerves.
- When a concomitant drug administration is suspected and when the method of administration is "drink spiking."

Therefore, congeners and other biomarkers should be included in what could be called "Alcohol testing of the 21st century."[77]

4. ALCOHOL AND DFC (DFSA): EPIDEMIOLOGICAL STUDIES

4.1 Methodology

Because the most prevalent DFC is DFSA and because a whole chapter of this book is dedicated to "Epidemiology of drug-facilitated crimes," we have limited our review of epidemiological studies to "alcohol and DFSAs." Papers were selected and reviewed based on a comprehensive PubMed search for articles about "Alcohol and DFSA" in English, as published to date. A final selection was made with the following additional keywords: blood alcohol levels, BAC and alcohol testing.

Finally, four studies[78–81] that fulfilled all the above criteria were selected.

4.2 Prevalence of Positive Alcohol Testing

All four studies showed a high frequency of positive alcohol testing. This high prevalence of alcohol itself is not surprising because most of the alleged

TABLE 4.5 Positive Alcohol Testing as a Function of the Time Interval between the Incident and the Test

Number of Cases (n)	Period of Study	Time Delay (hours)	Alcohol Positive n and (%)	Reference
1014	2000–2002 (3 years)	<24	470[46]	78
391	2000–2002 (3 years)	<12	316[81]	79
434	2002–2003 (1 year)	median: 20 range: 2–106	161[37]	80
291	1999–2005 (7 years)	–	163[56]	81
105		>12	54[51]	
137		<12	97[64]	

DFSAs were associated with social situations, such as at a public house, bar, night-club or party, where it is expected that alcohol would be consumed. The data from the four studies have been rearranged so that the results could be compared; these data are presented in Table 4.5.

The results in the table clearly show that the rate of positive alcohol testing is a function of the time delay, which represents the number of elapsed hours from the alleged assault to the examination and blood sampling. For a time delay >12 hours, the mean rate of positive alcohol testing was 45% ($n = 3$, 37, 46 and 51%), and for a time delay <12 hours, it was 72% ($n = 2$, 63–81%). The last value provides the best figure relating to alcohol consumption before the alleged assault, because 77% of the subjects self-reported that they had consumed alcohol.[80]

4.3 Back-calculated Blood Alcohol Concentrations

Two studies [79,81] proposed back calculations for finding the complainants' blood alcohol concentration (BAC) at the time of the alleged assault. Only data for time delay <12 hours were considered for the evaluation. The calculation method, as previously presented (see 2.6), was used with a $\beta_{60} = 0.18$ g/kg per hour.

The first study[79] evaluated the blood alcohol concentrations in 316 cases of alleged DFSAs between January 2000 and December 2002. A large majority of these cases (60%) had a back-calculated BAC higher than 1.5‰ or g/kg. In 36% of cases, the back-calculated BACs were very high, at over 2.0‰ or g/kg, which is sufficient to cause heavy drunkenness in a social drinker. It is worth noting that for the cases in which ethanol was measured in the urine sample only, a ratio UAC/BAC of 1.33 was used to convert the level to the equivalent blood alcohol concentration.

The second study[81] addressed the blood alcohol concentrations in 97 cases of alleged DFSAs from 1999 to 2005 (7 years). The authors calculated the average BAC for each year (mean value: 1.95‰ or g/kg, range: 1.68−2.18‰ or g/kg). The estimated overall range for the seven years was 0.96 to 4.06 g/kg.

Although these calculations were based on a number of assumptions and should be regarded as a guide, these data highlighted surprisingly high blood alcohol levels in complainant samples for cases of alleged DFSA. However, from these data, it is not possible to conclude whether all of the alcohol detected was consumed voluntarily or without the victim's consent.

4.4 Advice

The results of these epidemiological studies caused alarm for the health and safety of certain populations regarding their increased vulnerability to sexual assault and emphasized the need for education on the dangers of excessive alcohol consumption in some social settings.

Media interest in DFSA has focused on hypnotic, sedative or anesthetic drugs that could be used for this type of crime and on recommendations about how to avoid being drugged. However, advice regarding alcohol consumption itself[79] will be provided as follows:

Drinking slowly and moderately, not drinking on an empty stomach and avoiding of mixing large quantities of alcoholic drinks.

5. CONCLUSIONS

In recent years, there has been a notable increase in the number of reports of DFCs. Usually, victims report that they were robbed or assaulted while incapacitated by drugs. Most often, these drugs have the ability to produce an effect that leaves the victim in a semiconscious or even unconscious state. Epidemiological studies have demonstrated that ethanol is the most common drug in alleged DFCs, along with cannabis. However, in contrast to other drugs, ethanol can play either an active or a passive role in DFCs.

Ethanol itself can serve as a direct marker of alcohol consumption. When the time elapsed between the crime and blood sampling is not short and when the measured blood alcohol concentration is still 0.15 g/kg or more, a retrospective calculation of the blood alcohol concentration (BAC) at the moment of the crime is possible. However, when the time between the alleged crime and blood sampling is greater than 8 hours or when the BAC is close to 0 g/kg, collecting one urine sample and measuring the ethanol therein is recommended. In this case, the BAC at the moment of the crime could be determined using the UAC/BAC ratio.

Using similar assumptions, some epidemiological studies have highlighted the surprisingly high blood alcohol levels found in complainant samples in cases of alleged DFSAs, even if it is not possible to estimate the amount of alcohol consumed voluntarily or without the victim's consent.

Biomarker measurement is suitable for determining previous alcohol abuse for diagnostic improvement in DFC investigations. Among the different biomarkers presented in this chapter, ethyl glucuronide in hair is a powerful tool, allowing one of the largest retrospective time windows for the detection of alcohol consumption. By using the 30 pg/mg cut-off recommended by the Society of Hair Testing, excellent diagnostic performance in detecting heavy drinkers has been described.

Finally, even if the determination is limited to the cases in which a blood sample has been collected within 3 hours after drinking cessation, an analysis of ingredient congeners from the type of beverage consumed might constitute a helpful tool when a concomitant drug has been added to an alcoholic beverage by "drink spiking."

In conclusion, blood, urine and hair are standard matrices that should be collected in the cases of ethanol and drug-facilitated crime.

LIST OF ABBREVIATIONS

ACA	alcohol congener analysis
ADH	alcohol dehydrogenase
ADP	adenosine 5′diphosphate
ALDH	acetaldehyde dehydrogenase
BAC	blood alcohol concentration
BMI	body mass index
CA	alcohol congener
CE	capillary electrophoresis
CO_2	carbon dioxide
DBS	dried blood spots
DFC	drug-facilitated crime
DFSA	drug-facilitated sexual assault
ELSD	evaporative light scattering detector
EtG	ethyl glucuronide
EtS	ethyl sulfate
FAEE	fatty acid ethyl ester
FID	flame ionization detector
GC	gas chromatography
H_2O	water
HPLC	high performance liquid chromatography
HS	headspace (injector)
LC	liquid chromatography

LOD	limit of detection
LOQ	limit of quantification
MEOS	microsomal oxidation system
MS	mass spectrometry
MS-MS	tandem mass spectrometry
NCI	negative chemical ionization
PAPS	3'phosphoadenosine 5'phosphosulfate
PEth	phosphatidylethanol
PLD	phospholipase D
SULTs	sulfotransferases
TLC	thin layer chromatography
UGTs	UDP-glucuronyl transferases
UDP	uridine 5'diphosphate

REFERENCES

1. Shbair MKS, Ejabour S, Lhermitte M. Drugs involved in drug-facilitated crimes: Part I: Alcohol, sedative-hypnotic drugs, gamma-hydroxybutyrate and ketamine. A review. *Ann Pharmaceutiques Françaises* 2010;**68**:275−85.

2. Shbair MKS, Ejabour S, Bassyoni I, Lhermitte M. Drugs involved in drug-facilitated crimes: Part II: drugs of abuse, prescription and over-the-counter medications. A review. *Ann Pharmaceutiques Françaises* 2010;**68**:319−31.

3. Shbair MKS, Lhermitte M. Drug-facilitated crimes: definitions, prevalence, difficulties et recommendations. A review. *Ann. Pharmaceutiques Françaises* 2010;**68**:136−47.

4. Papadodima SA, Athanaselis A, Spiliopopoulou C. Toxicological investigation of drug-facilitated sexual assaults. *Int J Clin Pract* 2007;**61**:259−64.

5. Testa M, Livingston JA, Collins RL. The role of women's alcohol consumption in evaluation of vulnerability to sexual aggression. *Exp Clin Psychopharmacol* 2000;**8**:185−91.

6. Morel I, Anger JP. Alcool éthylique et éthylisme. In: Kintz P. *Traité de toxicologie médico-judiciaire*. 2e ed. 2012. pp. 279−98.

7. *WHO Global status report on alcohol and health*. Geneva: World Health Organization; 2011.

8. Wills S. *Alcohol. Drugs of abuse*. 2nd ed. Pharmaceutical Press; 2005. pp. 303−23.

9. Widmark EMP. *Principles and applications of medicolegal alcohol determination*. Davis, CA: Biomedical Publications; 1981 (English translation of Widmark's 1932 monograph).

10. Machata G. The routine examination of blood alcohol concentration using a gas chromatograph. *Microchim Acta* 1962;**50**:691−700.

11. Machata G. About the gas chromatographic determination of blood alcohol. Analysis of the vapor phase. *Microchim Acta* 1964;**50**:262−71.

12. Tarnoski G, Hayashi T, Igarashi K, Ochi H, Matoba R. Misidentification of ethyl chloride in the routine GC-FID analysis for alcohol. *Forensic Sci Int* 2009;**188**:e7−9.

13a. OFROU. Directives pour le calcul rétrospectif et le calcul théorique de l'alcoolémie. Annexe 4 des Instructions concernant la constatation de l'incapacité de conduire dans la circulation routière. *French Transl.* 2008;19−22.

13b. Augsburger M, Giroud C, Esseiva P, Staub C. Course for the master of advanced studies in toxicology. *Module Forensic Toxicol* 2012.

14. Jones AW. Ethanol distribution ratios between urine and capillary blood in controlled experiments and in apprehended drinking drivers. *J Forensic Sci* 1992;**37**:21−34.

15. Jones AW. Reference limits for urine/blood ratios of ethanol in two successive voids from drinking drivers. *J Anal Toxicol* 2002;**26**:333−9.

16. Jones AW, Kugelberg FC. Relationship between blood and urine alcohol concentrations in apprehended drivers who claimed consumption of alcohol after driving with and without supporting evidence. *Forensic Sci Int* 2010;**194**:97−102.

17. Foti RS, Fisher MB. Assessment of UDP-glucuronosyltransferase catalyzed formation of ethyl glucuronide in human liver microsomes and recombinant UGTs. *Forensic Sci Int* 2005;**153**:109−16.

18. Kharbouche H, Sporkert F, Staub C, Mangin P, Augsburger M. Ethyl glucuronide: a biomarker of alcohol consumption. *Praxis* 2009;**98**:1299−306.

19. Stephanson N, Dahl H, Helander A, Beck O. Direct quantification of ethyl glucuronide in clinical urine samples by liquid chromatography-mass spectrometry. *Ther Drug Monit* 2002;**24**:645−51.

20. Wojcik MH, Hawtorne J. Sensitivity of commercial ethylglucuronide (EtG) testing in screening for alcohol abstinence. *Alcohol Alcohol* 2007;**42**:317−20.

21. Dahl H, Stephanson N, Beck O, Helander A. Comparison of urinary excretion characteristic of ethanol and ethyl glucuronide. *J Anal Toxicol* 2002;**26**:201−2004.

22. Hoiseth G, Bernard JP, Stephanson N, Normann PT, Christophersen AS, Mørland J, et al. Comparison between the urinary alcohol markers EtG, EtS, and GTOL/5-HIAA in a controlled drinking experiment. *Alcohol Alcohol* 2008;**43**:187−91.

23. Schmitt G, Droenner P, Skopp G, Aderjan R. Ethyl glucuronide concentration in serum of human volunteers, teetotalers, and suspected drinking drivers. *J Forensic Sci* 1997;**42**:1099−102.

24. Helander A, Bottcher M, Fehr C, Dahmen N, Beck O. Detection times for urinary ethyl glucuronide and ethyl sulfate in heavy drinkers during alcohol detoxification. *Alcohol Alcohol* 2009;**44**:55−61.

25. Thierauf A, Gnann H, Wohlfarth A, Auwärter V, Perdekamp MG, Buttler KJ, et al. Urine tested positive for ethyl glucuronide and ethyl sulphate after the consumption of "non-alcoholic" beer. *Forensic Sci Int* 2010;**202**:82−5.

26. Arndt T, Grüner J, Scröfel S, Stemmerich K. False-positive ethyl glucuronide immunoassay screening caused by a propyl alcohol-based hand sanitizer. *Forensic Sci Int* 2012;**223**:359−63.

27. Janda I, Alt J. Improvement of ethyl glucuronide determination in human urine and serum samples by solid-phase extraction. *J Chromatogr B Biomed Sci Appl* 2001;**758**:229−34.

28. Albermann ME, Musshoff F, Doberentz E, Heese P, Banger M, Madea B. Preliminary investigations on ethyl glucuronide and ethyl sulfate cutoffs for detecting alcohol consumption on the basis of an ingestion experiment and on data from withdrawal treatment. *Int J Legal Med* 2012;**126**:757−64.

29. Weinmann W, Schaefer P, Thierauf A, Schreiber A, Wurst FM. Confirmatory analysis of ethylglucuronide in urine by liquid-chromatography/electrospray ionization/tandem mass spectrometry according to forensic guidelines. *J Am Soc Mass Spectrom* 2004;**15**:188−93.

30. Wurst FM, Yegles M, Alling C, Aradottir S, Dierkes J, Wiesbeck GA, et al. Measurement of direct ethanol metabolites in a case of a former driving under the influence (DUI) of alcohol offender, now claiming abstinence. *Int J Legal Med* 2008;**122**:235−9.

31. Beyer J, Vo Tu N, Gerostamoulos D, Drummer OH. Validated method for the determination of ethylglucuronide and ethylsulfate in human urine. *Anal Bioanal Chem* 2011;**400**:189−96.

32. Helander A, Kenan N, Beck O. Comparison of analytical approaches for liquid chromatography/mass spectrometry determination of the alcohol biomarker ethyl glucuronide in urine. *Rapid Commun Mass Spectrom* 2010;**24**:1737−43.

33. Hegstad S, Helland A, Hagemann C, Michelsen L, Spigset O. EtG/ETS in urine from sexual assault victims determined by UPLC-MS-MS. *J Anal Toxicol* 2013;**37**:227−32.

34. Kummer N, Wille S, Di Fazio V, Lambert W, Samyn N. A fully validated method for the quantification of ethyl glucuronide and ethyl sulphate in urine by UPLC-ESI-MS/MS applied in a prospective alcohol self-monitoring study. *J Chromatogr B* 2013;**929**:149−54.

35. Schmitt G, Aderjan R, Keller T, Wu M. Ethyl glucuronide: an unusual ethanol metabolite in humans. Synthesis, analytical data, and determination in serum and urine. *J Anal Toxicol* 1995;**19**:91−4.

36. Caslavska J, Jung B, Thormann W. Confirmation analysis of ethyl glucuronide and ethyl sulfate in human serum and urine by CZE-ESI-MS(n) after intake of alcoholic beverages. *Electrophoresis* 2011;**32**:1760−4.

37. Redondo AH, Körber C, König S, Längin A, Al-Ahmad A, Weinmann W. Inhibition of bacterial degradation of EtG by collection as dried urine spots (DUS). *Anal Bioanal Chem* 2012;**402**:2417−24.

38. Jurado C, Soriano T, Gimenez MP, Menendez M. Diagnosis of chronic alcohol consumption. Hair analysis for ethyl-glucuronide. *Forensic Sci Int* 2004;**145**:161−6.

39. Appenzeller BM, Agirman R, Neuberg P, Yegles M, Wennig R. Segmental determination of ethyl glucuronide in hair: a pilot study. *Forensic Sci Int* 2007;**173**:87−92.

40. Kharbouche H, Sporkert F, Troxler S, Ausburger M, Mangin P, Staub C. Development and validation of a gas chromatography-negative chemical ionization tandem mass spectrometry method for the determination of ethyl glucuronide in hair and its application to forensic toxicology. *J Chromatogr B* 2009;**877**:2337−43.

41. Kharbouche H, Faouzi M, Sanchez N, Deappen JB, Augsburger M, Mangin P, et al. Diagnostic performance of ethyl glucuronide in hair for the investigation of alcohol drinking behavior: a comparison with traditional biomarkers. *Int J Legal Med* 2012;**126**:243−50.

42. Boscolo-Berto R, Viel G, Montisci M, Terranova C, Favretto D, Ferrara SD. Ethyl glucuronide concentration in hair for detecting heavy drinking and/or abstinence: a meta-analysis. *Int J Legal Med* 2013;**127**:611−9.

43. Kummer N, Wille S, Lambert W, Nele S. Determination of ethylglucuronide in hair: optimization of the extraction process and validation of an UPLC-ESI-MS/MS procedure. *Poster presented at the 18th Scientific Meeting of the SOHT*. Geneva, Switzerland; 2013.

44. Helander A, Beck O. Mass spectrometric identification of ethyl sulfate as an ethanol metabolite in humans. *Clin Chem* 2004;**50**:936−7.

45. Morini L, Marchei E, Vagnarelli F, Garcia Algar O, Groppi A, et al. Ethyl glucuronide and ethyl sulfate in meconium and hair-potential biomarkers of intrauterine exposure to ethanol. *Forensic Sci Int* 2010;**196**:74−7.

46. Lang LG, Sobel B. Mitochondrial dysfunction induced by fatty acid ethyl esters, myocardial metabolites of ethanol. *J Clin Invest* 1986;**72**:724−31.

47. Laposata EA, Lange LG. Presence of nonoxidative ethanol metabolism in human organs commonly damaged by ethanol abuse. *Science* 1986;**31**:497−9.

48. Borucki K, Schreiner R, Dierkes J, Jachau K, Krause D, Westphal S, et al. Detection of recent ethanol intake with new markers: comparison of fatty acid ethyl esters in serum and of ethyl glucuronide and the ratio of 5-hydroxytryptophol to 5-hydroxyindole acetic acid in urine. *Alcohol Clin Exp Res* 2005;**29**:781−7.

49. Auwarter V, Sporkert F, Hartwig S, Pragst F, Vater H, Diefenbacher A. Fatty acid ethyl esters in hair as markers of alcohol consumption. Segmental hair analysis of alcoholics, social drinkers, and teetotalers. *Clin Chem* 2001;**47**:2114−23.

50. Pragst F, Auwaerter V, Sporkert F, Spiegel K. Analysis of fatty acid ethyl esters in hair as possible markers of chronically elevated alcohol consumption by headspace solid-phase microextraction (HS-SPME) and gas chromatography-mass spectrometry (GC-MS). *Forensic Sci Int* 2001;**121**:76–88.

51. De Giovani N, Donadio G, Chiarotti M. The reliability of fatty acid ethyl esters (FAEE) as biological markers for the diagnosis of alcohol abuse. *J Anal Toxicol* 2007;**31**:93–7.

52. Suesse S, Selavka CM, Mieczkowski T, Pragst F. Fatty acid ethyl ester concentrations In hair and self-reported alcohol consumption in 644 cases from different origin. *Forensic Sci Int* 2010;**196**:111–7.

53. SOHT. *Consensus of the Society of Hair Testing on hair testing for chronic excessive alcohol consumption.* <http://www.soht.org/pdf/Consensus_EtG_2009.pdf>; 2009.

54. Suesse S, Pragst F, Mieczkowski T, Selavka CM, Elian A, Sachs H, et al. Practical experiences in application of hair fatty acid ethyl esters and ethyl glucuronide for detection of chronic alcohol abuse in forensic cases. *Forensic Sci Int* 2012;**218**:82–91.

55. Alling C, Gustavsson L, Anggard E. An abnormal phospholipid in rat organs after ethanol. *FEBS Lett* 1983;**152**:24–8.

56. Gustavsson L, Alling C. Formation of phophatidylethanol in rat brain by pospholipase D. *Biochem Biophys Res Commun* 1987;**142**:958–63.

57. Gustavsson L. ESBRA 1994 award lecture. Phosphatidylethanol formation: specific effects of ethanol mediated via phospholipase D. *Alcohol Alcohol* 1995;**30**:391–406.

58. Isaksson A, Whalther L, Hansson T, Andersson A, Alling C. Phosphatidylethanol in blood (B-PEth): a marker for alcohol use and abuse. *Drug Test Anal* 2011;**3**:195–200.

59. Varga A, Hansson P, Johnson G, Alling C. Normalization rate and cellular localization of phosphatidylethanol in whole blood from chronic alcoholics. *Clin Chim Acta* 2000;**299**:141–50.

60. Wurst FM, Thon N, Aradottir S, Hartmann S, Wiesbeck GA, Lesch O, et al. Phosphatidylethanol: normalization during detoxification, gender aspects and correlation with other biomarkers and self-reports. *Addict Biol* 2010;**15**:88–95.

61. Wurst FM, Thon N, Weinmann W, Tippetts S, Marques P, Hahn JA, et al. Characterization of sialic acid index of plasma apolipoprotein J and phosphatidylethanol during alcohol detoxification—a pilot study. *Alcohol Clin Exp Res* 2012;**36**:251–7.

62. Gnann H, Weinmann W, Thierauf A. Formation of phosphatidylethanol and its subsequent elimination during an extensive drinking experiment over 5 days. *Alcohol Clin Exp Res* 2012;**36**:1507–11.

63. Gnann H, Engelmann C, Skopp G, Winkler M, Auwärter V, Dresen S, et al. Identification of 48 homologues of phosphatidylethanol in blood by LC-ESI-MS/MS. *Anal Bioanal Chem* 2010;**396**:2415–23.

64. Rusconi M. Thesis for master of advanced studies in toxicology. Method development for the detection of the direct ethanol biomarker phosphatidylethanol and its application in forensic toxicology. *Univ Geneva* 2013;1–37.

65. Sarri E, Servitja JM, Picatoste F, Claro E. Two phosphatidylethanol classes separated by thin layer chromatography are produced by phospholipase D in rat brain hippocampal slices. *FEBS Lett* 1996;**393**:303–6.

66. Varga A, Nilsson S. Non aqueous capillary electrophoresis for analysis of the ethanol consumption biomarker phosphatidylethanol. *Electrophoresis* 2008;**29**:1667–71.

67. Yon C, Hans JS. Analysis of trimethylsilyl derivatization products of phosphotidylethanol by gas chromatography-mass spectrometry. *Exp Mol Med* 2000;**32**:243–5.

68. Nissinen AE, Mäkelä SM, Vuoristo JT, Liisanantti MK, Hannuksela ML, Hörkkö S, et al. Immunological detection of in vitro formed phosphatidylethanol—an alcohol biomarker—with monoclonal antibodies. *Alcohol Clin Exp Res* 2008;**32**:921—8.

69. Viel G, Boscolo-Berto R, Cecchetto G, Fais P, Nalesso A, Ferrara SD. Phosphatidylethanol in blood as a marker of chronic alcohol use: a systematic review and meta-analysis. *Int J Mol Sci* 2012;**13**:14788—812.

70. Rodda LN, Beyer J, Gerostamoulos D, Drummer OH. Alcohol congener analysis and the source of alcohol: a review. *Forensic Sci Med Pathol* 2013;**9**:194—207.

71. Greizerstein HB. Congener contents of alcoholic beverages. *J Stud Alcohol* 1981; **42**:1030—7.

72. Machata G, Prokop L. About accompanying substances in the blood of alcoholic beverages. *Blutalkohol* 1971;**8**:349—53.

73. Bonte W. *Congener analysis. Encyclopedia of forensic sciences. Duesseldorf.* Academic Press; 2000. pp. 93—102.

74. Schulz K, Klaus Mueller R, Engewld W, Graefe A, Dressler J. Determination of aroma compounds from alcoholic beverages in spiked blood samples by means of dynamic headspace GC-MS. *Chromatographia* 2007;**66**:879—86.

75. Shulz K, Bertau M, Schlenz K, Malt S, Dressler J, Lachenmeier DW. Headspace solid-phase microextraction-gas chromatography-mass spectrometry determination of the characteristic flavourings menthone, isomenthone, neomenthol and menthol in serum samples with and without enzymatic cleavage to validate post-offense alcohol drinking claims. *Anal Chim Acta* 2009;**646**:128—40.

76. Intelmann D, Haseleu G, Hofmann T. LC-MS/MS quantitation of hop-derived bitter compounds in beer using the ECHO technique. *J Agric Food Chem* 2009;**57**:1172—82.

77. Kelly AT, Mozayani A. An overview of alcohol testing and interpretation in the 21st century. *J Pharm Pract* 2012;**25**:30—6.

78. Scott-Ham M, Burton FC. Toxicological findings in cases of alleged drug-facilitated sexual assault in the United Kingdom over a 3-year period. *J Clin Forensic Med* 2005;**12**:175—86.

79. Scott-Ham M, Burton FC. A study of blood and urine alcohol concentrations in cases of alleged drug-facilitated sexual assault in the United Kingdom over a 3-year period. *J Clin Forensic Med* 2006;**13**:107—11.

80. Hurley M, Parker H, Wells DL. The epidemiology of drug facilitated assault. *J Clin Forensic Med* 2006;**13**:181—5.

81. Hall J, Goodall EA, Moore T. Alleged drug facilitated sexual assault (DFSA) in Northern Ireland from 1999 to 2005. A study of blood alcohol levels. *J Forensic Legal Med* 2008;**15**:497—504.

Chapter 5

Memory Impairment after Drug-Facilitated Crimes

Elodie Saussereau, Michel Guerbet, Jean-Pierre Anger and
Jean-Pierre Goullé

In recent years, drug-facilitated crimes (DFCs) have received widespread
media coverage. To facilitate their crimes, the perpetrators commonly use
pharmaceutical drugs such as sedative-hypnotic drugs due to their amnestic
properties. Therefore, memory impairment is a major problem after a DFC.
This chapter describes the mechanism of memory process, the new molecular
biology of memory and memory impairment after drug exposure.

It is useful to recall a number of definitions which are mainly taken from
Kandel[1]:

- **Episodic memory (EM)** is the memory of one's own biographical events
  that can be precisely related in time, location and associated emotions.
  Thus, it is the collection of past personal and specific experiences that
  occurred at a particular time and place.
- **Semantic memory (SM)** is the memory of meanings, understandings and
  concepts related to facts, information and general knowledge about the
  world. The semantic memory gives meaning to otherwise meaningless
  words and sentences and enables learning based on past experiences.
  Semantic memory is abstracted from actual experience and is therefore
  said to be conceptual, that is, generalized and without reference to any
  specific experience.
- **Short-term memory (STM)** is the capacity to keep a small amount of
  information in mind in an active, readily available state for a short period
  of time. Short-term memory should be distinguished from working memory, which is broader and more general because it refers to structures and
  processes used for temporarily stored and manipulated information.
- **Working memory (WM)** is the system that actively maintains some
  amount of information in the mind to enable its manipulation for further
  information processing. This encompasses verbal and nonverbal tasks

Toxicological Aspects of Drug-Facilitated Crimes. DOI: http://dx.doi.org/10.1016/B978-0-12-416748-3.00005-0

involved in reasoning and comprehension. The information processing produced by the working memory system consists of manipulations of elements recalled by short-term memory activities.

- **Intermediate-term memory (ITM)** is a step between STM and long-term memory (LTM) and has two phases: an early intermediate memory and a late intermediate memory.[2]

- **Long-term memory (LTM)** refers to the unlimited, continuing memory store that can hold information over lengthy periods of time, even for an entire lifetime, as memory consolidation is a continuous process. Long-term memory is mainly preconscious and unconscious. Information in LTM is to a great extent outside of our awareness, but can be called into working memory to be used when needed. Some of this information is easy to recall, whereas some information is much more difficult to access.

- LTM is usually divided into *declarative or explicit memory* and *procedural or implicit memory*. Declarative memory includes all information that is available in the consciousness. It is located in the hippocampus and the adjacent medial temporal lobe (MTL) structures. Declarative or explicit memory can be further divided into *episodic memory* (past personal and specific experiences) and *semantic memory* (conceptual/generalized and without reference to any specific experience). *Procedural or implicit memory* is information about the pattern of body movement and procedures for using objects in the environment. It involves a number of different brain locations: the cerebellum, the striatum and the amygdala.

- **Autobiographical memory** contains information about specific personal, experienced events and personal facts. It refers to a person's history.

1. THEORY OF FORGETTING AND AMNESIA

Recent models postulate that memories show an initial dependence on the hippocampus that diminishes with time. This process of becoming independent is often referred to as memory consolidation.[3] It is typically assumed that repeated reinstatement of a hippocampal—neocortical representation drives this systems-level consolidation process, which seems to take place during sleep.[4] It is assumed that these processes are all able to hold a memory for a certain time period, from ultra-brief to very long.[4] Although the mechanisms of memory differ vastly in quality and scale, Murre et al.[4] hypothesized that all neural mechanisms involved in memory share two fundamental characteristics, which form the basis for the mechanism of abstraction. First, process memory strength diminishes over time. Second, as long as the memory has not been lost, it continues to generate or induce more permanent memory processes in a higher-level store. For example, as long as neural assemblies are firing, synaptic enhancement may take place: one process induces another, more permanent process. According to Murre et al.[4] these two fundamental properties operate on all time scales in roughly the same manner. These authors assumed that memory processes (neurobiological processes and structures) can be decomposed into a number of processes that contain memory representations which consist of one or more traces, any of which suffices to retrieve the memory. This type of memory trace could, for example, be a neural pathway that has been strengthened by long-term potentiation (LTP) so that upon its activation a learned response will be elicited. During the period of measurement, a newly learned memory will engage one or more of the processes, which are chained in a feed forward manner. Each trace in a process generates traces of its representation in the next higher process, for example through LTP in the hippocampus or neocortex.[5] A trace has a probability of being lost, for example because it is overwritten by different traces or because of neural noise. All traces in a process share the same loss probability. Once a trace is lost, it can no longer generate new traces in higher processes. Higher processes in the chain have lower decline rates, so that the process sketched here is one of rapidly declining processes trying to salvage their representations by generating traces in more slowly declining processes.

2. MEMORY MECHANISMS

There have been major advances in the study of the mechanisms of memory in the past few years. Memory research has progressed more in the last 6 years than in the preceding 50 years![6] According to Furini et al.[6] the most salient are:

1. the recent and major discovery of a role of an atypical isoform of protein kinase C (PKC), protein kinase M-zeta (PKMzeta), in memory consolidation and persistence[7,8];
2. the wide acceptance and extension of the mechanism known as "synaptic tagging" or "synaptic tagging and capture (STC)"[9] to a variety of memory forms,[10,11] including extinction[12];
3. the demonstration that extinction, now generally recognized not as forgetting but just as another form of learning,[13,14] can be modulated by several systems and procedures.[14]

   None of these discoveries would have been possible without perhaps the final agreement that LTP is indeed the basis of memory consolidation at the cellular level in the hippocampus.[15–17] This had been repeatedly proposed by many authors to be the case and work on *in vitro* LTP models was widely hailed as representing work on the actual mechanisms of memory formation in vertebrates, which eventually proved true.[6]

3. THE RECENT MOLECULAR BIOLOGY OF MEMORY

Memory processes are very complex. They can be decomposed into a number of various processes ranging from extremely short-term memory (milliseconds) to short-term memory (hours) and finally to long-term memory (days) or very long-term memory (decades).[4]

Memory consolidation is known to be a continuous process. Marra et al.[2] have studied the susceptibility of memory consolidation during lapses in recall. It is known that memories that can be recalled several hours after learning may paradoxically become non-accessible for brief periods after their formation. This raises major questions about the function of these early memory lapses in the structure of memory consolidation. These questions are difficult to investigate due to the lack of information on the precise timing of lapses. Marra et al.[2] have used electrophysiological and behavioral experiments in *Lymnaea* to solve this problem, which reveal lapses in memory recall at 30 minutes and 2 hours post-conditioning. These authors demonstrate that only during these lapses is consolidation of LTM susceptible to interruption by external disturbance. They show that these shared time points of memory lapse and susceptibility correspond to major transitions between separate phases of memory that have different and specific change in molecular mechanisms only during the early stages of memory formation. So it seems that recall of memory becomes more difficult when there are changes in molecular dependencies indicating that distinct molecular pathways are responsible for the different phases of memory formation.[18] Their previous experiments revealed that these essential changes in molecular requirements are initiated following a single training trial during an early stage of memory consolidation.[19,20] Subsequent downstream mechanisms cause recall between STM and early ITM (at 30 minutes) and between early and late ITM (at 2 hours) to become inherently weaker and susceptible. Marra et al.[2] used the training paradigm leading to uninterrupted memory to test for mechanisms of recall failure at the critical times in their pharmacological blocking experiments. This raised the question whether the two training paradigms result in memories using similar or distinct molecular processes. They demonstrated that both training paradigms induced the same translation but not transcription-dependent ITM at 3 hours and protein and RNA synthesis-dependent LTM at 4 and 24 hours. During the identification of different phases of memory, they demonstrated that[2]:

- the memory at 10 minutes is STM as characterized by the lack of requirement for protein and RNA synthesis;
- the memory at 1 hour is ITM as characterized by the requirement for protein synthesis and the lack of requirement for new RNA synthesis;
- the 4 hour memory trace is LTM because it requires both protein and RNA synthesis.

They proposed that during periods of molecular transition, memory recall is weakened, allowing novel sensory cues to block the consolidation of LTM.

In a review dedicated to the molecular biology of memory, Kandel[21] stated that the contributions to synaptic plasticity and memory have recruited the efforts of many laboratories over the world. There are six key steps in the molecular biological delineation of STM and its conversion to LTM for both implicit (procedural) and explicit (declarative) memory: cAMP (cyclic adenosine monophosphate), PKA (protein kinase A), CRE (cAMP response element), CREB-1 (cAMP response element binding protein-1), CREB-2 (cAMP response element binding protein-2) and CPEB (cytoplasmic polyadenylation element binding protein).

In this major review,[21] Kandel recalls the emergence of a molecular biology of memory-related synaptic plasticity and the delineation of cAMP and PKA in STM storage; and that classical conditioning involves both pre- and postsynaptic mechanisms of plasticity. He then developed the molecular biology of learning-related long-term synaptic plasticity. As previously stated, the formation of LTM requires the synthesis of new protein. An increase in the level of cAMP leads to longer lasting forms of synaptic plasticity. This more robust pattern of stimulation causes the catalytic subunit of PKA to recruit p42 MAPK (mitogen activated protein kinase) and both then move to the nucleus where they phosphorylate transcription factors and activate gene expression required for the induction of LTM. Various synaptic protein phosphatases act as inhibitors of memory formation as they locally counteract the activity of PKA, and the equilibrium between kinase and phosphorylase activities can regulate both memory storage and retrieval.[22] In this review, Kandel[21] explains the activation of nuclear transcription factors, how long-term synaptic changes are governed by both positive and negative regulators, and that the transition from short-term facilitation (STF) to long-term facilitation (LTF) requires the simultaneous removal of transcriptional repressors and activation of transcriptional activators. These transcriptional repressors and activators can interact with each other both physically and functionally.

For Kandel,[21] it is likely that the transition is a complex process involving temporally distinct phases of gene activation, repression and regulation of signal transduction. As reported in the literature, the CREB-mediated response to extracellular stimuli can be modulated by kinases (PKA, CaMKII or calcium calmodulin-dependent protein kinases II, MAPK, PKC, etc.) and phosphatases (phosphoprotein phosphatase 1 or PP1 and calcineurin). The CREB regulatory unit may therefore serve to integrate signals from various signal transduction pathways. This ability to integrate signaling, as well as to mediate activation or repression, may explain why CREB is so central to memory storage. Chromatin alteration and epigenetic changes in gene expression have been observed with memory storage: integration of LTM-related synaptic plasticity involves bidirectional regulation of gene expression and chromatin structure.[23]

Although, epigenetic mechanisms have been widely known to be involved in the formation and long-term storage of cellular information in response to transient environmental signals, the discovery of their putative relevance in adult brain function is relatively recent.[23,24]

The epigenetic marking of chromatin, such as histone modification, chromatin remodeling and the activity of retro transposons, may thus have long-term consequences in the transcriptional regulation of specific loci involved for long-term synaptic changes.[25] LTM fundamentally differs from the short-term process in involving the growth of new synaptic connections. For Kandel[21] the growth of new synapses may represent the final and perhaps most stable phase of LTM storage, raising the possibility that the persistence of the long-term process might be achieved, at least in part, because of the relative stability of synaptic structure. The fundamental difference between the storage of LTM and short-term changes is the requirement for the activation of gene expression. LTF and the associated synaptic changes are synapse specific and require CREB-1. For synaptic capture, there is not only a retrograde signaling from the synapse back to the nucleus, but also antero-grade signaling from the nucleus to the synapse. The molecular mechanism of synaptic capture involves many factors such as PKA, CPEB that activates mRNA and CRE.[21]

4. MEMORY ARCHIVE IN THE BRAIN OR CONSOLIDATION IN THE HIPPOCAMPAL CA1 REGION: MAJOR ROLE OF A PROTEIN KINASE: PKMzeta[6]

Hippocampal LTP is at the center of the initial, post-acquisition process of memory consolidation.[15–17] It has been shown to be one of the very few attributes of memory that is partly modulated by cholinergic transmission,[26] which explains the effect of pro-cholinergic drugs on memory impairments in particular. Memory consolidation is the process of formation of a memory archive in the brain. This takes place initially in the hippocampus, often with the concomitant participation of the entorhinal, of the posterior cortex and of the basolateral amygdala (BLA). The process takes 1–6 hours and involves activation of several protein kinase systems located in the hippo-campus.[15] The resulting stimulation of diverse cellular proteins, including nuclear transcription factors, triggers DNA transcription, and is followed by protein synthesis in ribosome,[27] which uses pre-existent mRNAs.[28] The system is also triggered by protein kinases and brain-derived neurotrophic factor (BDNF), and produces the GluR1 (glutamate receptor 1) subunit of the glutamate alpha-amino-3-hydroxy-5-methyl-4-isoxazolepropionic acid receptor (AMPAR), which is necessary for consolidation.[28] Due to its localization near synapses, the system is thought to play a key role in the processing of recent information by specific synapses, as is believed to happen in memory consolidation, which is accompanied and motivated by morphological synaptic changes.[15]

The processes summarized above (protein kinase activation, protein synthesis, synaptic change) integrate what is now called "cellular consolidation" and cannot be delayed without loss; it has to occur immediately following acquisition.[6] An additional consolidation process, termed "systems consolidation," which is initiated simultaneously, takes place in the prefrontal cortex and other cortical regions, lasts for many weeks or even years, and frequently results in changes in the content of each memory, which can in many cases become falsified.[29] After memories are consolidated in the hippocampal CA1 region, they are stored in a long-lasting form (days, weeks, years) elsewhere, but not in the hippocampus, as attested by studies of humans or animals with anatomical or biochemical lesions of the hippocampus and its surrounding areas.[6] Other studies suggest that the secondary somatosensory cortex and some prefrontal and parietal regions,[29,30] but not the hippocampus,[29] are sites of long-term memory storage. And further studies have implicated the hippocampus in the initiation of "permanent" memory storage, through local biochemical changes.[31,32] These biochemical changes involve the production of local BDNF[33] and/or the local activation of hippocampal MAPK activity and cAMP[34] and/or the release of a dual muscarinic and nicotinic cholinergic mechanism within the hippocampus[35] or the participation of a hippocampal β-noradrenergic mechanism activated by mild stress, presumably that of the training experience.[32]

As suggested by Sacktor et al.,[8] an atypical PKC isoform, PKMzeta, could be involved in both memory consolidation and persistence. PKCs, including PKMzeta, are involved in the phosphorylation of a wide number of proteins, including membrane proteins, other kinases, receptors and nuclear transcription factors. During LTP and memory formation, PKMzeta is synthesized *de novo* as a constitutively active kinase. In fact, the persistent activity of the PKMzeta is both necessary and sufficient for maintaining LTP; as blocking PKMzeta activity by pharmacological or dominant negative inhibitors disrupts previously stored LTM in a variety of neural circuits, including spatial and trace memories in the hippocampus, aversive memories in the BLA, appetitive memories in the nucleus accumbens, habit memory in the dorsal lateral striatum, and elementary associations, extinction and skilled sensorimotor memories in the neocortex.[8] For Sacktor, PKMzeta is the "working end" of LTP.

5. METAPLASTICITY GOVERNS SYNAPTIC TAGGING AND CAPTURE: THE ROLE OF PLASTICITY RELATED PROTEINS (PRPs)

As activity-dependent synaptic plasticity is widely accepted to be the cellular correlate of learning and memory, associativity between different synaptic inputs can transform short-lasting forms of synaptic plasticity (<3 hours) to long-lasting ones; STC might explain this heterosynaptic support, with local mechanisms of synaptic tags and synthesis of PRPs.[36] Sajikumar and Korte[36] demonstrate that priming stimulation through the activation of glutamate receptors increases the "range of threshold" for functional plasticity by producing PKMzeta as a PRP through local protein synthesis. For these authors, BDNF is also implicated as a PRP which is mandatory for establishing cross-capture between synaptic strengthening and weakening, whereas the newly generated PKMzeta specifically establishes synaptic tagging of long-term potentiation.[36] They show that STC are confined to specific dendritic compartments and that these compartments contain "synaptic clusters" with different plasticity thresholds; these clusters will then prepare the synaptic network to form LTM.[36] Their results suggest that within a dendritic compartment itself, a homeostatic process exists to adjust plasticity thresholds.[36]

6. SYNAPTIC PLASTICITY, THE ROLE OF OTHER POSSIBLE MECHANISMS

In contrast, for Furini et al.,[6] a role of PKMzeta or PKC in consolidation would mingle with its role in promoting persistence, and if this were so, the other mechanisms that have been postulated (BDNF-mediated, MAPK/CaMKII-dependent, noradrenergic, cholinergic) may simply be accessory or alternative. Three neurotransmitters play an important role in the chemicals pathways: two are exciters—acetylcholine (ACh) and glutamate (Glu)—and one is inhibitory—gamma-aminobutyric acid (GABA). The excitatory neurotransmitter ACh has been extensively studied, in particular, due to its prominent role in attention, learning and synaptic plasticity.[37] Synaptic plasticity is often considered the cellular and molecular correlate of learning and memory. In this context, electrophysiological data for the role of ACh in hippocampal synaptic plasticity are also mixed. Under a variety of *in vitro* and *in vivo* conditions, ACh either facilitates or directly causes hippocampal LTP or depression (LTD),[38] implicating a role for cholinergic input in synaptic plasticity but leaving open the questions of exactly how and by what mechanisms.

In addition to a role in synaptic plasticity, it has been proposed that cholinergic septohippocampal projections are critical for generating and phasing hippocampal theta and gamma oscillatory activity, therefore playing a central role in processes associated with learning and memory consolidation.[39] Septohippocampal projections encompass immunohistochemically distinct cholinergic, GABAergic and glutamatergic neurons.[39] Lecourtier et al.[39] have shown that GABAergic and cholinergic septohippocampal neurons both contribute to memory stabilization, and could do so in a sequential way: GABAergic processes could be engaged at an earlier stage than cholinergic ones during system consolidation of a spatial memory.[39] Finally, the anatomical organization gives rise to the septohippocampal system, a long-range feedback loop between the hippocampus and medial septum. This feedback loop allows cholinergic, GABAergic and glutamatergic neuronal populations to interact and modulate rhythmic activity and synaptic plasticity in the hippocampus.[40]

7. KEY ROLE OF SEROTONERGIC NEURONS IN SYNAPTIC TRANSMISSION

The serotonergic system consists of a small number of neurons that are born in the ventral regions of the hindbrain. Serotonergic neurons project to virtually all regions of the central nervous system and are consequently involved in many critical physiological functions such as memory and many other functions; serotonin release and serotonergic neuronal activity are controlled and modulated by interacting brain circuits to adapt to specific emotional and environmental states, in which the G protein-coupled receptors (GPCRs) and ion channels are also involved in the regulation of this system.[41] 5-Hydroxytryptamine (5-HT) neurons are located in the rostral raphe nuclei (RRN), such as the dorsal raphe nucleus (DRN) and the median raphe nucleus (MRN). The GPCRs and ion channels are located at somatodendritic and presynaptic regions of 5-HT neurons in the DRN and MRN that contribute to the modulation of 5-HT neuronal activity and 5-HT release.[41] Both DRN 5-HT neurons and MRN 5-HT neurons innervate areas involved in memory, the prefrontal and temporal cortex, and the lateral and medial septum, as well as the dorsal and ventral hippocampus.[41] Afferent projections to the raphe nuclei are diverse and include ACh from the laterodorsal tegmental nucleus, dopamine from the substantia nigra and ventral tegmentum area, histamine from tuberomammillary hypothalamic nucleus, noradrenaline from the locus coeruleus, serotonin itself from the raphe nuclei and several neuropeptides as well as excitatory glutamatergic and inhibitory GABAergic inputs.[41]

8. A VERY RECENT THEORY OF HIPPOCAMPAL FUNCTIONS IN MEMORY

Cheng[42] challenges the standard model of hippocampal plasticity and has proposed CRISP as an alternative theory. CRISP is based on Context Reset by dentate gyrus (DG), Intrinsic Sequences in hippocampal CA3, and Pattern completion in hippocampal CA1. Compared to previous models, CRISP uses a radically different mechanism for storing episodic memories in the hippocampal neural sequences intrinsic to CA3, and inputs are mapped onto these intrinsic sequences through synaptic plasticity in the feed forward projections of the hippocampus, hence, CRISP does not require plasticity in the recurrent CA3 synapses during the storage process. As in other theories, DG and CA1 play supporting roles; however, their function in CRISP has distinct implications. For instance, CA1 performs pattern completion in the absence of CA3 and DG contributes to episodic memory retrieval, increasing the speed, precision and robustness of retrieval.

9. AMNESIA OR LOSS OF MEMORY IS DIVIDED INTO TWO GROUPS

9.1 Anterograde Amnesia[43]

Anterograde amnesia is characterized by either impairment of information acquisition or impairment of consolidation and storage, or both. Acute events may lead to anterograde amnesia: cardiac arrest, asphyxia, cranial traumatism, as well as many pharmaceuticals including sedative-hypnotic drugs, some histamine H_1-antagonists, neuroleptics, anesthetics such as gamma-hydroxybutyric acid (GHB) or ketamine, drugs of abuse, etc. In addition, small quantities of alcohol may potentiate memory impairment of pharmaceuticals or drugs of abuse, and large amounts of alcohol alone will not only produce anterograde amnesia but will also greatly interfere with performance. It is significant that, in the vast majority of case reports, anterograde amnesia involves people not remembering behaviors that are a part of their normal daily routine (e.g. talking to people, buying food, driving a car, sex, performing professional activities).[44] In other words, the large majority of these reports indicate that people are functioning perhaps "automatically" but are not performing actions beyond their normal daily routine. Furthermore, despite the anterograde amnesia, people are able to perform rather routine complex tasks, such as driving a car or a physician practicing medicine.[44] This is in contrast to large quantities of alcohol, which can not only cause anterograde amnesia but also greatly interfere with performance. Finally, it is noteworthy that in most of the reports of anterograde amnesia secondary to pharmaceuticals, outside observers including physicians could not detect any abnormal behavior in people suffering from amnesia. Drug abuse may lead to "automatism amnesia" syndrome with behavior impairment, confusion, consent attitude, suggestibility and automatic behavior followed by partial or total anterograde amnesia.[45] In some cases the subjects were keenly aware of their invincibility.[43]

9.2 Retrograde Amnesia[43]

During retrograde amnesia, early memories are lost. Retrograde amnesia has been associated with cerebral injuries, senile dementia or Alzheimer's disease. It has been suggested that retrograde amnesia associated with drug action occurs only when sedation has been sufficiently deep to cause some degree of cerebral hypoxia.[46] Usually, retrograde amnesia is not observed with pharmaceuticals.

10. PHARMACEUTICALS AND ANTEROGRADE AMNESIA

As explained above, the feedback loop allows cholinergic, GABAergic, glutamatergic and serotonergic neuronal populations to interact and modulate rhythmic activity and synaptic plasticity in the hippocampus necessary for memorization, therefore all pharmaceuticals that interact with these neuronal populations are likely to produce anterograde amnesia.

10.1 Pharmaceuticals and GABAergic Neuronal Populations

Sedative-hypnotic drugs and nonsedative-hypnotic drugs, particularly benzodiazepines, are known to act on the GABA-A receptors.[43] Activation of the GABA receptor causes membrane chloride channels to open, increasing the influx of negative chloride ions through the cell membrane and cell hyperpolarization, thereby preventing depolarization of the neuron. The GABA-receptor complex is directly affected by barbiturates, ethanol and other drugs or drugs of abuse, and their wide distribution in the central nervous system accounts, in part, for the relatively broad sedative effects of these agents. Benzodiazepines appear to potentiate GABA-mediated inhibition in a more selective manner by increasing the affinity of GABA for its receptor, rather than by producing a direct effect. While the GABA system plays a regulatory role in neurotransmission, benzodiazepines may represent an evolutionary fine-tuning of inhibition by acting as a parent regulator of the GABA system.[43] Fast synaptic inhibition in the brain is largely mediated by the activation of GABA-A receptors, which are heteromeric GABA-gated chloride channels.[47] Their opening frequency is enhanced by agonists of the benzodiazepine site, which is the basis of their therapeutic effectiveness but also of their undesired side effects. For benzodiazepines, the sedation, the seizure protection and the amnesia properties were mainly attributed to α1-containing GABA-A receptor subtypes, while the anxiolysis, the myorelaxation, the motor impairment and the ethanol potentiation were attributed to the α2-, α3-, α5-containing GABA-A receptor subtypes.[48] In their study, Rudolph et al.[48] demonstrated the specificity of the GABA-A α1 receptor in mediating diazepam-induced amnesia. The most prescribed nonbenzodiazepine hypnotics such as zolpidem and zopiclone exert the same effects in impairing attention and memory as they are positive allosteric modulators of the subclass of GABA-A receptors.[43] Many other drugs such as general anesthetics (propofol, etomidate and barbiturates) produce profound amnesia and hypnosis, but weak immobility, by enhancing the activity of the GABA-A receptors. Propofol has been shown to enhance two types of GABAergic inhibition: a synaptic form (phasic inhibition) regulating neural excitability via the activation of postsynaptic GABA-A receptors by intermittent GABA release from presynaptic terminals; and a persistent tonic form (tonic inhibition) generated by continuous activation of extrasynaptic GABA-A receptors by low concentrations of ambient GABA.[49]

10.2 A New Class of Hypnotic Drugs without Action on the GABA-A Receptors, the Orexin Receptor Antagonists

The orexin or hypocretin system was recently discovered, and a number of experimental observations have suggested that this system plays an important role in the sleep–wake cycle.[50] These observations have spurred considerable interest in the development of orexin receptor antagonists as a potential new treatment for insomnia. In contrast to GABA, widely distributed in the brain structures, orexin A and B are almost synthesized in the lateral hypothalamus and projected to brain regions primarily involved in sleep.[51] The selective dual orexin receptor antagonists (DORAs), such as suvorexant and almorexant, have been shown to promote sleep onset and maintenance in clinical trials for patients with insomnia. In an effort to develop better tolerated medicines, Uslaner et al.[51] have identified DORAs that promote sleep in preclinical animal models and humans. In 2013, they compared sleep-promoting doses to the cognitive-impairing doses of orally administered eszopiclone, zolpidem and diazepam to the dual orexin receptor antagonist DORA-22. At doses that produce equivalent amounts of sleep in animals, sleep drugs currently in use significantly disrupted attention and memory, whereas DORA-22 promoted sleep at doses that did not exert effects on disrupted attention and memory.[51] Subsequently, DORAs do not seem to be a good candidate for DFC!

10.3 Pharmaceuticals and Cholinergic Neuronal Populations

Scopolamine, an alkaloid of *Datura* and an acetylcholine receptor antagonist, has been reported to impair cognitive performances, especially spatial learning and memory,[52] as well as vigilance. These effects have been known since the eighteenth century when robbers gave to their victims snuff tobacco containing *Datura* powder to sedate them and obtain anterograde amnesia. Scopolamine exerts an amnesic effect equally in various memory behavioral models. Among pharmaceuticals, many neuroleptics exert anticholinergic properties, particularly H_1-antihistaminic. These compounds were primarily modifications of those synthesized as cholinergic antagonists and originate from diverse chemical entities, ethanolamines, ethylene diamines, alkylamines, piperazines, piperidines and phenothiazines. The first-generation antihistamines had poor receptor selectivity and significant unwanted side effects, particularly central nervous system and anticholinergic effects with impaired memory. The residual effects of poor sleep, including impairment of attention, vigilance, working memory and sensory-motor performance, are still present the next morning.[53]

10.4 Pharmaceuticals, Drugs of Abuse and Glutamatergic Neuronal Populations

A general anesthetic, ketamine may produce amnesia. Although ketamine blocks NMDA receptors of the glutamatergic neurons as an open channel blocker, it was shown that ketamine inhibits hyperpolarization-activated cationic currents and enhances GABA-induced currents in $\alpha6$-GABA receptors, which suggests that ketamine has multiple molecular targets in hypnotic, analgesic and amnestic actions.[49] Another anesthetic, notorious among addicts, is GHB, which disrupts the acquisition of spatial learning and memory in adolescent rats. GHB is known to interact with several neurotransmitter systems that have been implicated in cognitive functioning. As previously described in this chapter, the NMDA type of glutamate receptor is considered to be an important target for spatial learning and memory.

As molecular mechanisms governing the neuroadaptations following repeated GHB treatment remain unknown, Sircar et al.[54] examined the role of NMDA receptors in adolescent rat GHB-induced cognitive deficit. Their findings support the hypothesis that adolescent GHB-induced cognitive deficits in rats are associated with neuroadaptations in glutamatergic transmission, particularly NMDA receptor functioning in the frontal cortex.[54] Cannabis and cannabinoid CB1 agonists are also candidates among the chemicals that interfere with the NMDA receptors of the glutamatergic neurons. Ghiasvand et al.[55] demonstrated that amnesia induced by cannabinoid CB1 agonists in rats is at least partly mediated through an NMDA receptor mechanism in the central amygdala.

Memory impairment has also been reported in many studies in humans. Indlekofer et al.[56] reported memory and attention performance in a population-based sample of young adults with a moderate lifetime use of cannabis, ecstasy (MDMA) and alcohol. In their study, cognitive functioning was examined in 284 young participants, between 22 and 34 years of age. In general, their lifetime drug experience was moderate. Participants completed a neuropsychological test battery, including measures for verbal learning, memory and various attentional functions. MDMA and cannabis use were significantly related to poorer episodic memory function in a dose-related manner. The results were consistent with decrements of memory and attentional performance described in previous studies. These effects are relatively small; however, it must be kept in mind that this study focused on assessing young adults with moderate drug use from a population-based study. In a precedent Internet survey, Rodgers et al.[57] showed that cannabis was associated with subjective STM problems and internally cued prospective memory, whereas MDMA use was more related to subjective LTM problems, which were more related to storage and retrieval difficulties.

10.5 Amphetamines and Serotonergic Toxicity

Amphetamine and MDMA are known as serotonin releasers. Serotonergic neurotoxicity following MDMA is well established in laboratory animals, and neuroimaging studies have found lower serotonin transporter (SERT) binding in abstinent MDMA users. Declarative memory, prospective memory and higher cognitive skills are often impaired. Neurocognitive deficits are associated with reduced SERT in the hippocampus, parietal cortex and prefrontal cortex.[58] In an overview of 25 years of empirical research, Parrott[59] observed that recreational MDMA users show deficits in retrospective memory, prospective memory, higher cognition, problem solving and social intelligence. He concluded that: "The damaging effects of Ecstasy/MDMA are far more widespread than was realized a few years ago, with new neuropsychobiological deficits still emerging." In another study, Becker et al.[60] using functional neuroimaging studies with cross-sectional designs reported altered memory-related hippocampal functioning in ecstasy-polydrug users, suggesting specific effects of MDMA use on memory-related hippocampal functioning. In a review of 23 articles published between 2002 and 2010 with an explicit focus on the combination, or administration, of MDMA and cannabis or cannabinoid agents, Schultz[61] found that recent retrospective studies on cognitive functions in long-term drug abusers point to an additive negative effect on different types of memory, as well as a cannabis-independent decrease in learning and decision making in MDMA users. As a neural mechanism underlying these changes, an interaction between the cannabinoid system, especially CB1 receptor, and the serotonergic and dopaminergic system in the prefrontal cortex, nucleus accumbens and hippocampus is suggested.

10.6 The Effect of Cocaine on Memory

The effects of cocaine on memory are controversial. Furthermore, the psychostimulant action of cocaine can be a critical issue in the interpretation of its effects on learning/memory models. The effects of a single administration of cocaine on memory were investigated by Niigaki et al.[62] during the presence of motor stimulating effect or just after termination. When cocaine was injected 30 minutes pre-training, the drug did not modify motor activity, but produced marked amnestic effects at all doses tested. This amnesia induced by cocaine given 30 minutes pre-training was not related to a state-dependent learning because it was not abolished by pre-test administration of the drug. Post-training cocaine administration did not induce memory deficits either. These results suggest that the post-stimulant phase is the critical moment for cocaine-induced memory deficit in a discriminative task in mice. Two rare reports of cocaine hippocampi ischemic strokes involving memory impairment have been reported.[63]

REFERENCES

1. Kandel ER. *In search of memory: the emergence of a new science of mind*. New York: Norton & Company; 2007.
2. Marra V, O'Shea M, Benjamin PR, Kemenes I. Susceptibility of memory consolidation during lapses in recall. *Nat Commun* 2013;**4**:1578 <http://refhubelsevier.com/B978-0-12-416748-3.00005-0/sbref2>.
3. Meeter M, Murre JMJ. Consolidation of long-term memory: evidence and alternatives. *Psychol Bull* 2004;**130**:843−57.
4. Murre JMJ, Chessa AG, Meeter M. A mathematical model of forgetting and amnesia. *Front Psychol* 2013;**4**:76 <http://refhub.elsevier.com/B978-0-12-416748-3.00005-0/sbref4>.
5. Abraham WC. How long will long-term potentiation last?. *Philos Trans R Soc Lond BBiol Sci* 2003;**358**:735−44.
6. Furini CR, Myskiw JC, Benetti F, Izquierdo I. New frontiers in the study of memory mechanisms. *Rev Bras Psiquiatr* 2013;**35**:173−7.
7. Pastalkova E, Serrano P, Pinkhasova D, Wallace E, Fenton AA, Sacktor TC. Storage of spatial information by the maintenance mechanism of LTP. *Science* 2006;**313**:1141−4.
8. Sacktor TC. Memory maintenance by PKMzeta an evolutionary perspective. *Mol Brain* 2012;**18**:5−31.
9. Frey S, Frey JU. "Synaptic tagging" and "cross-tagging" and related associative reinforcement processes of functional plasticity as the cellular basis for memory formation. *Prog Brain Res* 2008;**169**:117−43.
10. Ballarini F, Moncada D, Martinez MC, Alen N, Viola H. Behavioral tagging is a general mechanism of long-term memory formation. *Proc Natl Acad Sci USA* 2009;**106**:14599−604.
11. Moncada D, Ballarini F, Martinez MC, Frey JU, Viola H. Identification of transmitter systems and learning tag molecules involved in behavioral tagging during memory formation. *Proc Natl Acad Sci USA* 2011;**108**:12931−6.
12. Myskiw JC, Benetti F, Izquierdo I. Behavioral tagging of extinction learning. *Proc Natl Acad Sci USA* 2013;**110**:1071−6.
13. Milad MR, Quirk GJ. Fear extinction as a model for translational neuroscience: ten years of progress. *Annu Rev Psychol* 2012;**63**:129−51.
14. Fiorenza NG, Rosa J, Izquierdo I, Myskiw JC. Modulation of the extinction of two different fear-motivated tasks in three distinct brain areas. *Behav Brain Res* 2012;**232**:210−6.
15. Izquierdo I, Bevilaqua LR, Rossato JI, Bonini JS, Medina JH, Cammarota M. Different molecular cascades in different sites of the brain control consolidation. *Trends Neurosci* 2006;**229**:496−505.
16. Whitlock JR, Heynen AJ, Shuler MG, Bear MF. Learning induces long-term potentiation in the hippocampus. *Science* 2006;**313**:1093−7.
17. Clarke JR, Cammarota M, Gruart A, Izquierdo I, Delgado-García JM. Plastic modifications induced by object recognition memory processing. *Proc Natl Acad Sci USA* 2010;**107**:2652−7.
18. Crow T, Xue-Bian JJ. Proteomic analysis of short- and intermediate-term memory in Hermissenda. *Neuroscience* 2011;**192**:102−11.
19. Fulton D, Kemenes I, Andrew RJ, Benjamin PR. A single time-window for protein synthesis-dependent long-term memory formation after one-trial appetitive conditioning. *Eur J Neurosci* 2005;**21**:1347−58.

20. Fulton D, Kemenes I, Andrew RJ, Benjamin PR. Time-window for sensitivity to cooling distinguishes the effects of hypothermia and protein synthesis inhibition on the consolidation of long-term memory. *Neurobiol Learn Mem* 2008;**90**:651—4.

21. Kandel ER. The molecular biology of memory: cAMP, PKA, CRE, CREB-1, CREB-2, and CPEB. *Mol Brain* 2012;**5**:14 <http://refhubelsevier.com/B978-0-12-416748-3.00005-0/sbref21>.

22. Sharma SK, Bagnall MW, Sutton MA, Carew TJ. Inhibition of calcineurin facilitates the induction of memory for sensitization in Aplysia: requirement of mitogen-activated protein kinase. *Proc Natl Acad Sci USA* 2003;**100**:4861—6.

23. Guan Z, Giustetto M, Lomvardas S, Kim JH, Miniaci MC, Schwartz JH, et al. Integration of long-term memory-related synaptic plasticity involves bidirectional regulation of gene expression and chromatin structure. *Cell* 2002;**111**:483—93.

24. Levenson JM, Sweatt JD. Epigenetic mechanisms in memory formation. *Nat Rev Neurosci* 2005;**6**:108—18.

25. Hsieh J, Gage FH. Chromatin remodeling in neural development and plasticity. *Curr Opin Cell Biol* 2005;**17**:664—71.

26. Martyn AC, De Jaeger X, Magalhães AC, Kesarwani R, Gonçalves DF, Raulic, et al. Elimination of the vesicular acetylcholine transporter in the forebrain causes hyperactivity and deficits in spatial memory and long-term potentiation. *Proc Natl Acad Sci USA* 2012;**109**:17651—6.

27. Igaz LM, Vianna MR, Medina JH, Izquierdo I. Two time periods of hippocampal mRNA synthesis are required for memory consolidation of fear-motivated learning. *J Neurosci* 2002;**22**:6781—9.

28. Slipczuk L, Bekinschtein P, Katche C, Cammarota M, Izquierdo I, Medina JH. BDNF activates mTOR to regulate GluR1 expression required for memory formation. *PLoS One* 2009;**4**:e6007 <http://refhubelsevier.com/B978-0-12-416748-3.00005-0/sbref28>.

29. Squire LR, Wixted JT. The cognitive neuroscience of human memory since H.M. *Annu Rev Neurosci* 2011;**34**:259—88.

30. Eichenbaum H. What H.M. taught us? *J Cogn Neurosci* 2013;**25**:14—21.

31. Bekinschtein P, Cammarota M, Igaz LM, Bevilaqua LR, Izquierdo I, Medina JH. Persistence of long-term memory storage requires a late protein synthesis- and BDNF-dependent phase in the hippocampus. *Neuron* 2007;**53**:261—77.

32. Parfitt GM, Barbosa ÂK, Campos RC, Koth AP, Barros DM. Moderate stress enhances memory persistence: are adrenergic mechanisms involved? *Behav Neurosci* 2012;**126**:729—34.

33. Bekinschtein P, Cammarota M, Katche C, Slipczuk L, Rossato JI, Goldin A, et al. BDNF is essential to promote persistence of long-term memory storage. *Proc Natl Acad Sci USA* 2008;**105**:2711—6.

34. Eckel-Mahan KL, Phan T, Han S, Wang H, Chan GC, Scheiner ZS, et al. Circadian oscillation of hippocampal MAPK activity and cAmp: implications for memory persistence. *Nat Neurosci* 2008;**11**:1074—82.

35. Parfitt GM, Campos RC, Barbosa AK, Koth AP, Barros DM. Participation of hippocampal cholinergic system in memory persistence for inhibitory avoidance in rats. *Neurobiol Learn Mem* 2012;**97**:183—8.

36. Sajikumar S, Korte M. Metaplasticity governs compartmentalization of synaptic tagging and capture through brain-derived neurotrophic factor (BDNF) and protein kinase Mzeta (PKMzeta). *Proc Natl Acad Sci USA* 2011;**108**:2551—6.

37. Micheau J, Marighetto A. Acetylcholine and memory: a long, complex and chaotic but still living relationship. *Behav Brain Res* 2011;**221**:424—9.

38. Sugisaki E, Fukushima Y, Tsukada M, Aihara T. Cholinergic modulation on spike timing-dependent plasticity in hippocampal CA1 network. *Neuroscience* 2011;**192**:91−101.

39. Lecourtier L, De Vasconcelos AP, Leroux E, Cosquer B, Geiger K, Lithfous S, et al. Septohippocampal pathways contribute to system consolidation of a spatial memory: sequential implication of GABAergic and cholinergic neurons. *Hippocampus* 2011;**21**: 1277−89.

40. Teles-Grilo Ruivo LM, Mellor JR. Cholinergic modulation of hippocampal network function. *Front Synaptic Neurosci* 2013. <http://refhub.elsevier.com/B978-0-12-416748-3.00005-0/sbref40>.

41. Maejima T, Masseck OA, Mark MD, Herlitze S. Modulation of firing and synaptic transmission of serotonergic neurons by intrinsic G protein-coupled receptors and ion channels. *Front Integr Neurosci* 2013. <http://refhub.elsevier.com/B978-0-12-416748-3.00005-0/sbref41>.

42. Cheng S. The CRISP theory of hippocampal function in episodic memory. *Front Neural Circuits* 2013. <http://refhub.elsevier.com/B978-0-12-416748-3.00005-0/sbref42>.

43. Goullé JP, Anger JP. Drug-facilitated robbery or sexual assault: problems associated with amnesia. *Ther Drug Monit* 2004;**26**:206−10.

44. Rothschild AJ. Disinhibition, amnestic reactions, and other adverse reactions secondary to triazolam: a review of the literature. *J Clin Psychiatry* 1992;**53**:69−79.

45. Salvaggio J, Jacob C, Schmitt C, Orizet C, Ruel M, Lambert H. Consommation abusive de flunitrazépam par les toxicomanes aux opiacés. *Ann Med Interne* 2000;**151**:A6−9.

46. MacKay AC, Dundee JW. Effect of oral benzodiazepine on memory. *Br J Anaesth* 1980;**52**:1247−57.

47. Barnard EA, Skolnick P, Olsen RW, Mohler H, Sieghart W, Biggio G, et al. International Union of Pharmacology. XV. Subtypes of gamma-aminobutyric acidA receptors: classification on the basis of subunit structure and receptor function. *Pharmacol Rev* 1998;**50**:291−313.

48. Rudolph U, Crestani F, Benke D, Brünig I, Benson JA, Fritschy JM, et al. Benzodiazepine actions mediated by specific gamma-aminobutyric acid(A) receptor subtypes. *Nature* 1999;**401**:796−800.

49. Nishikawa K. Roles of glutamatergic and GABAergic nervous system in hypnotic and analgesic actions of general anesthetics. *Masui* 2011;**60**:534−43.

50. de Lecea L, Kilduff TS, Peyron C, Gao X, Foye PE, Danielson PE, et al. The hypocretins: hypothalamus-specific peptides with neuroexcitatory activity. *Proc Natl Acad Sci USA* 1998;**95**:322−7.

51. Uslaner JM, Tye SJ, Eddins DM, Wang X, Fox SV, Savitz AT, et al. Orexin receptor antagonists differ from standard sleep drugs by promoting sleep at doses that do not disrupt cognition. *Sci Transl Med* 2013. <http://rcfhub.clscvicr.com/B978-0-12-416748-3.00005-0/sbref51>.

52. Saraf MK, Prabhakar S, Khanduja KL, Anand A. Bacopa monniera Attenuates Scopolamine-Induced Impairment of Spatial Memory in Mice. *Evid Based Complement Alternat Med* 2011;**2011**:236186 <http://refhubelsevier.com/B978-0-12-416748-3.00005-0/sbref52>.

53. Church DS, Church MK. Pharmacology of antihistamines. *World Allergy Organ J* 2011;**4**: S22−7.

54. Sircar R, Wu LC, Reddy K, Sircar D, Basak AK. GHB-induced cognitive deficits during adolescence and the role of NMDA receptor. *Curr Neuropharmacol* 2011;**9**:240−3.

55. Ghiasvand M, Rezayof A, Zarrindast MR, Ahmadi S. Activation of cannabinoid CB1 receptors in the central amygdala impairs inhibitory avoidance memory consolidation via NMDA receptors. *Neurobiol Learn Mem* 2011;**96**:333−8.

56. Indlekofer F, Piechatzek M, Daamen M, Glasmacher C, Lieb R, Pfister H, et al. Reduced memory and attention performance in a population-based sample of young adults with a moderate lifetime use of cannabis, ecstasy and alcohol. *J Psychopharmacol* 2009;**23**:495−509.

57. Rodgers J, Buchanan T, Scholey AB, Heffernan TM, Ling J, Parrott A. Differential effects of Ecstasy and cannabis on self-reports of memory ability: a web-based study. *Hum Psychopharmacol* 2001;**16**:619−25.

58. Parrott AC. MDMA, serotonergic neurotoxicity, and the diverse functional deficits of recreational "Ecstasy" users. *Neurosci Biobehav Rev* 2013;**37**:1466−84.

59. Parrott AC. Human psychobiology of MDMA or "Ecstasy": an overview of 25 years of empirical research. *Hum Psychopharmacol* 2013;**4**:289−307.

60. Becker B, Wagner D, Koester P, Bender K, Kabbasch C, Gouzoulis-Mayfrank E, et al. Memory-related hippocampal functioning in ecstasy and amphetamine users: a prospective fMRI study. *Psychopharmacology* 2013;**225**:923−34.

61. Schulz S. MDMA & cannabis: a mini-review of cognitive, behavioral, and neurobiological effects of co-consumption. *Curr Drug Abuse Rev* 2011;**4**:81−6.

62. Niigaki ST, Silva RH, Patti CL, Cunha JL, Kameda SR, Correia-Pinto JC, et al. Amnestic effect of cocaine after the termination of its stimulant action. *Prog Neuropsychopharmacol Biol Psychiatry* 2010;**34**:212−8.

63. Morales Vidal SG, Hornik A, Morgan C. Cocaine induced hippocampi infarction. *BMJ Case Rep* Jul 3, 2012.

Chapter 6

Cannabis and Drug-Facilitated Crimes

Bertrand Brunet and Patrick Mura

1. INTRODUCTION

Cannabis is the most commonly used illicit drug worldwide, with an estimated annual prevalence of about 163 million or about 3.9% of the global
population aged 15 years or above in 2000/2001.[1] For example, almost 17
million Americans were users of cannabis in 2009, as illustrated in
Figure 6.1. An estimated 15.4 million young Europeans (aged 15−34)
(11.7% of this age group) used cannabis in 2012, with 9.2 million of them
aged 15−24 (14.9%). Cannabis use is generally higher among males.[2] In
France in 2010, of adults aged 18 to 64, approximately one-third (33%)
stated having consumed cannabis during their life.[3] This experimentation
takes place more often among men than women (41% versus 25%). Of people aged 18−64, current use (i.e. use in the last 12 months) ranges between
4% and 8%. This use pertains mainly to younger generations: 18% of males
and 9% of females aged 18−25 are general users, 9% and 4%, respectively,
are regular users.

Cannabis is an important public health problem in the world and may
induce serious consequences in a number of circumstances, such as road
accidents[4−7] and accidents at work.[8−11] This drug of abuse is also considered as a doping agent in sports,[12,13] particularly where participants need to
be relaxed, for instance, in accuracy specialties such as archery, rifle shoot-
ing and horse riding.[14] Cannabis use contributes to aggressive and violent
behavior including intimate partner violence.[15,16] There is also some evidence that heavy use has adverse effects on mental health and involvement
in drug-related crimes.[17]

The aim of this chapter is to answer the following questions. What is
the occurrence of cannabis in drug-facilitated sexual assault? Is cannabis a
good candidate for chemical submission and why? How can it be demonstrated that cannabis has been used for this purpose? Concerning analytical

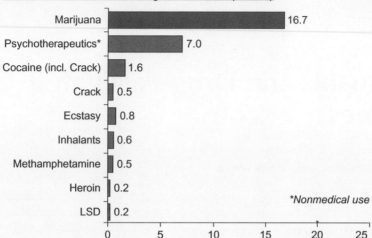

Number of Past Month Users, Aged 12 or Older (Millions)

Source: SAMHSA, *2009 National Survey on Drug Use and Health* (September 2010).

FIGURE 6.1 Number of current users of psychoactive substances in the USA.

investigations, which biological fluids or tissues should be analyzed and how are the results interpreted?

2. CANNABIS PLANT

The cannabis plant has two main subspecies, *Cannabis indica* and *Cannabis sativa*, which can be differentiated by their physical and chemical characteristics. *C. indica*-dominant strains are short plants with broad, dark green leaves. *C. sativa*-dominant strains are usually taller and have thin leaves with a pale green color.[18]

The hemp plant *C. sativa* var. *indica* grows throughout the world and flourishes in most temperate and tropical regions; Asia, Africa and Latin America are the major producers of illicit cannabis. Names for cannabis products include marijuana (from the Mexican Spanish "marihuana"), hashish, charas, bhang and ganja.

C. sativa var. *indica* is a complex plant with over 400 compounds and a total of more than 60 cannabinoids,[19] including delta-9-tetrahydrocannabinol (THC, the principal psychoactive constituent), cannabidiol (CBD), cannabinol (CBN), tetrahydrocannabivarin (THCV) and cannabigerol (CBG). *C. sativa* var. *indica* may have a CBD/THC ratio 4–5 times that of *C. sativa*. Cannabis preparations are largely derived from the female plant and the THC content is highest in the flowering tops,[20] declining in the lower leaves, stems and seeds of the plant.

3. CANNABIS PRODUCTS

The three main forms of cannabis products are the flower, resin (hashish) and oil (hash oil).

"Cannabis" or "marijuana" refers generally to the dried flowers and subtending leaves and stems of the female plant. This is the most widely consumed form.

As delta-9-THC is the main ingredient that causes the desired "stoned" effect, users prefer the strains of the plant with higher THC content. Particularly over the last 15 years, such variants of the plant have been more widely available on the street "market." A French study has revealed that the THC level found in cannabis products (resin and herbal samples available on the street market) has constantly increased (by a factor of 2) between 1993 and 2004, with 32% of samples analyzed containing more than 10% in 2004.[21] In recent years this evolution and the occurrence of high THC levels in cannabis products has also been reported in many countries. In Japan, the analysis of 335 samples of fresh seedless buds has revealed an average of 11.2% and a maximum of 22.6% THC.[22] In Italy, 4000 samples of cannabis products were analyzed over the period 2010−2012. Overall median THC content showed an increasing trend over the study period from 6.0% to 8.1%. The variation in the THC content of individual samples was very large, ranging from 0.3% to 31% for cannabis resin and from 0.1% to 19% for herbal cannabis.[23] A very recent study performed in Australia[24] on 206 cannabis samples showed very high mean THC content (14.88%) and very low mean CBD content (0.14%).

The word "kief" or "kif" is derived from Arabic "kayf" and means well-being or pleasure. Kief is a powder, rich in trichomes, which can be drifted from the leaves and flowers of cannabis plants and either consumed in powder form or compressed to reduced hashish cakes.

Hashish or "hash" is a concentrated resin cake or ball produced from pressed kief. It varies in color from black to golden brown depending upon purity and coloring agent used.[25] It can be smoked or taken orally. Marijuana butter or "bud butter" is the most frequent way to incorporate cannabis in foods such as chocolate cakes. Indeed, when cooking with hashish and when a rapid psychoactive effect is required, it is very important for consumers to use fat (oil, butter or milk) because THC is fat soluble and not water soluble.

Hash oil is obtained from the cannabis plant by solvent extraction, and contains the cannabinoids present in cannabis flowers and leaves. The solvent is evaporated to obtain a very concentrated oil. Hash oil potencies vary considerably, generally around 17% THC[26] but may reach 60%. However, very low THC levels were found in commercially available hemp seed oil products (11.5 to 117.5 mg/g).[27] Hash oil may be consumed by smoking (by placing drops on a tobacco cigarette), vaporizing or eating (by adding to food).

Cannabis infusions are also used. The plant material is mixed with a non-volatile solvent (usually cocoa butter, dairy butter, cooking oil or glycerin) and then pressed and filtered to express the oils of the plant. Depending on the solvent, these may be added to foods.

4. CANNABIS CONSUMPTION

Cannabis may be consumed by:

- Smoking using small pipes, bongs, paper-wrapped joints, tobacco leaf-wrapped blunts or roach clips.
- Using a vaporizer, which heats herbal cannabis to 330–375°F (166–191°C) causing the active ingredients to evaporate into a vapor without burning the plant material.
- Eating: cannabis (hashish or hash oil) is incorporated in food such as "space-cakes." In this way, cannabis may be administered unbeknownst to somebody for criminal purposes.

5. MECHANISMS OF ACTION[28]

Evidence gathered up to the mid-1980s led to the hypothesis that THC and other cannabinoids act via a pharmacologically distinct set of receptors. Howlett and coworkers[29] demonstrated that THC inhibited the intracellular enzyme adenylate cyclase and that such inhibition required the presence of a G-protein complex. Central (CB1) and peripheral (CB2) cannabinoid receptors have been characterized, endogenous ligands (e.g. anandamide and 2-arachidonyl glycerol) have been identified and specific CB1 and CB2 receptor antagonists have been synthesized. CB1 receptor activation inhibits striatal dopamine release or leads to a decrease in serotonin release in the hippocampus.[30] In addition, activation of CB1 receptor results in inhibition of the enzyme adenylate cyclase through an inhibitory G-protein. The resulting decrease in cyclic AMP (cAMP) leads to a decrease in phosphorylation by protein kinase A of liganded ion channels triggering inhibition of calcium channels and activation of potassium channels. Potassium ions can exit the neuron, and, ultimately, the release of neurotransmitters such as glutamate is inhibited.[28]

The CB1 receptors are particularly expressed in the basal ganglia, cerebellum, frontal cortex, hippocampus and the amygdala, a distribution pattern which accounts for the cognitive, affective and motor effects of cannabis. In the same way, THC has been found in important concentrations in these same areas.[31]

6. ACUTE EFFECTS IN HUMANS

The central nervous system (CNS) effects of THC in humans vary with dose, route of administration, experience of the user, vulnerability to psychoactive effects and setting of use.[32] The effects of cannabis are dose dependent.

Behavioral effects include feelings of euphoria and relaxation, altered time perception, lack of concentration, impaired memory, and mood changes such as panic reactions and paranoia. Cannabis's spectrum of behavioral effects is unique, preventing classification of the drug as a stimulant, sedative, tranquilizer or hallucinogen.[33] Acute cannabis consumption may impair cognitive and performance tasks, including reaction time, motor coordination, perception, attention and memory. Acute and non-acute effects of cannabis have been described regarding human memory function. Neuroimaging studies have shown that cannabis use is associated with a pattern of increased activity and a higher level of deactivation in different memory-related areas.[34] Cannabis users exhibit deficits in prospective memory[35] and executive function, which persist beyond acute intoxication. Impairment of working memory is now considered as one of the most important deleterious effects of cannabis intoxication in humans. It has been recently demonstrated that the impairment of working memory by marijuana and cannabinoids is due to the activation of astroglial CB1R and is associated with astroglia-dependent hippocampal LTD *in vivo*.[36] A case of transient global amnesia in a young boy intoxicated with cannabis has been reported.[37]

During the period of cannabis intoxication, there is also impairment of cognitive functions, perception and reaction time. Impairment of coordination and tracking behavior has been reported to persist for several hours beyond the perception of the high. Specific effects of cannabis on behavioral disinhibition, associated with euphoria and relaxing effects, have been reported by several authors.[38–40]

Depersonalization is also described as a possible direct consequence of cannabis use.[41,42]

All these effects are enhanced when cannabis is associated with other psychoactive drugs such as alcohol, other drugs of abuse, benzodiazepines, antidepressants and in a general manner all substances that affect the CNS.

7. METABOLISM AND TOXICOKINETICS

From the kinetic point of view, cannabis is far from the ideal substance of choice used by perpetrators of drug-facilitated crimes (DFCs). Mostly due to its lipophilicity and metabolism, THC has long-lasting effects and remains in the organism for several days. When cannabis is smoked, THC is rapidly absorbed and bioavailability ranges from 18% to 50% depending on the subject's smoking habits.[43,44] THC appears within seconds after inhalation in the bloodstream and plasma peak concentrations are usually reached before the last puff.[45] Maximum concentrations after smoking a 6.8% THC-containing joint are in the range 13 to 63 ng/mL with a median of 50 ng/mL. After 1 hour the concentrations have dropped to a median of 10 ng/mL and are in the ng/mL range 6 hours after the end of smoking.[46]

Although inhalation is the most usual way of consumption of cannabis, ingestion is also possible and could be a way of surreptitiously administering cannabis to a victim. Cookies and pastries are the most employed vehicle for ingested cannabis. But of course there is a longer delay before the appearance of the effects (about 1 to 1.5 hours). Those effects last longer than when cannabis is smoked and can be observed for 4 to 6 hours after ingestion of dronabinol.[47] More than one peak is usually detected in the kinetic of THC after ingestion; this can be due to a fractional absorption along the gastrointestinal system or enterohepatic recirculation.[48] Bioavailability after ingestion is reduced to 4−20%,[49] partly due to degradation in the stomach and first-pass metabolism. This latest phenomenon is responsible for the elevated concentrations of the active metabolite 11-hydroxy-tetrahydrocannabinol (11-OH-THC) observed after ingestion. Plasma concentrations of 11-OH-THC usually represent about 10% of THC concentrations after inhalation but can reach 50% to 100% after ingestion.[50] 11-OH-THC is equipotent to THC, and the effects observed after oral administration can be perceived as more important than after inhalation. Moreover, prevalence of cannabis acute psychosis seems to be greater after ingestion of cannabis compared to the smoking route.[47]

After absorption, THC is widely distributed into the organism. All the tissues and especially the brain are rapidly filled with the drug. THC has a large volume of distribution of 10 L/kg, reflecting its lipophilicity.[51] High lipid content of some tissues such as brain and fat is at the origin of a retention or accumulation of the drug. It has been proven that THC can be detected in brain longer than in blood[52,52] and prolonged retention in fat tissue also has been demonstrated in animals and humans.[53,54] Other highly perfused organs such as lungs are also more importantly exposed to THC.[55]

THC undergoes extensive metabolism by hepatic cytochrome P450 enzymes mainly on the carbon at the position 11 (Figure 6.2). The primary metabolite is the 11-OH-THC previously mentioned, but this metabolite has a relatively short half-life and is further oxidized to 11-oxo-THC, which is a reactive intermediate immediately transformed into an acidic metabolite 11-nor-9-carboxy-delta-9-tetrahydrocannabinol (THC-COOH).[56] The latest is the phase 1 terminal metabolite in humans. THC-COOH is the most abundant cannabinoid in blood as soon as 30 minutes after inhalation or 1 hour after ingestion of cannabis. Before being excreted in urine THC-COOH undergoes phase 2 metabolism by conjugation with glucuronic acid. Glucuronidation can occur on two different positions, either on the phenolic or acidic moiety. The ester and ether glucuronide of THC-COOH react differently to hydrolysis with beta-glucuronidase.[57] Outside of the liver, some

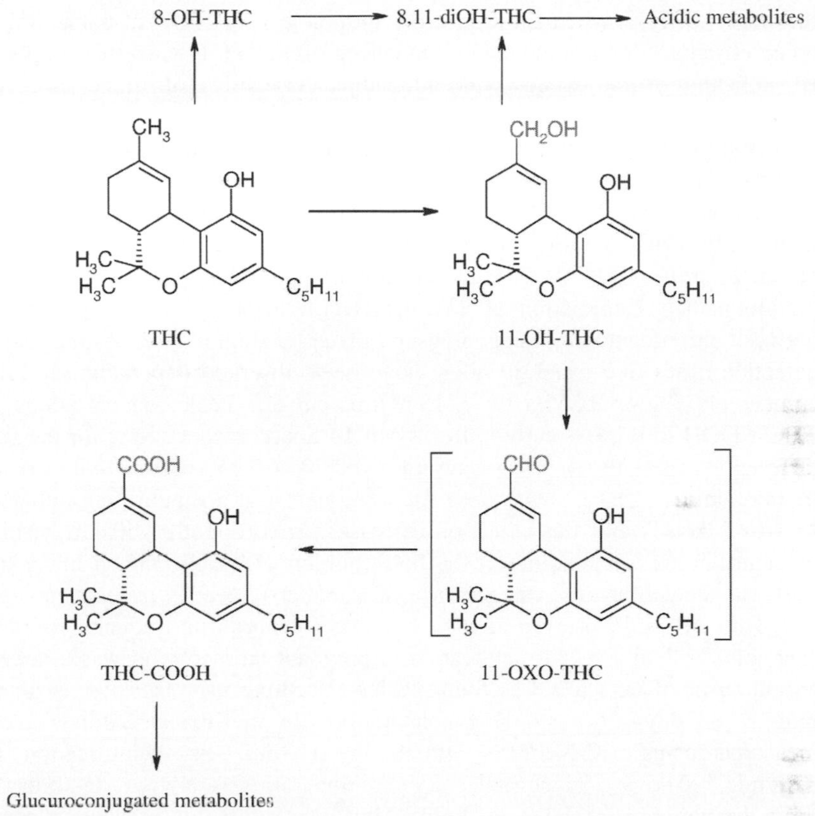

FIGURE 6.2   Major pathways of THC metabolism.

other organs can participate in the metabolism of THC to a lesser extent. Lungs, brain and the intestine possess the isoenzymes of cytochrome P450 necessary for metabolizing THC, but it is usually a minor pathway that is favored. In those organs, production of 8-OH-THC is increased compared to 11-OH-THC; di-hydroxyl metabolites are also common but are inactive.[58]

The metabolism of cannabis has been known since the 1970s but more recent advances have been made concerning the enzymes involved in the different pathways. Bornheim et al. were the first to suggest that an isoenzyme belonging to the CYP2C9 subfamily was responsible for the formation of 11-OH-THC.[59] It was further confirmed that the minor pathway leading to the formation of 8-OH-THC was catalyzed by CYP3A4.[60] A possibility of interaction between phenytoin, another substrate of CYP2C, and THC has been described, meaning that THC could be at the origin of the inefficiency of this epilepsy medication.[61] Recently, it has been discovered that a polymorphism of CYP2C9 could lead to a three-fold increase in the area under the curve of THC when subjects carry the allele CYP2C9 3*3 compared to other variants.[62] This could lead to enhanced effects of THC in this subpopulation, adding to the already wide intersubject variability of effects observed after cannabis consumption.

Elimination of cannabinoids occurs slowly, mainly in the feces (>65%) and in urine (20%). Minor routes of elimination also include sweat and breast milk.[50] 11-OH-THC and 8-11-diOH-THC are predominant in feces along with THC-COOH. Those compounds are found either free or conjugated. In urine, THC-COOH and its glucuronidated conjugate are largely predominant.[63] Elimination of THC-COOH in urine is extremely variable between infrequent and frequent users. After a single dose of marijuana, detection times of 34 and 89 hours have been observed depending on THC content (1.75% or 3.55%) for a 15 ng/mL cut-off. Peak concentrations of THC-COOH in urine occurred after 8 and 14 hours, respectively, for the two different doses with mean concentrations of 90 and 153 ng/mL.[64] It is commonly admitted that a single dose for infrequent users should be eliminated in 3 to 5 days.[65] But this detection increases proportionally with the history of cannabis use. Depending on the body burden of THC retained in fat tissues, this detection time can increase in a matter of weeks or even months. Half-lives of 16, 19 or even 32 days have been reported in frequents users of cannabis.[66–68] In a recent publication, a pregnant woman who was a heavy, chronic user of cannabis was found to have positive urine specimens for as long as 84 days after stopping consumption of marijuana. Samples were measured using LC-MS/MS with a lower limit of quantification of 3 ng/mL.[68] The use of normalized creatinine ratios is advised in order to limit the variability related to diuresis but even with this precaution some subjects can have positive urine specimens interspersed with negative results without being indicative of new cannabis consumption.[68] The very long terminal half-life of THC-COOH can be an advantage for the detection of an administration of cannabis to a victim of DFC, meaning that it will be detectable for several days; but if the victim has used cannabis in the previous days before the offense it will be more difficult to prove the incapacitated crime.

8. INTERPRETATIONS OF CANNABIS ANALYSIS

Given the particular metabolism and the slow elimination of THC, interpretation of a positive or negative result can lead to different conclusions for the biological sample concerned. The different matrices detailed hereafter are from the shortest detection time window (oral fluid) to the longest (hair). For cannabis, like any other substance involved in a DFC or DFSA (drug-facilitated sexual assault), the analytical gold standard is chromatographic separation coupled to mass spectrometric detection, therefore immunoassay tests will not be discussed in the following section.

Oral fluid has recently gained interest as an alternative matrix since the implementation of on-site detection of drugs of abuse in the workplace or driving under the influence programs. The sample is easy to collect, non-invasive and collection can be supervised directly reducing the opportunity for adulteration.[69] Oral fluid offers a short detection window that makes it ideal for detecting recent cannabis use. On the other hand, the concentrations of cannabinoids in oral fluid are low, require sensitive analytical techniques and the amount of sample available can be limited. Advances in analytical techniques have allowed the detection and quantification of THC-COOH in oral fluid, which is the only analyte available in order to exclude the possibility of passive inhalation. The detection time window of cannabinoids in oral fluid depends on the sensitivity of the analytical method employed. One study has shown that THC was found to be positive in oral fluid for up to 13 hours in frequent and occasional users after smoking a 6.8% THC cigarette. Cannabidiol and cannabinol showed a shorter detection time with a maximum of 4 and 8 hours, respectively. THC-COOH was found to be present between 0 and 24 hours in oral fluid of occasional users and to persist over 30 hours in frequent cannabis smokers.[70] In DFCs, oral fluid is not a specimen of choice but it could be a good alternative matrix in order to distinguish between a recent intake of cannabis and a consumption that occurred before the alleged facts. Of course, if this sample is not taken shortly after the facts (6−12 hours) it will be inadmissible.

The most commonly analyzed specimen in cases of DFCs is blood and it is the best sample to prove that a subject was under the influence of drugs of abuse or medication at the time of sampling. With the analytical methods currently available, the detection and quantification of cannabinoids in blood by means of GC-MS or LC-MS/MS is easily performed. If the analytical part is not an issue, the interpretation of a positive result is still a difficult task.[33] A wide intersubject variability exists in the rate of elimination of cannabis, and the extent of this variability can be disappointing when occasional and chronic users are compared. General knowledge of cannabis excretion suggests that recent exposure (6−8 hours) is linked to THC concentrations over 2−3 ng/mL.[71] Time of detection for THC varies from 3 to 12 hours after smoking one 1.75% THC cigarette or from 6 to 27 hours after smoking a 3.55% THC cigarette[45] and the limit of quantification of the method was 0.5 ng/mL in that study. For THC-COOH in plasma, mean detection times were 84 and 152 hours after smoking, respectively, the low and high dose THC cigarette. Sensitivity is a critical point when determining the detection time window of cannabinoids, and studies employing the best sensitivity have always reported the longest elimination half-lives for THC. For example, a study using deuterium-labeled THC reported a terminal half-life for THC of 4.1 days.[72] This relatively old study was conducted on chronic users, and in the light of recent publications the extended terminal half-life for chronic abusers of cannabis seems to be confirmed.[73] Bergamaschi et al.

published a study in which most participants were still THC positive after 15 days of monitored abstinence ($N = 18$, LOQ = 0.25 ng/mL). Ninety-one percent of the participants were also positive for THC-COOH in blood after 28 days of monitored abstinence ($N = 11$, LOQ = 0.25 ng/mL).[74] Finally, the best analyte to characterize a recent intake of cannabis was 11-OH-THC, which was only positive in blood for 3 days for all the participants ($N = 28$, LOQ = 0.5 ng/mL). These recent publications have prompted us to reconsider our knowledge in terms of the detection time window for THC. In occasional users the generally accepted window of 12−24 hours for THC is probably still valid, but in frequent users the detection time can be extremely longer. This applies also for THC-COOH, the body burden of THC; storage in fat and other tissues is responsible for the slow release in blood.

The general rules that apply for blood are also true for urine. There will be a great difference in excretion of cannabinoids in urine between occasional and frequent cannabis users. The major analyte searched for in urine is THC-COOH. Its detection is indicative of cannabis exposure but does not provide information on the route of administration, the amount, the time of exposure or the degree of impairment.[33] Mean detection times for occasional users were, respectively, 34 and 89 hours after smoking a single 1.75% or 3.55% THC cigarette using a 15 ng/mL threshold.[75] This time can be extended to weeks or even months when dealing with heavy, chronic abusers of marijuana. THC and 11-OH-THC are also present in urine mostly as glucuronides but their detection time window is shorter and probably more indicative of recent use. The analysis of those two analytes in urine is not done on a routine basis. In cases of DFC, a positive urine result will prove consumption but it will be difficult to estimate when this exposure took place.

In the specific situation of DFCs, hair analysis can give important information about the victim's or offender's past drug abuse or use of prescription medicine. Various analytes can be detected in hair such as THC, cannabinol, cannabidiol and THC-COOH. The first three analytes can be easily quantified since their concentrations are in the range of 10 to 1000 pg/mg depending on the cannabis consumption. For carboxy-THC, the concentrations in hair range from 0.1 to 10 pg/mg making it more difficult to detect. Reaching these limits will need the use of very powerful instruments, the gold standard currently being GC-MS/MS, but the most recent LC-MS/MS is also usable. Nevertheless, THC-COOH is the analyte recommended to demonstrate cannabis consumption. As THC-COOH is not present in cannabis smoke, it is the only analyte that rules out passive exposure. Since THC, cannabinol and cannabidiol are present in cannabis smoke, passive deposition on hair from the environment cannot be totally excluded. Cut-off concentrations have been proposed by the Society of Hair Testing to demonstrate cannabis consumption, e.g. THC >100 pg/mg and THC-COOH >0.2 pg/mg.[76] It has been demonstrated that detection of THC-COOH at an LOQ of 0.1 pg/mg would detect more drug users than using an LOQ of 1 pg/mg for THC.[77] In DFCs, the benefit of analyzing cannabis in hair would be to confirm a positive finding in blood or urine. Hair analysis will determine if the victim was a regular user of cannabis or not. A cannabis-positive urine or blood specimen associated with a negative result in hair (since for cannabis a single exposure will not be detectable) will be easier to interpret as a drug-facilitated or incapacitated crime.

9. IMPLICATION OF CANNABIS IN DRUG-FACILITATED CRIMES

Among substances regularly implicated in DFCs, cannabis has a special place. Along with alcohol, cannabis is not the typical substance that the offender will use by itself to commit the crime. The surreptitious administration of cannabis can probably be considered as marginal. Thus, two other scenarios should be evoked. The first one consists of the use of cannabis as an adjuvant to potentiate the effects of other drugs to be administered. The second and probably the most common case is when cannabis is shared by the victim and the offender and later the offender will take advantage of the impaired victim. In the last scenario, it will be considered as an opportunistic crime rather than a proactive DFC.[78] The majority of cannabis cases fall in the first category. By themselves, alcohol and cannabis have enough potential psychoactive effects to impair a victim, especially when the victim is not used to consuming these substances. The synergistic effects of cannabis with other xenobiotics (alcohol, drugs of abuse or prescription medications) have already been described. The particular situation of cannabis with regards to DFC has unfortunately prevented the implementation of epidemiologic studies concerning this specific substance. Data on marijuana use in DFCs are scarce and usually disseminated in larger studies dealing with drug or drugs of abuse findings in DFCs.

The prevalence of cannabis occurrence in cases of DFC is obviously linked to the prevalence of use in the general population. For instance, cannabis use in Scandinavian countries is lower than in Mediterranean or Eastern European countries and it is reflected in studies of drugs involved in DFCs. Occurrence of cannabis in blood or urine of female victims of alleged sexual assault was about 5.5% in Sweden between 2003 and 2007,[79] slightly over the 4.8% occurrence of amphetamines. Even if cannabis was the most frequently detected illicit drug,[80] these numbers are much less than those for the occurrence of cannabis in DFC in France or the United States. More than 1000 cases have been compiled in 1999 coming from all over the USA, and cannabis was found to be the most frequently detected drug after alcohol with an occurrence of 18.5%. Of the 1179 urine samples, 218 tested positive for THC-COOH at a 50 ng/mL threshold.[81] It is interesting to note that carboxy-THC was the most frequently detected analyte, even more than alcohol, when the samples were taken after more than 24 hours of the alleged crime. This result underlies the long elimination half-life of cannabis compared to other drugs involved in DFC.

In a continuing study until 2001, the prevalence of positive cannabinoids in urine was 18.6% in a sample set of 3303 urine analyses; cannabis was detected in 30.3% of the positive cases with only alcohol being more frequent.[82] In France, a case series reexamining previously negative urine results found that benzodiazepines were the most frequent analytes detected (49%) followed by cannabis with 17%.[83] It is not easy to report the true prevalence of cannabis occurrence in DFC because in the oldest studies it was not always considered as a drug that needed real focus in such cases in contrast to GHB or benzodiazepines. The marginality of spiked drink cases has led to reconsideration of the importance of alcohol, cannabis and other drugs of abuse in DFCs. In the UK, in a study of over 1000 DFC cases, the authors concluded that deliberate spiking could be identified in approximately 2% of the positive cases, whereas alcohol was involved in 46% and illicit drugs in 34%. Cannabis (26% of the total cases) and cocaine (11%) were the most common drugs of abuse detected.[84] It is interesting to note that only 63 out of the 260 subjects tested positive for cannabis (24%) admitted to using the drug.

In France, a yearly survey on chemical submission shows year after year that cannabis is still the most frequently encountered drug of abuse in cases of drug-facilitated or incapacitated crimes. This national survey was set up in 2002 after reports of case series involving GHB and benzodiazepines in France. Since then each year, regional centers of study and information on dependency collect and send to the ANSM (French agency for the security of medications) all cases related to DFCs. Alcohol and cannabis were until 2012 always the most common findings in the various biological samples analyzed all over the French territory. In 2011, 457 cases were notified; among those 273 were classified as verified chemical submission and another 102 were stated as chemical vulnerability. In the first category, five cases involved cannabis and in the second category, 22 cases were related to cannabis use.[85] Since 2007, the report of this national survey has made a clear distinction between DFCs (or so-called chemical submission in France), where the drug is surreptitiously administered to the victim, and incapacitated crimes (chemical vulnerability), where the drug is offered by the offender and shared with the victim or might even be consumed only by the victim. Legal consequences for the offender are not the same between the two and a case of incapacitated crime might be more difficult to plead for the victim.

Given that victims of sexual assault report higher prevalence of drug and alcohol use compared to non-assault victims, Resnick et al. studied the prevalence of assault-related marijuana or alcohol use among women seeking post-rape medical care. Alcohol use was reported by 54% of the women while cannabis use at the time of the assault was reported by only 12% of the participants.[86] This last number appears low in reference to the previously cited studies but when use of cannabis pre-assault (during the last 6 weeks prior to assault) is examined the number increases to 29%, relatively close to the generally reported prevalence of cannabis use in DFCs. This means that about two-thirds of the cannabis-positive findings (especially when urine is the tested biological material) might be related to anterior use of marijuana. The detection of this consumption not related to the offense might also be a negative factor for the victim when trying to get the case prosecuted. While it is socially acceptable to drink alcohol (except in Muslim countries), the consumption of marijuana is prohibited in most of countries around the world and use of drugs of abuse tends to discredit the victim. It has been proven that consumption of drugs of abuse and particularly cannabis is a factor associated with violence, arguments or fights especially among young people who frequent the nightlife culture and for those seeking for opportunities for sex.[87] Thus, use of cannabis by the offender and/or the victim may be a facilitator of the offense to be committed.

Nevertheless, it is difficult to find in the literature a single well-described case of DFC or sexual assault involving only cannabis (with or without alcohol). In France, a specific study has been made on a series involving 27 DFSA cases positive for THC-COOH in urine. In 10 cases (seven victims and three offenders), THC-COOH but not THC or 11-OH-THC was detected in blood, meaning that the subjects were not under the influence at the time of blood sampling. These cases are difficult to conclude because of the delay between the facts and the time of sampling. In the other 17 cases, the active molecules THC and 11 OH-THC were found in the blood of the subjects (14 victims and three offenders). Among the 21 victims, hair was analyzed for 12 of them and chronic use of cannabis was proven for 11. Only one case showed the absence of THC in hair and its presence in blood, suggesting that this could be called a case of cannabis-facilitated sexual assault. For the nine remaining cases where hair could not have been analyzed, the interpretation will remain inconclusive. In their conclusion the authors insist on the necessity of sampling hair in order to determine if the victim was a regular cannabis user or not; the presence of THC in blood only is not enough to support a DFC accusation.[88]

In 2004 in France, a case involving multiple patients intoxicated with cannabis was reported.[89] The case concerned a surreptitious administration of cannabis to 12 persons of the same company. An intern wanting to make fun of his coworkers prepared a cake containing hashish and made them eat it during a coffee-break. Two hours after eating the cake some of the employees were feeling nauseous, with trembling and weakness in the lower limbs. Three hours after eating the cake, when the intern revealed the truth, they were all admitted to the emergency room. Three of the 12 patients presented more serious signs of intoxication. The first one had excessive sweating, tremors and increased heart rate, and the second had increased blood pressure and dizziness. The last one showed a Wolff—Parkinson—White syndrome consisting of arrhythmia that could have led to ventricular fibrillation. In the three cases the symptoms resolved in 6 to 8 hours. At admission, urine samples of the 12 patients were collected showing positive results for 11 of them. For the three more seriously intoxicated patients, blood samples were drawn at admission and 3 hours after. All blood samples at any time were positive for THC, 11-OH-THC and THC-COOH. For five out of six samples, 11-OH-THC concentrations were greater than the THC concentrations, which is typical of the oral route of consumption of marijuana. It was not proven that the intern wanted to take advantage of the situation to commit any crime, so it was classified as administration of harmful substance rather than a DFC.[89]

10. CONCLUSION

The presence of cannabis in biological samples of subjects' victims of DFC is a common finding. The difficulty lies in the fact that this positive finding might or might not be related to the offense. THC has such a long elimination half-life that consumption from the last few days can be identified and determining when the exposure took place is very hazardous. Knowledge of the victim's history of drug use is crucial to interpret the results. Hair analysis is recommended to document the case, but ideal situations where cannabis is detected in blood or urine and not in the hair are not as common. Because of the high prevalence of marijuana use in the general population, most of the time a positive result for cannabis will be only incidental with no link to the actual case. Nevertheless, the psychoactive potential of cannabis must not be underestimated and its synergy of effects with alcohol and other CNS depressants should be kept in mind when interpreting cases of DFSAs or DFCs.

REFERENCES

1. United Nations. *Office on Drugs and Crime. Global illicit drug trends—2003*. Vienna, Austria: United Nations International Drug Control Programme Research Section; 2003.
2. European Drug Report 2013: Trends and development. EMCDDA, Lisbon, May 2013.
3. Beck F, Tovar ML, Guignard R, Spilka S, Richard JB. Levels of drug use in France in 2010. *Tendances* 2013;**76**:1–6.
4. Mura P, Kintz P, Ludes B, Gaulier JM, Marquet P, Martin-Dupont S, et al. Comparison of the prevalence of alcohol, cannabis and other drugs between 900 injured drivers and 900 control subjects: results of a French collaborative study. *Forensic Sci Int* 2003;**133**:79–85.
5. Laumon B, Gadegbeku B, Martin JL, Biecheler MB, SAM Group. Cannabis intoxication and fatal road crashes in France: population based case—control study. *BMJ* 2005;**331**:1371.

6. Drummer OH, Gerostamoulos J, Batziris H, Chu M, Caplehorn JR, Robertson MD, Swann P. The incidence of drugs in drivers killed in Australian road traffic crashes. *Forensic Sci Int* 2003;**134**:154–62.

7. Legrand SA, Silverans P, de Pacpe P, Buylaert W, Verstraete AG. Presence of psychoactive substances in injured Belgian drivers. *Traffic Inj Prev* 2013;**14**:461–8.

8. Reisfield GM, Shults T, Demery J, Dupont R. A protocol to evaluate drug-related workplace impairment. *J Pain Palliat Care Pharmacother* 2013;**27**:43–8.

9. Mura P, Saussereau E, Brunet B, Goullé JP. Workplace testing of drugs of abuse and psychotropic drugs. *Ann Pharm Fr* 2012;**70**:120–32.

10. Macdonald S, Hall W, Roman P, Stockwell T, Coghlan M, Nesvaag S. Testing for cannabis in the work-place: a review of the evidence. *Addiction* 2010;**105**:408–16.

11. Lhermitte M, Frimat P, Labat L, Haguenoer JM. Use of illicit substances in the workplace. *Ann Pharm Fr* 2012;**70**:3–14.

12. Campos DR, Yonamine M, de Moraes Moreau RL. Marijuana as doping in sports. *Sports Med* 2003;**33**:395–9.

13. Bergamashi MM, Crippa JAS. Why should cannabis be considered doping in sports? *Front Psychiatry* 2013;**15**:32.

14. Mura P, Trouvé R, Mauco G. Is cannabis a doping substance? *Ann Toxicol Annal* 2000;**12**:43–8.

15. Fals-Stewart W, Golden J, Schumacher JA. Intimate partner violence and substance use: a longitudinal day-to-day examination. *Addict Behav* 2003;**28**:1555–15574.

16. Moore TM, Stuart GL, Meehan JC, Rhatigan DL, Hellmuth JC, Keen SM. Drug abuse and aggression between intimate partners: a meta-analytic review. *Clin Psychol Rev* 2008;**28**:247–74.

17. Hall W, Solowij N. Adverse effects of cannabis. *The Lancet* 1998;**352**:1611–6.

18. Turner CE, ElSohly MA, Boeren EG. Constituents of cannabis sativa L.XVII. A review of the natural constituents. *J Nat Prod* 1980;**43**:169–234.

19. Atakan Z. Cannabis, a complex plant: different compounds and different effects on individuals. *Ther Adv Psychopharmacol* 2012;**2(6)**:241–54.

20. Bruci Z, Papoutsis I, Athanaselis S, Nikolaou P, Pazari E, Spiliopoulou C, Vyshka G. First systematic evaluation of the potency of Cannabis sativa plants grown in Albania. *Forensic Sci Int* 2013;**222**:40–6.

21. Mura P, Brunet B, Dujourdy L, Paetzold C, Bertrand G, Sera B, et al. Cannabis of the past and cannabis today. Increase of THC contents from 1993 to 2004 in France. *Ann Toxicol Annal* 2006;**18**:3–6.

22. Tsumura Y, Aoki R, Tokieda R, Akutsu M, Kawase Y, Kataoka T, et al. A survey of the potency of Japanese illicit cannabis in fiscal year 2010. *Forensic Sci Int* 2012;**221**:77–83.

23. Zamengo L, Frison G, Bettin C, Sciarrone R. Variability of cannabis potency in the Venice area (Italy): a survey over the period 2010–2012. *Drug Test Anal* 2013.10.1002/dta.1515.

24. Swift W, Wong A, Li KM, Armold JC, McGregor IS. Analysis of Cannabis seizures in NSW, Australia: cannabis potency and cannabinoid profile. *PloS ONE* 2013;**8**:e70052.

25. Mura P, Dumestre-Toulet V. Cannabis sativa variété indica. In: Kintz P, editor. *Traité de toxicologie médico-judiciaire*. Issy les Moulineaux: Elsevier Masson; 2012. pp. 299–320.

26. Mehmedic Z, Chandra S, Slade D, Denham H, Foster S, Patel AS, et al. Potency trends of THC and other cannabinoids in confiscated cannabis preparations from 1993 to 2008. *J Forensic Sci* 2010;**55**:1209–17.

27. Bozy TZ, Cole KA. Consumption and quantitation of delta-9-tetrahydrocannabinol in commercially available hemp seed oil products. *J Anal Toxicol* 2000;**24**:562–6.

28. Julien RM. *A primer of drug action.* New York: W.H. Freeman and Company; 1997.
29. Howlett AC, Qualy JM, Khachatrian LL. Involvement of Gi in the inhibition of adenylate cyclase by cannabimimetic drugs. *Mol Pharmacol* 1986;**29**:307−13.
30. Paldy E, Bereczki E, Santha M, Wenger T, Borsodi A, Zimmer A, Benyhe S. CB2 cannabinoid receptor antagonist SR144528 decreases mu-opioid receptor expression and activation in mouse brainstem: role of CB2 receptor in pain. *Neurochem Int* 2008;**53**:309−16.
31. Mura P, Kintz P, Dumestre V, Raul S, Hauet T. THC can be detected in brain while absent in blood. *J Anal Toxicol* 2005;**29**:841−3.
32. O'Brien CP. Drug addiction and drug abuse. In: Hardman JC, Limbird LE, Molinoff PB, Ruddon RW, Gilman AG, editors. *The pharmacological basis of therapeutics.* New York: Macmillan; 1995.
33. Huestis M. Cannabis (Marijuana)—effects on human behavior and performance. *Forensic Sci Rev* 2002;**14**:15−59.
34. Bossong MG, Jager G, Bhattacharyya S, Allen P. Acute and non-acute effects of cannabis on human memory function: a critical review of imaging studies. *Curr Pharm Des* 2013. Epub ahead of print.
35. Riedel G, Davies SN. Cannabinoid function in learning, memory and plasticity. *Handb Exp Pharmacol* 2005;**168**:445−77.
36. Han J, Kesner P, Metna-Laurent M, Duan T, Xu L, Georges F, et al. Acute cannabinoids impair working memory through astroglial CB1 receptor modulation of hippocampal LTD. *Cell* 2012;**148**:1039−50.
37. Shukla PC, Moore UB. Marijuana-induced transient global amnesia. *South Med J* 2004;**97**:782−4.
38. Gillet C, Polard E, Mauduit N, Allain H. Acting out and psychoactive substances: alcohol, drugs, illicit substances. *Encephale* 2001;**27**:351−9.
39. Verdejo-Garcia A, Rivas-Perez C, Lopez-Torrecillas F, Perez-Garcia M. Differential impact of drug use on frontal behavioral symptoms. *Addict Behav* 2006;**31**:1373−82.
40. Wrege J, Schmidt A, Walter A, Smieskova R, Bendfeldt K, Radue EW, et al. Effects of cannabis on impulsivity: a systematic review of neuroimaging findings. *Curr Pharm Des* 2013. Epub ahead of print.
41. Peeters FP. Chronic depersonalisation following cannabis use. *Ned Tijdschr Geneeskd* 2005;**149**:1058−61.
42. Hürlimann F, Kupferschmid S, Simon AE. Cannabis-induced depersonalization disorder in adolescence. *Neuropsychobiology* 2012;**65**:141−6.
43. Agurell S, Halldin M, Lindgren JE, Ohlsson A, Widman M, Gillespie H, Hollister L. Pharmacokinetics and metabolism of delta 1-tetrahydrocannabinol and other cannabinoids with emphasis on man. *Pharmacol Rev* 1986;**38**:21−43.
44. Azorlosa JL, Greenwald MK, Stitzer ML. Marijuana smoking: effects of varying puff volume and breathhold duration. *J Pharmacol Exp Ther* 1995;**272**:560−9.
45. Huestis MA, Henningfield JE, Cone EJ. Blood cannabinoids. I. Absorption of THC and formation of 11-OH-THC and THCCOOH during and after smoking marijuana. *J Anal Toxicol* 1992;**16**:276−82.
46. Schwope DM, Karschner EL, Gorelick DA, Huestis MA. Identification of recent cannabis use: whole-blood and plasma free and glucuronidated cannabinoid pharmacokinetics following controlled smoked cannabis administration. *Clin Chem* 2011;**57**:1406−14.
47. Favrat B, Ménétrey A, Augsburger M, Rothuizen LE, Appenzeller M, Buclin T, et al. Two cases of "cannabis acute psychosis" following the administration of oral cannabis. *BMC Psychiatry* 2005;**5**:17−22.

48. Ménétrey A, Augsburger M, Rothuizen LE, Pin MA, Appenzeller M, Favrat B, et al. Profils cinétiques du Δ^9-tetrahydrocannabinol, du 11-hydroxy-Δ^9-tetrahydrocannabinol et de l'acide 11-nor-Δ^9-tetrahydrocannabinol-9-carboxylique chez le sujet volontaire sain après administration orale de décoctions de cannabis ou de dronabinol. *Ann Toxicol Anal* 2004;**15**:231−43.

49. Ohlsson A, Lindgren JE, Wahlen A, Agurell S, Hollister LE, Gillespie HK. Plasma delta-9 tetrahydrocannabinol concentrations and clinical effects after oral and intravenous adminis-tration and smoking. *Clin Pharmacol Ther* 1980;**28**:409−16.

50. Wall ME, Sadler BM, Brine D, Taylor H, Perez-Reyes M. Metabolism, disposition, and kinetics of delta-9-tetrahydrocannabinol in men and women. *Clin Pharmacol Ther* 1983;**34**:352−63.

51. Hunt CA, Jones RT. Tolerance and disposition of tetrahydrocannabinol in man. *J Pharmacol Exp Ther* 1980;**215**:35−44.

52. Giroud C, Michaud K, Sporkert F, Eap C, Augsburger M, Cardinal P, Mangin P. A fatal over-dose of cocaine associated with coingestion of marijuana, buprenorphine, and fluoxetine. Body fluid and tissue distribution of cocaine and its metabolites determined by hydrophilic interaction chromatography-mass spectrometry (HILIC-MS). *J Anal Toxicol* 2004;**28**:464−74.

53. Johansson E, Norén K, Sjövall J, Halldin MM. Determination of delta 1-tetrahydrocannabinol in human fat biopsies from marihuana users by gas chromatography-mass spectrometry. *Biomed Chromatogr* 1989;**3**:35−8.

54. Brunet B, Doucet C, Venisse N, Hauet T, Hébrard W, Papet Y, et al. Validation of Large White Pig as an animal model for the study of cannabinoids metabolism: application to the study of THC distribution in tissues. *Forensic Sci Int* 2006;**161**:169−74.

55. Kudo K, Nagata T, Kimura K, Imamura T, Jitsufuchi N. Sensitive determination of delta 9-tetrahydrocannabinol in human tissues by GC-MS. *J Anal Toxicol* 1995;**19**:87−90.

56. Lemberger L, Crabtree RE, Rowe HM. 11-Hydroxy-9-tetrahydrocannabinol: pharmacology, disposition, and metabolism of a major metabolite of marihuana in man. *Science* 1972;**177**:62−4.

57. Abraham TT, Lowe RH, Pirnay SO, Darwin WD, Huestis MA. Simultaneous GC-EI-MS determination of delta9-tetrahydrocannabinol, 11-hydroxy-delta9-tetrahydrocannabinol, and 11-nor-9-carboxy-delta9-tetrahydrocannabinol in human urine following tandem enzyme-alkaline hydrolysis. *J Anal Toxicol* 2007;**31**:477−85.

58. Krishna DR, Klotz U. Extrahepatic metabolism of drugs in humans. *Clin Pharmacokinet* 1994;**26**:144−60.

59. Bornheim LM, Lasker JM, Raucy JL. Human hepatic microsomal metabolism of delta 1-tetrahydrocannabinol. *Drug Metab Dispos* 1992;**20**:241−6.

60. Watanabe K, Yamaori S, Funahashi T, Kimura T, Yamamoto I. Cytochrome P450 enzymes involved in the metabolism of tetrahydrocannabinols and cannabinol by human hepatic microsomes. *Life Sci* 2007;**80**:1415−9.

61. Bland TM, Haining RL, Tracy TS, Callery PS. CYP2C-catalyzed delta9-tetrahydrocannabi-nol metabolism: kinetics, pharmacogenetics and interaction with phenytoin. *Biochem Pharmacol* 2005;**70**:1096−103.

62. Sachse-Seeboth C, Pfeil J, Sehrt D, Meineke I, Tzvetkov M, Bruns E, et al. Interindividual variation in the pharmacokinetics of delta9-tetrahydrocannabinol as related to genetic poly-morphisms in CYP2C9. *Clin Pharmacol Ther* 2009;**85**:273−6.

63. Harvey DJ. Absorption, distribution, and biotransformation of the cannabinoids. In: Nahas GG, Sutin KM, Harvey DJ, Agurell S, editors. *Marijuana and medicine.* Totowa: Humana Press; 2001. p. 91.

64. Huestis MA, Mitchell JM, Cone EJ. Urinary excretion profiles of 11-nor-9-carboxy-delta 9-tetrahydrocannabinol in humans after single smoked doses of marijuana. *J Anal Toxicol* 1996;**20**:441−52.

65. Johansson E, Halldin MM. Urinary excretion half-life of delta 1-tetrahydrocannabinol-7-oic acid in heavy marijuana users after smoking. *J Anal Toxicol* 1989;**13**:218−23.

66. Lafolie P, Beck O, Blennow G, Boreus L, Borg S, Elwin CE, et al. Importance of creatinine analysis in urine when screening for abused drugs. *Clin Chem* 1991;**37**:1927−31.

67. Smith-Kielland A. Urinary excretion of 11-nor-9-carboxy-delta9-tetrahydrocannabinol: a case with an apparent long terminal half-life. *Scand J Clin Lab Invest* 2006;**66**:169−71.

68. Westin AA, Huestis MA, Aarstad K, Spigset O. Urinary excretion of 11-nor-9-carboxy-delta(9)-tetrahydrocannabinol in a pregnant woman following heavy, chronic cannabis use. *J Anal Toxicol* 2009;**33**:610−14.

69. Concheiro M, Lee D, Lendoiro E, Huestis MA. Simultaneous quantification of Δ(9)-tetrahydrocannabinol, 11-nor-9-carboxy-tetrahydrocannabinol, cannabidiol and cannabinol in oral fluid by microflow-liquid chromatography-high resolution mass spectrometry. *J Chromatogr A* 2013;**1297**:123−30.

70. Anizan S, Milman G, Desrosiers N, Barnes AJ, Gorelick DA, Huestis MA. Oral fluid cannabinoid concentrations following controlled smoked cannabis in chronic frequent and occasional smokers. *Anal Bioanal Chem* 2013. http://dx.doi.org/10:1007/s00216−013−7291-5.

71. Mason AP, McBay AJ. Cannabis: pharmacology and interpretation of effects. *J Forensic Sci* 1985;**30**:615−31.

72. Johansson E, Agurell S, Hollister LE, Halldin MM. Prolonged apparent half-life of delta 1-tetrahydrocannabinol in plasma of chronic marijuana users. *J Pharm Pharmacol* 1988;**40**:374−5.

73. Karschner EL, Schwilke EW, Lowe RH, Darwin WD, Pope HG, Herning R, et al. Do delta9-tetrahydrocannabinol concentrations indicate recent use in chronic cannabis users? *Addiction* 2009;**104**:2041−8.

74. Bergamaschi MM, Karschner EL, Goodwin RS, Scheidweiler KB, Hirvonen J, Queiroz RH, Huestis MA. Impact of prolonged cannabinoid excretion in chronic daily cannabis smokers' blood on per se drugged driving laws. *Clin Chem* 2013;**59**:519−26.

75. Huestis MA, Mitchell JM, Cone EJ. Detection times of marijuana metabolites in urine by immunoassay and GC-MS. *J Anal Toxicol* 1995;**19**:443−9.

76. SOHT. Recommendations for hair testing in forensic cases. *Forensic Sci Int* 2004;**145**:83−4.

77. Huestis MA, Gustafson RA, Moolchan ET, Barnes A, Bourland JA, Sweeney SA, et al. Cannabinoid concentrations in hair from documented cannabis users. *Forensic Sci Int* 2007;**169**:129−36.

78. Hall JA, Moore CB. Drug facilitated sexual assault—a review. *J Forensic Leg Med* 2008;**15**:291−7.

79. Jones AW, Holmgren A, Ahlner J. Toxicological analysis of blood and urine samples from female victims of alleged sexual assault. *Clin Toxicol (Phila)* 2012;**50**:555−61.

80. Jones AW, Kugelberg FC, Holmgren A, Ahlner J. Occurrence of ethanol and other drugs in blood and urine specimens from female victims of alleged sexual assault. *Forensic Sci Int* 2008;**181**:40−6.

81. ElSohly MA, Salamone SJ. Prevalence of drugs used in cases of alleged sexual assault. *J Anal Toxicol* 1999;**23**:141−6.

82. Hindmarch I, ElSohly M, Gambles J, Salamone S. Forensic urinalysis of drug use in cases of alleged sexual assault. *J Clin Forensic Med* 2001;**8**:197–205.

83. Boussairi A, Dupeyron JP, Hernandez B, Delaitre D, Beugnet L, Espinoza P, Diamant-Berger O. Urine benzodiazepines screening of involuntarily drugged and robbed or raped patients. *J Toxicol Clin Toxicol* 1996;**34**:721–4.

84. Scott-Ham M, Burton FC. Toxicological findings in cases of alleged drug-facilitated sexual assault in the United Kingdom over a 3-year period. *J Clin Forensic Med* 2005;**12**:175–86.

85. ANSM. Résultats de l'enquête nationale sur la soumission chimique 2011. Available from: URL: <http://ansm.sante.fr/var/ansm_site/storage/original/application/531d6b066b8fc67 a47a19e6feee3b093.pdf> [accessed 19.09.13].

86. Resnick HS, Walsh K, McCauley JL, Schumacher JA, Kilpatrick DG, Acierno RE. Assault related substance use as a predictor of substance use over time within a sample of recent victims of sexual assault. *Addict Behav* 2012;**37**:914–21.

87. Calafat A, Bellis MA, Fernández Del Rio E, Juan M, Hughes K, Morleo M, et al. Nightlife, verbal and physical violence among young European holidaymakers: what are the triggers? *Public Health* 2013;**10**:908–15.

88. Mura P, Visinoni P, Alvarez JC, Goullé JP, Kintz P. Cannabis: which occurrence in chemical submission? *Ann Toxicol Anal* 2002;**14**:412–16.

89. Brunet B, Rouffineau J, Papet Y, Bataillon S, Mura P. Données cliniques et biologiques de 13 cas de consommation de cannabis par voie orale ou…rectale. *Ann Toxicol Anal* 2004;**15**:175–6.

Chapter 7

Drugs Involved in Drug-Facilitated Crimes (DFC)

Analytical Aspects: 1—Blood and Urine

Luc Humbert, Guillaume Hoizey and Michel Lhermitte

In drug-facilitated crime (DFC) cases, apart from the complete clinical examination of the victim that must be done by a qualified health care professional, the systematic collection of biological specimens is also essential in the first phase of investigation. Blood and urine are the most usual matrices to document drug exposure. These specimens must be collected as soon as possible after the alleged assault and must be quickly refrigerated until analysis. The length of time that drugs used for DFC remain in urine or blood depends on a number of factors (e.g. the type and amount of drug ingested, patient body size, rate of metabolism, whether patients have a full stomach, and whether they have previously urinated). The sooner a blood and/or urine specimen is obtained after the alleged event, the greater is the chance of detecting drugs that are rapidly eliminated from the body.[1]

The body fluids collected from complainants for toxicological analysis should be submitted to a forensic toxicology laboratory that is capable of screening for a wide range of compounds with high sensitivity and specificity. A chain custody documentation including the victim's medical report and basic questionnaire must also accompany the specimens.

1. GENERAL CONSIDERATIONS REGARDING URINE AND BLOOD SAMPLING

1.1 Urine

Because drugs and metabolites are generally concentrated in the urine, they tend to be more readily detectable.[2] This fact allows toxicologists to detect their presence over longer periods of time than is the case with blood. Urine should be collected no later than 120 hours after the alleged drugging.

Toxicological Aspects of Drug-Facilitated Crimes. DOI: http://dx.doi.org/10.1016/B978-0-12-416748-3.00007-4

Indeed, most of the drugs encountered in DFC cases can be eliminated from urine in less than 4 to 5 days, although some with longer half-lives remain in urine at very low concentrations after that time.[1] Ideally, urine should be collected rapidly after the assault. The urine sample does not have to be a clean catch (e.g. bacteria in the urine will not compromise test results).[3] If patients must urinate before their arrival at the exam facility, first responders should ask them to provide a sample and bring it to the facility, documenting the chain of custody.[3] Urine should be transferred in at least two standard urine collection cups without preservative and stored at +4°C until analysis. One sample could be stored refrigerated in case further analysis is requested.

1.2 Whole Blood

Because blood, compared to urine, allows a shorter window of detection for drugs and/or metabolites commonly encountered in DFC cases, it should be collected preferably no later than 48 hours after the alleged event. In cases in which blood can be collected very shortly after drug ingestion, the combination of blood and urine specimens is essential to provide a clearer picture as to the window of exposure of the drug.[2] A few milliliters of whole blood are generally necessary and should be collected in sample vials containing preservative and anticoagulant. Similarly to urine sample, one blood sample could be stored in case of further investigations, such as a defense analysis.

The recent guidelines edited by the United Nations Office on Drugs and Crime (UNODC) for the forensic analysis of DFC and other criminal acts recommends a minimum of 50 mL of urine, collected in at least two sterile containers (with no preservative) and at least two 5 mL blood samples collected in tubes containing compounds such as sodium fluoride and potassium oxalate.[4] The French DFC protocol established in 2005 by the ANSM (Agence Nationale de Sécurité du Médicament et des produits de Santé) and the one proposed by the French Society of Analytical Toxicology (SFTA: Société Française de Toxicologie Analytique) recommend volumes of blood and urine relatively similar to those proposed by UNODC.[5,6]

Regarding blood and urine sampling, there are at least two factors which are out of the control of the forensic toxicologist: first, the rapid collection of blood and urine samples with a sufficient volume upon admission of the victim at the emergency or forensic unit, and second, one must be sure that samples are stored at the facility in a secure environment at the correct temperature.[4] As with any forensic evidence, the chain of custody must be maintained. The toxicologist may refer to the current *Forensic Toxicology Laboratory Guidelines* by the Society of Forensic Toxicologists and the American Academy of Forensic Sciences for detailed guidance on proper collection, labeling, handling, submission and analysis of toxicology samples.[7] These issues underline the great importance of a permanent communication between the forensic toxicologist, the clinician in charge of the victim and the investigating officers and/or the prosecutors.

2. GENERAL ANALYTICAL CONSIDERATIONS

One of the most important issues that need to be considered in a DFC investigation is the sensitivity and specificity of the analytical methods used, since most of the compounds are usually used at low doses.[8] This is complicated by the fact that victims of DFC often report the event some considerable time after drug ingestion, therefore limiting the chance of detecting substances that could have been potentially ingested in biological fluids. Amnesia, doubt about what may have happened or psychological considerations could be the reasons for late reporting.[6] Lack of experience among investigators, medical personnel, laboratory staff and prosecutors in handling such cases may also render investigations difficult.[4]

In this context, DFC-related substances in blood and urine must be analyzed by highly sensitive and selective methods developed in appropriately equipped forensic toxicology laboratories with good laboratory practices and well-trained staff. Over the years, specimens collected in investigations of DFC have at times been unnecessarily wasted because the specimens were sent to laboratories that did not have appropriate methods or instrumentation to carry out efficiently the toxicological analysis.[2,9] We must keep in mind that false-negative results due to the use of inadequate methods can be dissuasive for further investigation and may discourage the victim.[4] Consequently, it remains clear that the use of immunoassays and enzymatic techniques should be avoided, even discouraged. Nevertheless, if those methods are used in a laboratory, they must be strictly limited to a preliminary screening in urine, and the forensic toxicologist should ensure that the sample amount available is sufficient for further analyses by more sophisticated methods.

As for other forensic areas, the reliability of qualitative and quantitative analytical findings is essential for an accurate interpretation of the results.[4] In this context, analytical methods used in DFC cases must be fully validated following the classical parameters, such as low limit of detection, low limit of quantification, selectivity, linearity, accuracy, precision, stability, recovery and matrix effect (particularly for LC-MS techniques).

Sample preparation is undoubtedly a key step of the analytical procedure since high sensitivity is required (see below).

For blood and urine analyses, methodologies based on hyphenated chromatographic and spectroscopic techniques, such as LC-MS/MS and GC-MS or GC-MS/MS are today considered as a prerequisite to investigating a DFC case. For those reasons, it remains clear that specimens should only be submitted to qualified forensic laboratories for analysis. As Lebeau reminds us in an article in 2008, we should keep in mind that for investigators of DFCs, one of the frustrating aspects of toxicology results is the disparity in capabilities from one laboratory to another.[2] These differences are often the result of the diverse technologies available among independent laboratories. Discrepancies in results may also be related to failure to correctly determine the detection limits of analytical procedures. This can result in negative results that have no real meaning.[2] In order to evaluate their current capabilities in terms of limit of detection in urine for the most prevalent drugs and metabolites encountered in DFCs, laboratories are encouraged to consult the document edited by the Drug-Facilitated Sexual Assault Committee from the Society of Forensic Toxicologists (SOFT) to determine if they meet the recommended performance limits. This is a list of substances that should be targeted for the analysis of urine, with minimum required performance limits, including parent drugs and metabolites. It is specified that this list is not a complete list of drugs encountered in DFC, just the common ones. It is recommended by the committee for each laboratory to select the substances which are most commonly used in their region and/or country. This list is reported in Table 7.1.[10]

In summary, the following techniques are the main recommended ones for urine and blood analysis in DFC investigations[4]:

- Ethanol by GC-FID or HS-GC-FID.
- Ethylglucuronide and ethylsulfate by LC-MS/MS or GC-MS after derivatization.
- Non-volatile organic compounds: target analysis and screening for drugs and metabolites must be performed by chromatographic methods with mass spectrometry detection (LC or UHPLC-MS/MS, GC-MS and GC-MS/MS). More recently, high resolution mass spectrometry methods (LC-TOF/MS, LC-HR-MS) for the identification of unknown compounds have been successfully applied to cases of suspected DFC.

3. METHODOLOGY

Although the coupling of gas chromatography with mass spectrometry—GC-MS(/MS)—is still present and widely used in all toxicology laboratories, the emergence of coupling liquid chromatography with an increasing number of different mass spectrometry detectors—LC-MS(/MS)—has recently emerged. These last couplings have received major improvements regarding chromatographic separation, with the advent of devices capable of supporting much higher pressures (>1000 bar) to work with more powerful stationary phases of smaller sizes ($<2 \, \mu m$). The main limitation of LC was the lack of efficiency compared to GC. Using particles $<2 \, \mu m$ increases both efficiency and also the pressure in the system considerably. These new chromatographs support the increase of pressure, but allow drastic reduction in retention time with still good separation, hence the name of Fast LC.[11]

TABLE 7.1 Substances that should be Targeted for in the Analysis, with Minimum Required Performance Limits, Including Parent Drugs and Metabolites[10]

Target Drug/Metabolite	Recommended Maximum Detection Limit
Ethanol	0.1 g/L
Ethylglucuronide	100 µg/L
GHB	
Gamma-hydroxybutyrate	10 mg/L
Benzodiazepines	
Alprazolam and alpha-OH-alprazolam	10 µg/L
Bromazepam and OH bromazepam	10 µg/L
Chlordiazepoxide	10 µg/L
Clobazam	10 µg/L
Clonazepam and 7-aminoclonazepam	5 µg/L
Clotiazepam	10 µg/L
Diazepam	10 µg/L
Estazolam	10 µg/L
Flunitrazepam and 7-aminoflunitrazepam	5 µg/L
Loprazolam	10 µg/L
Lorazepam	10 µg/L
Lormetazepam	10 µg/L
Midazolam	10 µg/L
Nitrazepam and 7-aminonitrazepam	5 µg/L
Nordiazepam	10 µg/L
Oxazepam	10 µg/L
Phenazepam	5 µg/L
Prazepam	10 µg/L
Temazepam	10 µg/L
Tetrazepam	10 µg/L
Triazolam and 4-OH-triazolam	5 µg/L

(*Continued*)

TABLE 7.1 (Continued)

Target Drug/Metabolite	Recommended Maximum Detection Limit
Z-drugs	
Zaleplon	10 µg/L
Zolpidem and metabolites	10 µg/L
Zopiclone and metabolites	10 µg/L
Antihistamines, anti-depressants and others	
Aceprometazine	10 µg/L
Alimemazine	10 µg/L
Amitriptyline and nortriptyline	10 µg/L
Brompheniramine and desmethyl-B	10 µg/L
Carisoprodol and meprobamate	50 µg/L
Cetirizine	10 µg/L
Chlorpheniramine and desmethyl-C	10 µg/L
Citalopram and desmethylcitalopram	10 µg/L
Clonidine	10 µg/L
Cyamemazine	10 µg/L
Cyclobenzaprine	10 µg/L
Desipramine	10 µg/L
Diphenhydramine	10 µg/L
Doxepin and desmethyldoxepin	10 µg/L
Doxylamine and desmethyldoxylamine	10 µg/L
Fluoxetine and norfluoxetine	10 µg/L
Haloperidol	10 µg/L
Hydroxyzine	10 µg/L
Imipramine	10 µg/L
Niaprazine	10 µg/L
Oxomemazine	20 µg/L
Paroxetine	10 µg/L
Sertraline and norsertraline	10 µg/L
Valproic acid	50 µg/L

(Continued)

TABLE 7.1 (Continued)

Target Drug/Metabolite	Recommended Maximum Detection Limit
Street drugs and miscellaneous drugs	
Amobarbital	25 µg/L
Butalbital	25 µg/L
Pentobarbital	25 µg/L
Phenobarbital	25 µg/L
Secobarbital	25 µg/L
Narcotics and non-narcotics analgesics	
Codeine	10 µg/L
Dextromethorphan	10 µg/L
Dihydrocodeine	10 µg/L
Fentanyl	1 µg/L
Hydrocodone	10 µg/L
Hydromorphone	10 µg/L
Meperidine (pethidine)	10 µg/L
Methadone	10 µg/L
Morphine	10 µg/L
Oxycodone	10 µg/L
Propoxyphene and norpropoxyphene	10 µg/L
Street drugs and miscellaneous drugs	
Cannabinoids	
THC-COOH	10 µg/L
Opiates	
6-Mono-acetyl-morphine (MAM)	10 µg/L
Morphine	10 µg/L
Cocaine	
Benzoylecgonine	50 µg/L
Cocaine	50 µg/L
Cocaethylene	50 µg/L
Methylecgonine	50 µg/L

(Continued)

TABLE 7.1 (Continued)

Target Drug/Metabolite	Recommended Maximum Detection Limit
Amphetamines	
Amphetamine	10 µg/L
Methamphetamine	10 µg/L
MBDB	10 µg/L
MDA	10 µg/L
MDEA	10 µg/L
MDMA	10 µg/L
Ketamine and norketamine	1 µg/L
LSD	1 µg/L
Phencyclidine	10 µg/L
Piperazine group	10 µg/L
Scopolamine	10 µg/L

Interfaces have also improved considerably in their geometries, and different modes of ionization of molecules are now available, the most common being: electrospray ionization (ESI), atmospheric pressure chemical ionization (APCI) and atmospheric pressure photo ionization (APPI), which can alternate the acquisition in positive and negative mode.

The detection limit of the mass detector is constantly improving. New, more sensitive devices regularly appear on the market. The best sensitivity is still currently obtained by detectors called tandem mass (triple quadrupole or ion trap). However, mass spectrometers capable of acquiring the exact mass of molecules are currently expanding and appear to be of great interest for DFC investigations.

It was thought that these innovative technological developments would eliminate the various steps of sample pretreatment. This is obviously not the case, as the preparation of biological samples remains, and will remain, fundamental in the field of DFC investigation.

Blood and urine are complex biological matrices which contain a large number of endogenous compounds irrelevant to the toxicological analysis and which could affect the quality of the analysis (high background, ion suppression, etc.).

Characterization of a DFC case relies on both the identification of specific compounds that are known to be frequently used in DFC and the use of

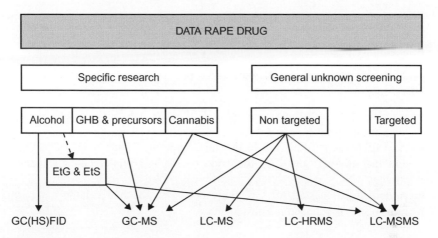

FIGURE 7.1   Different analytics approaches.

strategies that allow a more extensive research of substances that may affect alertness. Figure 7.1 shows the specific molecules to be searched for in the cases of DFC and the different strategies that should be used.

The identification of ethanol and its markers, as well as the detection of cannabinoids, is discussed in separate chapters dealing specifically with alcohol (Chapter 4) and cannabis (Chapter 6), respectively. Here, we will discuss the different methods of sample preparation, as well as the different analytical strategies that can be used to perform the most sensitive and extensive detection of psychoactive substances involved in DFCs.

3.1 Sample Preparation

Blood and urine both contain a multitude of endogenous substances in amounts superior to those of the compounds or metabolites of interest. The ideal sample preparation procedure should ensure the elimination of the maximum of those endogenous compounds, as well as the concentration of compounds potentially of interest. To lower the detection limit of analytical techniques, most published methods rely on the recovery of the sample extract by a lower volume.

The choice of the methods of extraction has to be adapted to the further screening strategy that will be applied, i.e. a unique, large and untargeted screening of compounds in a single acquisition mode and/or multiple targeted acquisitions to detect specific molecules or a family of molecules.

The choice and the development of an extraction method should take into account:

- Physicochemical properties of the analytes.
- Nature of the biological matrix.

- Stability of the analytes during the different (pre)analytical treatment steps.
- Solubility of the dry extract in the elution solvent.

Most often, the matrix-related sample preparation and the proposed analytical method will have to include:

- Hydrolysis of glucuronide compounds that are generally present in large amounts in urine.
- An extraction step that has to be chosen among a wide range of methods and that is best suited to the context and the implemented screening strategy.
- A derivatization step for GC analysis due to the non-volatile nature of most of the psychoactive substances.

3.1.1 Liquid/Liquid Extraction

Liquid/liquid extraction (LLE) is based on the partition of an analyte between two immiscible phases, one being the serum or the urine. It is often performed at a pH where the analyte is non-ionized to facilitate its migration into the organic phase.

This inexpensive and easy to implement method is still widely used. Nevertheless, it has the inconvenience of being time-consuming, difficult to automate, often consuming toxic solvents and less efficient for highly polar compounds. The solvent choice is based on its polarity; generally, polar solvents extract polar analytes more efficiently than do apolar analytes. Consequently, LLE cannot be specific for a particular analyte, as the solvent can extract all molecules from the matrix (endogenous and exogenous, i.e. xenobiotics) with similar physicochemical properties.

This type of method is used to extract groups or families of molecules, including benzodiazepines[12-14] and antidepressants,[15] for the screening of synthetic cannabinoids.[16,17]

Being able to extract a large number of analytes that are different regarding their structure and chemical nature requires a combination of solvents with various polarities. For that purpose, many authors have used mixtures combining four to five different solvents.[18-20]

3.1.2 Solid Phase Extraction (SPE)

Solid phase extraction is based on the partition of a solute between a mobile liquid phase (the biological matrix and various solvents) and a solid stationary phase. Since its introduction, many stationary phases have been developed, allowing more targeted extractions or adaptation for the extraction of a large number of chemicals of various types. The diversity of stationary phases allows the extraction of polar compounds that were previously difficult to extract by organic phases.[21]

3.1.2.1 Offline Solid Phase Extraction

The offline solid phase extraction procedure, which can be performed on cartridges or 96 well plates, consists of four main steps:

1. The conditioning of the stationary phase regenerates retention sites that are involved in the molecular interactions.
2. The sample loading.
3. Washing is not a systematic step; it aims to eliminate the weakly-retained molecules. The method is used to characterize a specific compound or a family of compounds, and, according to the nature of the stationary phase used, improvement of the sample purification can also be achieved by acting alternatively on the eluting force of the solvent or on the pH to modify the molecule ionization. In the case of an application for a large screening of compounds, this step will generally not be applicable.
4. An appropriate organic solvent is then used to elute the molecules.

Many procedures for offline SPE have been described for toxicological screenings. It has been successfully used for the extraction of groups or families of molecules including benzodiazepines,[22] cathinones[23] and phenethylamines.[24] Protocols for much larger screenings have been also reported.[25–27]

3.1.2.2 Online Solid Phase Extraction

The growing interest in SPE is due to its possibility for automation. For a few years, many methods of online preparation have been described, in particular due to the increasing use of coupling Fast LC-MS(/MS).[28]

The stationary phase which is contained in a small column (ca. 2 cm) is integrated into the chromatographic system (Figure 7.2). The system requires an additional pump for the loading of the sample onto the extraction column, as well as two valves for solvent selection in order to switch and control both pumps during the various steps.

The elution of the compounds of interest is achieved using a "backflush" mode towards the analytical column. Among the many advantages of this method are its greater robustness (independent of the operator), an increased sensitivity due to the injection of the whole prepared sample and the possibility of performing several specific extraction protocols consecutively by modifying loading or washing conditions. Many analytical methods using this technique have been published.[29–32]

3.1.3 Molecularly Imprinted Polymer Extraction (MIP)

New selective supports involving molecular recognition mechanisms have been developed. These use molecularly imprinted polymers (MIP) that have been processed using the molecular imprinting technique, which leaves cavities in the polymer matrix with an affinity to a chosen template molecule. The most

(a) Loading

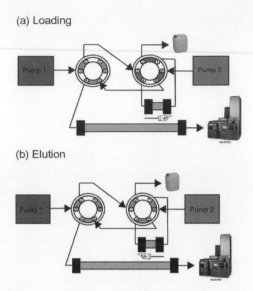

(b) Elution

FIGURE 7.2 Principle steps of *online* extraction.

interesting application in the context of the characterization of a DFC concerns LSD, which was detected at a urine concentration of 0.2 pg/mL.[33]

3.2 Instrumental Analysis

The analytical characterization of a DFC involves the identification of a psychoactive substance and/or of its specific metabolites in a biological matrix. As already mentioned, the substance is mostly administered as a single dose and has usually a short half-life. Furthermore, the molecule will be present at a concentration that will become lower as the delay between administration and sampling increases. The detection of the slightest trace of a psychoactive molecule is crucial for the investigation and can be helpful for the victim who has limited or no recollection of events.

Apart from the specific detection of ethanol or cannabis, the important challenge for the toxicologist is to have an analytical strategy that combines an exhaustive screening of xenobiotics at a high sensitivity. However, the analytical strategy must also guarantee specificity to avoid a false-positive result that would have deleterious consequences. Good control of sample preparation combined with the analyses done on recent and efficient equipment will guarantee the relevance of a result. The detection of molecules by mass spectrometry is the only current method that combines high sensitivity and specificity. The detection and separation of ions can be made by various types of analyzers that differ in their measurement of the m/z ratio, which can be:

- Dispersion of ions based on their time or kinetic energy (magnetic or electric sector instruments).

- Separation in time, based on the speed of the ions (time of flight).
- Ion transmission through an electrodynamic field (quadrupole).
- Periodic movement in a magnetic field or electrodynamic field (traps or ion traps).

The ability of these analyzers to separate the various ions classifies them into two categories. The first, called low-resolution (<5000) analyzers, can detect and separate nominal masses with a resolution called "unit mass" (quadrupole, ion trap). The second, called high resolution (>5000), are more efficient as they measure the exact mass of the ion (time of flight, Orbitrap).

To achieve the most complete screening possible, two types of approach are possible:

- A wide screening without information obtained by scanning detection.
- A series of targeted searches of a number of molecules usually belonging to the same family.
- The "full scan" mode is based on the continuous acquisition of a broad mass range (for example, from 50 to 1000 m/z). It can be carried out with mass detectors like single quadrupole, ion trap or high resolution analyzers. In the targeting mode, the analyzer is programmed permanently to detect specific masses during a relatively short time (a few milliseconds). The currently used analyzers are able to perform the acquisition of a large number of specific masses very quickly (every few milliseconds) during the chromatographic analysis.

3.2.1 Non-targeted Approaches using Low Mass Resolution

3.2.1.1 Gas Chromatography

GC-MS has long been widely used and is essential for the detection of certain molecules. The most used is the quadrupole analyzer and sometimes the ion trap. The most suitable ionization mode for toxicological screening is the electron impact mode creating a large amount of fragments, which is the chemical fingerprint of a molecule. The identification of a molecule is based on the comparison of its spectrum with commercial libraries of mass spectra. This method has the advantage of having at its disposal a number of libraries with many spectra; it is also possible to create its own libraries. Acquired spectra are independent of the origin of the analyzer, which is not the case for LC-MS.

The disadvantages of this approach are that it is limited to molecules that are thermally stable, volatile and of small molecular weight; the other molecules must be derivatized (methylation acetylation, trimethylsilylation, etc.) to make them more volatile.

Some authors have published extensive screening results for urine after derivatization with BSTFA and TMCS, which can detect many compounds at acceptable sensitivity with regards to the recommendations of the

SOFT.[25,26] Gamma hydroxybutyrate (GHB) is also detected using this approach.[34-36]

3.2.1.2 Liquid Chromatography

Liquid chromatography removes most of the disadvantages of gas chromatography, and is recognized as much more universal, hence its widespread use for conducting toxicological screening. The appearance of Fast-LC increased its appeal; it improves the selectivity and speed of analysis. Compared to GC-MS, the coupling of liquid chromatography with a mass detector is more complex, and requires an interface and different ionization techniques.

The most widely used ionization modes are ESI and APCI either in positive or negative ionization mode. The desolvation of the mobile phase, the ionization of solutes and the transfer of ions are carried out at atmospheric pressure in the interface between LC and the mass spectrometer. The geometry of the analyzer is specific to each manufacturer. These ionization methods are much softer than EI ionization in GC-MS.

Structural information can be obtained by rapidly chaining events within the interface. It is possible to adjust the parameters to change the acceleration of the ions and generate collision-induced dissociation (CID) creating fragments of variable size depending on the stability of the ions. It is possible to chain multiple speed acceleration to acquire simultaneously more specific spectra of a molecule. These fragmentation spectra are unfortunately not as universal compared to the GC-MS spectra and depend on the geometry of the source of each manufacturer.[37,38] Another drawback is that the fragments obtained in the interface resulting from the collision of all the molecules are eluted at the same time, reducing the specificity in the case of co-eluent compounds.

Most of the methods described use a quadrupole analyzer and continuously combine different conditions of acceleration in the source during chromatography. All the acquired spectra, most often associated with a retention time, allow the identification of the molecules.[20,39,40]

3.2.2 Non-targeted Approaches using High Mass Resolution

The coupling of liquid chromatography with mass analyzers measuring the exact so-called high resolution (LC-HRMS) has grown very rapidly on the market (time of flight, Orbitrap).[41-45] These instruments provide new fields of investigation for the toxicologist. Current devices measure an exact mass with a measurement uncertainty of about 2–3 ppm. From an exact mass, it is possible to identify one or more potential empirical formulas (the number depends on the molecular weight). Some devices can significantly reduce this list by calculating from each elemental composition their theoretical isotopic pattern, which is compared with the one of the unknown molecule. From the empirical formula, the good isomer can then be determined.

The price of these instruments is continually decreasing. Their acquisition has the huge advantage of operating in "full scan" mode. These devices alternate very quickly between acquisitions at low energy, without fragmentation, to obtain the protonated or deprotonated molecular ions, and acquisitions at high energy in order to obtain the molecular fragments that will confirm their presence. In this case, the spectral data are grouped into databases containing: name, molecular formula, chromatographic retention time and specific fragments. Some authors have created very large databases created from injections of compounds according to their analytical conditions; other compounds were added with partial data from the literature or the web.[46,47] Correct identification is made on the basis of accurate mass, an isotopic pattern, the presence of specific fragments and the retention time.

The method is now used by a growing number of laboratories for wide screening.[32,47–53] HRMS offers many more interesting possibilities. Urine still remains the standard for comprehensive screening of biosamples, generally in unknown cases. Many drugs in urine can be detected by the presence of their metabolites, and for some of them the metabolites are the only detectable compounds. The metabolites generally have longer half-lives, so they will be detectable for longer in the urine. The presence of metabolites significantly expands the detection window of a given substance.[54,55] However, available commercial or personal libraries only contain a very small number of metabolites; moreover, it is difficult to obtain pure substances (very expensive or non-synthetized). The number of searched for active psychotropic substances is important and some are extensively metabolized producing a number of potential metabolites to search for. Obviously not all of them are eliminated in the same quantity, so it is important to be able to detect two or three major metabolites. HRMS instruments have the capacity to find and characterize these metabolites *in silico*.

The metabolism of most psychoactive molecules to look for is known.

The instrument has specific software in order to facilitate the research of metabolites. For each molecule a list of metabolic pathways corresponding to a desired molecule has to be chosen. The software calculates the exact masses of potential metabolites (hydroxylation, demethylation, sulfoxylation, etc.) and researches them in the low energy acquisition function.

For each chromatographic peak with one of the identified accurate masses, the characterization of the presence of a potential metabolite is made from the analysis of different structural formulas of the desired metabolites and fragments obtained for the same chromatographic peaks from the function acquired at high energy.[56,57]

3.2.3 Targeted Screening Approaches

The majority of molecules involved in DFC are known and well characterized physicochemically as well as chromatographically. It is possible with mass spectrometers like the single quadrupole, triple quadrupole or hybrid triple quadrupole ion trap types to set up the acquisition differently in order to obtain the lowest possible limit of detection.

These modes are:

- Selected ion monitoring mode (SIR)
- Dependent data acquisition (DDA)
- MRM (multiple reaction monitoring)

SIR mode is used with a single quadrupole; the sequential detection of a list of two or three specific ions of each molecule is scheduled throughout the chromatography. With this method, the detector is focused longer on the presence of mass (m/z) belonging to the molecules of interest.[22,24]

Another approach uses a hybrid triple quadrupole instrument (QTRAP) in which the third quadrupole can be used as a linear ion trap (LIT). This was based on tandem MS data-dependent acquisition (DDA) using SRM as a survey scan and an enhanced product ion (EPI) scan. Identification of the obtained product ion spectra (PIS) was conducted by library search using the authors' EPI spectra libraries. As these spectra contain, in most cases, several fragment ions, these approaches provide better identification power than those using only one to three transitions. This technique has been well published and used by several laboratories.[30−31,40,58−60]

Acquisition in MRM (multiple reaction monitoring) mode is possible after the determination in "daughter scan" mode of the most intense and specific fragments obtained at different rates of acceleration for each of the molecules to search for. The parent ion is selected in the first quadrupole, fragmented in the collision cell and the third quadrupole is focused on one of its daughter ions. According to a European guideline, at least two MRM transitions should be used to identify a molecule.[61] This acquisition mode has a double selectivity (the parent ion and daughter ion). Both analyzers are set at constant and defined values over a longer period of time; the detection sensitivity is improved compared to other scanning modes, making MRM the most sensitive acquisition mode at present.

This technique has been widely used for the production of dedicated screening in many areas, including the characterization of DFC.[62,63,23]

The main disadvantages of these methods are:

- It is only possible to find what one is specifically looking for (other compounds may be missed).
- Any subsequent restatement is impossible.

3.3 General Considerations

Validation of screening methods should not be as comprehensive as quantitative methods, but should include tests for selectivity, matrix effect, recovery, detection limits, analyte carryover and stability.[45]

3.3.1 Ion Suppression

LC-MS coupling is known to be sensitive to matrix effects. During the process of ionization of molecules in the interface, competition between the ions of interest and co-eluent substances exist.[64-68] The matrix effect can either reduce or more rarely increase the response of an analyte. Ion suppression is due to the presence of less volatile compounds that can affect the efficiency of formation or droplet evaporation of the mobile phase, but also will depend particularly in positive ES mode of the proton affinity of each co-eluted molecule. This phenomenon affects negatively the detection limits of a method and significantly penalizes the search for traces. Matrix effect must be systematically evaluated in the development of a new method. If for some compounds suppression ion is important, analytical changes should be considered (extraction method, chromatographic conditions, ionization mode).

3.3.2 Quality Control

It is very important to continuously ensure that the methods used to search for psychoactive substances are efficient. It is preferable to use one or more internal standards in these studies. Their detection during the analysis of the chromatograms ensures that the extraction and also the analysis by GC-MS (MS) or LC-MS (MS) or LC-HRMS were properly made.

Each laboratory should consider adhering to external quality controls adapted to the context of the DFC (for example, the SFTA[69] propose for its members an EQC in blood and urine).

3.3.3 Evaluation Comparative

All the described analytical approaches offer many possibilities from which it is sometimes difficult to choose. The laboratory equipment will of course be an important element to consider and will be a prerequisite to carry out research as part of DFC. Table 7.2 summarizes the various strengths and weaknesses of the different technologies.

4. CONCLUSION

The characterization of DFC in blood or urine is difficult; it should detect the largest number of psychoactive substances possible. A large and growing number of molecules should be searched for with an ultimate sensitivity (drugs, narcotics, new psychoactive substances, etc.). The quality of the analysis will depend on the availability of diversified and highly efficient analytical equipment and the preparation of effective and appropriate protocols to be used in sample research. A good physicochemical and pharmacological knowledge of the involved molecules and their elimination mechanism is necessary. For better efficiency, metabolite detection should be performed in urine.

TABLE 7.2 Strengths and Weaknesses of the Different Technologies

	GCMS	LCMS	LCMSMS	LCHRMS
Detection limit	+	+	+ + +	+ +
Specificity	+ + +	+ + +	+ + +	+ + +
Reference libraries	+ + +	+	Not applicable	+ + +
Broad search	+ +	+ + +	+	+ + +
Retreatment	+ + +	+ + +	Not applicable	+ + +
On line extraction	+	+ + +	+ + +	+ + +
Matrix effects	+	+ + +	+ + +	+ + +
Cost	+	+	+ +	+ + +

Still nowadays, MRM acquisition is and will always be the most sensitive mode. But in recent years, there has been a growing interest in exact mass measurement detectors. The acquisition of full spectral data enables an increase in the number of compounds without compromising sensitivity; it also allows more information to be obtained from each sample with the use of software to identify unknowns or other metabolites and transformation products. This approach is and will be an excellent complementary tool for toxicological screening in biological matrices.

REFERENCES

1. Lebeau M, Andollo W, Hearn WL, Baselt R, Cone E, Finkle B, et al. Recommandations for toxicological investigations of drug-facilitated sexual assaults. *J Forensic Sci* 1999;**44**:227−30.
2. Lebeau MA. Guidance for improved detection of drugs used to facilitate crimes. *Ther Drug Monit* 2008;**30**:229−33.
3. A national protocol for sexual assault medical forensic examinations—adults/adolescents. Second Edition. DNA Initiative. Available from <https://www.ncjrs.gov/pdffiles1/ovw/241903.pdf>;2013 [accessed 3.05.13].
4. Guidelines for the forensic analysis of drugs facilitating sexual assault and other criminal acts. UNODC. Available from <http://www.unodc.org/documents/scientific/forensic_analys_of_-drugs_facilitating_sexual_assault_and_other_criminal_acts.pdf>;2011 [accessed 13.04.13].
5. Agence Nationale de Sécurité du Médicament et des produits de Santé (ANSM). Enquête soumission chimique. Annexe 3: conduite à tenir pour les prélèvements biologiques. ANSM website, Available from <http://ansm.sante.fr/>;2005 [accessed 2.05.13].
6. Kintz P. Toxicological investigations in case of drug-facilitated crimes. *Ann Toxico Anal* 2003;**15**:239−42.

7. Forensic Toxicology Laboratory Guidelines. Society of Forensic Toxicology/American Academy of Forensic Sciences. Available from <http://www.soft-tox.org/files/Guidelines_2006_Final.pdf>;2006 [accessed 6.05.13].

8. Negrusz A, Gaensolen RE. *Drug-facilitated sexual assault. Clarkes's analytical forensic toxicology*. London: Pharmaceutical Press; 2008.

9. Shbair MKS, Lhermitte M. Drug-facilitated crimes: definitions, prevalence, difficulties and recommendations. A review. *Ann Pharm Fran* 2010;**68**:136—47.

10. Recommended Maximum Detection Limits for common DFSA drugs and metabolites in urine samples. Drug-Facilitated Sexual Assault Committee. Society of Forensic Toxicology. Available from <http://www.soft-tox.org/>;2012 [accessed 3.05.13].

11. Kintz P. *Traité de toxicologie médico-judiciaire méthodes analytiques*. 2nd ed. Issy-les-Moulineaux: Elsevier Masson; 2012.

12. ElSohly MA, Gul W, ElSohly KM, Avula B, Khan IA. LC-MS-(TOF) analysis method for benzodiazepines in urine samples from alleged drug-facilitated sexual assault victims. *J Anal Toxicol* 2006;**30**:524—38.

13. Hayashida M, Takino M, Terada M, Kurisaki E, Kudo K, Ohno Y. Time-of-flight mass spectrometry (TOF-MS) exact mass database for benzodiazepine screening. *Leg Med (Tokyo)* 2009;**11**(Suppl. 1):423—5.

14. Remane D, Meyer MR, Wissenbach DK, Maurer HH. Ultra high performance liquid chromatographic-tandem mass spectrometric multi-analyte procedure for target screening and quantification in human blood plasma: validation and application for 31 neuroleptics, 28 benzodiazepines, and Z-drugs. *Anal Bioanal Chem* 2011;**401**:1341—52.

15. Remane D, Meyer MR, Wissenbach DK, Maurer HH. Full validation and application of an ultra high performance liquid chromatographic—tandem mass spectrometric procedure for target screening and quantification of 34 antidepressants in human blood plasma as part of a comprehensive multi-analyte approach. *Anal Bioanal Chem* 2011;**400**:2093—107.

16. Dresen S, Kneisel S, Weinmann W, Zimmermann R, Auwärter V. Development and validation of a liquid chromatography-tandem mass spectrometry method for the quantitation of synthetic cannabinoids of the aminoalkylindole type and methanandamide in serum and its application to forensic samples. *J Mass Spectrom* 2011;**46**:163—71.

17. Kneisel S, Auwärter V. Analysis of 30 synthetic cannabinoids in serum by liquid chromatography-electrospray ionization tandem mass spectrometry after liquid-liquid extraction. *J Mass Spectrom* 2012;**47**:825—35.

18. Mueller CA, Weinmann W, Dresen S, Schreiber A, Gergov M. Development of a multi-target screening analysis for 301 drugs using a QTrap liquid chromatography/tandem mass spectrometry system and automated library searching. *Rapid Commun Mass Spectrom* 2005;**19**:1332—8.

19. Lee HK, Ho CS, Iu YP, Lai PS, Shek CC, Lo YC, Klinke HB, Wood M. Development of a broad toxicological screening technique for urine using ultra-performance liquid chromatography and time-of-flight mass spectrometry. *Anal Chim Acta* 2009;**649**:80—90.

20. Humbert L, Grisel F, Richeval C, Lhermitte M. Screening of xenobiotics by ultra-performance liquid chromatography-mass spectrometry using in-source fragmentation at increasing cone voltages: library constitution and an evaluation of spectral stability. *J Anal Toxicol* 2010;**34**:571—80.

21. Humbert L. Extraction en phase solide (SPE): théorie et applications. *Ann Toxicol Anal* 2010;**22**:61—8.

22. Ishida T, Kudo K, Hayashida M, Ikeda N. Rapid and quantitative screening method for 43 benzodiazepines and their metabolites, zolpidem and zopiclone in human plasma by liquid

chromatography/mass spectrometry with a small particle column. *J Chromatogr B: Analyt Technol Biomed Life Sci* 2009;**877**:2652−7.

23. Swortwood MJ, Boland DM, DeCaprio AP. Determination of 32 cathinone derivatives and other designer drugs in serum by comprehensive LC-QQQ-MS/MS analysis. *Anal Bioanal Chem* 2013;**405**:1383−97.

24. Kerrigan S, Banuelos S, Perrella L, Hardy B. Simultaneous detection of ten psychedelic phenethylamines in urine by gas chromatography-mass spectrometry. *J Anal Toxicol* 2011;**35**:459−69.

25. Juhascik M, Le NL, Tomlinson K, Moore C, Gaensslen RE, Negrusz A. Development of an analytical approach to the specimens collected from victims of sexual assault. *J Anal Toxicol* 2004;**28**:400−6.

26. Adamowicz P, Kala M. Simultaneous screening for and determination of 128 date-rape drugs in urine by gas chromatography-electron ionization-mass spectrometry. *Forensic Sci Int* 2010;**198**:39−45.

27. Birkler RI, Telving R, Ingemann-Hansen O, Charles AV, Johannsen M, Andreasen MF. Screening analysis for medicinal drugs and drugs of abuse in whole blood using ultra-performance liquid chromatography time-of-flight mass spectrometry (UPLC-TOF-MS)—toxicological findings in cases of alleged sexual assault. *Forensic Sci Int* 2012;**222**:154−61.

28. Marquet P. LC-MS vs. GC-MS, online extraction systems, advantages of technology for drug screening assays. *Methods Mol Biol* 2012;**902**:15−27.

29. Sturm S, Hammann F, Drewe J, Maurer HH, Scholer A. An automated screening method for drugs and toxic compounds in human serum and urine using liquid chromatography-tandem mass spectrometry. *J Chromatogr B Analyt Technol Biomed Life Sci* 2010;**878**:2726−32.

30. Mueller DM, Duretz B, Espourteille FA, Rentsch KM. Development of a fully automated toxicological LC-MS(n) screening system in urine using online extraction with turbulent flow chromatography. *Anal Bioanal Chem* 2011;**400**:89−100.

31. Mueller DM, Rentsch KM. Online extraction toxicological MS(n) screening system for serum and heparinized plasma and comparison of screening results between plasma and urine in the context of clinical data. *J Chromatogr B Analyt Technol Biomed Life Sci* 2012;**883−884**:189−97.

32. Guale F, Shahreza S, Walterscheid JP, Chen HH, Arndt C, Kelly AT, Mozayani A. Validation of LC-TOF-MS screening for drugs, metabolites, and collateral compounds in forensic toxicology specimens. *J Anal Toxicol* 2013;**37**:17−24.

33. Chapuis-Hugon F, Pichon V. Utilisation d'outils sélectifs pour l'analyse de traces dans des échantillons complexes. *Ann Toxicol Anal* 2010;**22**:97−101.

34. Elian AA. GC-MS determination of gamma-hydroxybutyric acid (GHB) in blood. *Forensic Sci Int* 2001;**122**:43−7.

35. Villain M, Cirimele V, Ludes B, Kintz P. Ultra-rapid procedure to test for gamma-hydroxybutyric acid in blood and urine by gas chromatography-mass spectrometry. *J Chromatogr B Analyt Technol Biomed Life Sci* 2003;**792**:83−7.

36. Paul R, Tsanaclis L, Kingston R, Berry A, Guwy A. GC-MS-MS determination of gamma-hydroxybutyrate in blood and urine. *J Anal Toxicol* 2006;**30**:375−9.

37. Jansen R, Lachatre G, Marquet P. LC-MS/MS systematic toxicological analysis: comparison of MS/MS spectra obtained with different instruments and settings. *Clin Biochem* 2005;**38**:362−72.

38. Wissenbach DK, Meyer MR, Weber AA, Remane D, Ewald AH, Peters FT, Maurer HH. Towards a universal LC-MS screening procedure—can an LIT LC-MS(n) screening

approach and reference library be used on a quadrupole-LIT hybrid instrument? *J Mass Spectrom* 2012;**47**:66−71.

39. Venisse N, Marquet P, Duchoslav E, Dupuy JL, Lachâtre G. A general unknown screening procedure for drugs and toxic compounds in serum using liquid chromatography-electrospray-single quadrupole mass spectrometry. *J Anal Toxicol* 2003;**27**:7−14.

40. Sauvage FL, Saint-Marcoux F, Duretz B, Deporte D, Lachatre G, Marquet P. Screening of drugs and toxic compounds with liquid chromatography-linear ion trap tandem mass spectrometry. *Clin Chem* 2006;**52**:1735−42.

41. Peters FT. Recent advances of liquid chromatography-(tandem) mass spectrometry in clinical and forensic toxicology. *Clin Biochem* 2011;**44**:54−65.

42. Jiwan JL, Wallemacq P, Hérent MF. HPLC-high resolution mass spectrometry in clinical laboratory? *Clin Biochem* 2011;**44**:136−47.

43. Himmelsbach M. 10 years of MS instrumental developments—impact on LC−MS/MS in clinical chemistry. *J Chromatogr B* 2012;**883−884**:3−17.

44. Wu AH, Gerona R, Armenian P, French D, Petrie M, Lynch KL. Role of liquid chromatography-high-resolution mass spectrometry (LC-HR/MS) in clinical toxicology. *Clin Toxicol (Phila)* 2012;**50**:733−42.

45. Maurer HH. What is the future of (ultra) high performance liquid chromatography coupled to low and high resolution mass spectrometry for toxicological drug screening? *J Chromatogr A* 2013;**1292**:19−24.

46. Polettini A, Gottardo R, Pascali JP, Tagliaro F. Implementation and performance evaluation of a database of chemical formulas for the screening of pharmaco/toxicologically relevant compounds in biological samples using electrospray ionization-time-of-flight mass spectrometry. *Anal Chem* 2008;**80**:3050−7.

47. Broecker S, Herre S, Wüst B, Zweigenbaum J, Pragst F. Development and practical application of a library of CID accurate mass spectra of more than 2,500 toxic compounds for systematic toxicological analysis by LC-QTOF-MS with data-dependent acquisition. *Anal Bioanal Chem* 2011;**400**:101−17.

48. Kolmonen M, Leinonen A, Pelander A, Ojanperä I. A general screening method for doping agents in human urine by solid phase extraction and liquid chromatography/time-of-flight mass spectrometry. *Anal Chim Acta* 2007;**585**:94−102.

49. Lee HK, Ho CS, Iu YP, Lai PS, Shek CC, Lo YC. Development of a broad toxicological screening technique for urine using ultra-performance liquid chromatography and time-of-flight mass spectrometry. *Anal Chim Acta* 2009;**649**:80−90.

50. de Castro A, Gergov M, Ostman P, Ojanperä I, Pelander A. Combined drug screening and confirmation by liquid chromatography time-of-flight mass spectrometry with reverse database search. *Anal Bioanal Chem* 2012;**403**:1265−78.

51. Ojanperä I, Kolmonen M, Pelander A. Current use of high-resolution mass spectrometry in drug screening relevant to clinical and forensic toxicology and doping control. *Anal Bioanal Chem* 2012;**403**:1203−20.

52. Marin SJ, Hughes JM, Lawlor BG, Clark CJ, McMillin GA. Rapid screening for 67 drugs and metabolites in serum or plasma by accurate-mass LC-TOF-MS. *J Anal Toxicol* 2012;**36**:477−86.

53. Strano Rossi S, Anzillotti L, Castrignanò E, Frison G, Zancanaro F, Chiarotti M. UHPLC-MS/MS and UHPLC-HRMS identification of zolpidem and zopiclone main urinary metabolites and method development for their toxicological determination. *Drug Test Anal* 2013;**19** Epub ahead of print.

54. Richeval C, Rifflet A, Humbert L, Imbenotte M, Houssin R, Lhermitte M. Élargissement de la fenêtre de détection du zolpidem par la recherche de ses métabolites urinaires dans le cadre de la soumission chimique. *Ann Toxicol Anal* 2008;**20**:79−83.

55. Johansen SS, Dahl-Sørensen R. A drug rape case involving triazolam detected in hair and urine. *Int J Legal Med* 2012;**126**:637−43.

56. Pelander A, Tyrkkö E, Ojanperä I. In silico methods for predicting metabolism and mass fragmentation applied to quetiapine in liquid chromatography/time-of-flight mass spectrometry urine drug screening. *Rapid Commun Mass Spectrom* 2009;**23**:506−14.

57. Meyer MR, Maurer HH. Current applications of high-resolution mass spectrometry in drug metabolism studies. *Anal Bioanal Chem* 2012;**403**:1221−31.

58. Jansen R, Lachatre G, Marquet P. LC-MS/MS systematic toxicological analysis: comparison of MS/MS spectra obtained with different instruments and settings. *Clin Biochem* 2005;**38**:362−72.

59. Mueller CA, Weinmann W, Dresen S, Schreiber A, Gergov M. Development of a multi-target screening analysis for 301 drugs using a QTrap liquid chromatography/tandem mass spectrometry system and automated library searching. *Rapid Commun Mass Spectrom* 2005;**19**:1332−8.

60. Dresen S, Ferreiros N, Gnann H, Zimmermann R, Weinmann W. Detection and identification of 700 drugs by multi-target screening with a 3200 Q TRAP LC-MS/MS system and library searching. *Anal Bioanal Chem* 2010;**396**:2425−34.

61. Rivier L. Criteria for the identification of compounds by liquid chromatography-mass spectrometry and liquid chromatography-multi mass spectrometry in forensic toxicology and doping analysis. *Anal Chim Acta* 2003;**926**:199−209.

62. Villain M, Chèze M, Tracqui A, Ludes B, Kintz P. Windows of detection of zolpidem in urine and hair: application to two drug facilitated sexual assaults. *Forensic Sci Int* 2004;**143**:157−61.

63. Deveaux M, Chèze M, Pépin G. The role of liquid chromatography-tandem mass spectrometry (LC-MS/MS) to test blood and urine samples for the toxicological investigation of drug-facilitated crimes. *Ther Drug Monit* 2008;**30**:225−8.

64. Müller C, Schäfer P, Störtzel M, Vogt S, Weinmann W. Ion suppression effects in liquid chromatography-electrospray-ionisation transport-region collision induced dissociation mass spectrometry with different serum extraction methods for systematic toxicological analysis with mass spectra libraries. *J Chromatogr B Analyt Technol Biomed Life Sci* 2002;**773**:47−52.

65. Annesley TM. Ion suppression in mass spectrometry. *Clin Chem* 2003;**49**:1041−4.

66. Liang HR, Foltz RL, Meng M, Bennett P. Ionization enhancement in atmospheric pressure chemical ionization and suppression in electrospray ionization between target drugs and stable-isotope-labeled internal standards in quantitative liquid chromatography/tandem mass spectrometry. *Rapid Commun Mass Spectrom* 2003;**17**:2815−21.

67. Dams R, Huestis MA, Lambert WE, Murphy CM. Matrix effect in bio-analysis of illicit drugs with LC-MS/MS: influence of ionization type, sample preparation, and biofluid. *J Am Soc Mass Spectrom* 2003;**14**:1290−4.

68. Saar E, Gerostamoulos D, Drummer OH, Beyer J. Comparison of extraction efficiencies and LC-MS-MS matrix effects using LLE and SPE methods for 19 antipsychotics in human blood. *Anal Bioanal Chem* 2009;**393**:727−34.

69. Société Française de Toxicologie Analytique (SFTA). <http://sfta.org/presentation/main/main_accueil.php> [accessed 20.09.13].

Chapter 8

Drugs Involved in Drug-Facilitated Crimes (DFC)

Analytical Aspects: 2—Hair

Marjorie Chèze and Jean-Michel Gaulier

1. INTRODUCTION

In drug-facilitated crimes (DFCs), particularly in drug-facilitated sexual assault (DFSA), it is not unusual for the delay between facts and biological samplings to exceed several days or weeks.[1] In 56% of cases in a study from 2010, due to the long length of time that elapsed between the offenses and the opportunity to obtain samples for analysis, scalp hair was the only matrix able to establish the involvement of drugs in the crimes.[2] Indeed, in such situations, hair is generally of interest for toxicological investigations owing to its large detection window. Taking into account that the mean growth rate of human scalp hair is approximately 1 cm/month (range from 0.7 to 1.4 cm/month with a mean of about 1 cm/month accepted by the scientific community),[3] administration of a single dose can be confirmed by the detection of the psychotropic drug in the corresponding hair segment, with no presence in the preceding and subsequent ones. In addition, segmental analysis makes it possible to assess the possibility of repeated offenses on a long-term basis, as well as to distinguish chronic treatment from a single exposure in the case of psychoactive drug presence in blood and/or urine samples. As a consequence, hair analysis has become an essential and necessary tool in forensic and clinical toxicology in DFC cases (as well as in other contexts; i.e. addiction monitoring).[4] As a result, toxicology laboratories are frequently asked to collect and analyze hair from DFSA victims in order to reveal the supposedly administered drugs.

After a single dose intake, the expected concentration in hair is generally in the low picogram/milligram range for most psychotropic drugs. Therefore, the use of highly sensitive instrumental techniques, such as gas or liquid chromatography coupled to tandem mass spectrometry (GC or LC-MS/MS)

Toxicological Aspects of Drug-Facilitated Crimes. DOI: http://dx.doi.org/10.1016/B978-0-12-416748-3.00008-6

or liquid chromatography coupled to high resolution mass spectrometry (LC-HRMS), is today obligatory when investigating DFC.[5–7]

The list of substances (and metabolites) to screen in cases of DFC has been broadly discussed in the previous chapters. The compounds or therapeutic classes potentially used are numerous and diverse because the expected effects can be obtained by many neuropharmacological mechanisms or combinations of mechanisms. Nevertheless, among various groups of psychotropic drugs, several benzodiazepines and related compounds are highly involved in DFC, especially in DFSA: a) they may be used to modify a person's behavior, and may cause anterograde amnesia, b) they have advantageous pharmacological properties (low blood concentrations, short elimination half-life, etc.) and c) for practical reasons (availability, galenic forms, etc.).[1,8,9] Benzodiazepines and analogs (zolpidem, zopiclone) are still the most frequently used DFC drugs in France[7,10] and these drugs were also reported to be widely used in the United States.[11,12] Consecutively, analytical methods for hair analysis in DFC cases found in the literature mainly concern benzodiazepines, although unusual compounds can sometimes be observed.[1,13,14]

The aim of this chapter is to examine the analytical aspects of hair analysis in DFC cases (Figure 8.1) in a nonexhaustive way and with a special focus on hypnotic-sedative drugs, especially benzodiazepines and related compounds.

2. PHYSIOLOGY OF HAIR GROWTH AND INCORPORATION OF DRUGS IN HAIR

2.1 Physiology of Hair Growth

Hair is a matrix displaying a cylindrical structure, with the cuticle forming an outer protective layer around the cortical cells.[15] The distribution and nature of pigments (melanin is the most important) determines the color of hair. It is produced by melanocytes, mostly located in the basal layer of the cortex.[16] The innermost region of hair is the medulla, and consists of a framework of spongy keratin and hair spaces, which can be discontinuous or absent. The germination center around the hair bulb papilla is formed by matrix cells (keratinocytes and melanocytes) present on the basement membrane. The matrix cell cycle is one of the most rapid of all human tissues. Rapid mitosis forces a migration of the upper zones into the direction of the hair root mouth. Cortex and cuticle cells follow different paths of development. Cortex cells change from spherical shape at the germinative level to a spindle-like form, and protein filaments are synthesized, which fill the cell and fuse together. In the zone of hardening, disulfide bonding, resorption and dehydration, all cytoplasmic organelles, disappear with cellular residue coupled by membrane structures. Cuticle cells originate from matrix cells of

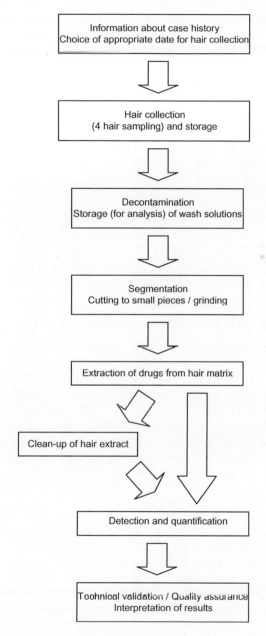

FIGURE 8.1   Analytical aspects of hair analysis in DFC cases.

the outer sphere of the papilla. These cells change to a shingle-like structure and contain amorphous protein, and their membrane complex consists of proteins and a protein–lipid complex originating from previous cell membranes.[16] This part of hair is most vulnerable to chemical and mechanical attack and is the primary diffusion point for the incorporation and elimination of drugs.

Hair follicles are embedded in the epidermal epithelium of the skin, 3 to 5 mm below the skin surface, and include the sebaceous and apocrine glands, which directly secrete into the hair follicle, while the sweat glands secrete near the exit of the hair follicle. Sebaceous glands are located over the entire surface of the body while apocrine glands are localized in the eyelids, underarms, the external auditory meatus and the perineal region. Three types of hair are usually described[15,16]:

- Vellus hair, produced by non-sexual hair follicles, is not influenced by hormones and is short, fine and non-pigmented. It is found on the eyelids, forehead and on the body of children and adults.
- Terminal hair is coarse, long and pigmented. It is found on the scalp, beard, eyebrow, eyelash, armpit and pubic areas.
- Intermediate hair has characteristics of both vellus and terminal hair. It is found on the arms and legs of adults and has characteristics of both vellus and terminal hairs.

The hair growth cycle is segmented in three stages[15,16]:

- The anagen phase: around 85% of the hairs on the human scalp are involved by this stage, during which metabolic activity, cell division and growth are increased. This phase can last between 4 and 8 years.
- The catagen phase: this transition stage concerns less than 1% of the hairs on the human scalp. Cell division stops, the hair shaft becomes fully keratinized and the bulb begins to degenerate. This phase generally lasts a few weeks.
- The telogen phase: around 15% of adult scalp hair is in this final stage. There is no more hair growth, the follicle is short and can be easily removed by pulling. This phase can last between 4 and 6 months, and the duration of this phase depends on the hair type and increases with age.

The anagen/telogen hair ratio varies with the anatomical sites, race, sex, age and state of health. Scalp hair growth ranges from 0.6 to 3.36 cm per month, with an average growth rate of 1 cm generally described, and it takes between 7 and 10 days for the growing hair to reach the surface of the scalp. Hair sampled from the vertex region of the scalp is recommended for toxicological investigations, especially in DFC cases, owing to the fastest growth rate and the highest proportion of follicles in the anagen phase in this region.

2.2 Drug Incorporation

Exact mechanisms of drug incorporation are not yet fully understood, but some notions are already well known.

   The main routes of incorporation are from the blood supply, by passive diffusion from blood capillaries into growing cells, and also sebum, sweat and external contamination.[15] The final concentration of analytes in hair would result in a combination of these different routes of incorporation. Thus, as it would be logical to assume that hair concentration is proportional to blood concentration, metabolic profiles between these two matrices do not match this hypothesis, and there is no linear relationship between dose and hair concentration.[15,16] For example, cocaine, heroin and 6-monoacetylmorphine are far more easily detected in hair than in blood. It has been proved that sweat and sebum contain drugs, and contribute to incorporation. External passive contamination may result from being within the same environment as individuals smoking drugs, handling drugs directly or touching surfaces contaminated before touching one's own hair. In addition to these contamination routes, unborn children can also be exposed during the latter months of gestation if the mother continues to use drugs during pregnancy.[16]

   Hair color plays also a role in drug incorporation, and the binding mechanisms may be different for each drug. Factors affecting the incorporation and binding include pKa, non-protein-bound drug molecules, size, lipophilicity, structure and melanin affinity.[16] It is assumed that basic and lipophilic drugs (amphetamines and cocaine) incorporate more into hair than neutral or acidic drugs (benzodiazepines and cannabinoids), and basic drugs possess a higher affinity to melanin, thus they are more incorporated into dark hair than into light colored or non-pigmented hair. On the contrary, incorporation of neutral and acidic compounds does not seem to be impacted by hair color. In most cases, drug metabolism leads to molecules with increased hydrophilicity, which explains lower hair levels of metabolites like benzoylecgonine, morphine or amphetamine than their lipophilic precursors (cocaine, 6-monoacetylmorphine and methamphetamine).[15,16]

   Compounds incorporated in hair remain relatively stable for months and even years, unlike in blood, urine or other conventional biological matrices used in forensic toxicology. The levels of drugs in hair may depend on the environment in which hair has been kept. The diffusion of drugs in the presence of water, into and out of hair, provides a route for external contamination or loss of drug concentration. Moreover, exposure to sunlight, weather conditions, heat and chemical treatments (dyeing, perming and bleaching) may alter and even damage the structure of hair, and generally leads to a decrease in drug levels. It has been proved that cannabinoids are sensitive to sunlight, and particularly to UV light.[15,16] Although shampooing does not significantly affect drug concentrations, it is assumed that hydrophilic compounds (i.e. ethyl glucuronide) might be washed out by such regular hygiene measures.[17]

3. HAIR ANALYSIS FOR DRUG-FACILITATED CRIME

3.1 Case Background

In the case of alleged DFC, the multisectional analysis strategy of hair as well as the kind of drugs to research depends on case history. Besides, the time elapsed between the incident and the report is essential to determine the appropriate date(s) of sample collection. The recommendations of the Society of Hair Testing (SoHT)[18] are to wait for 4 to 6 weeks after the alleged incident and, in case of a positive result, to collect a second hair sample to corroborate the findings. In addition, cosmetic treatments may have a deleterious effect on the drug concentration in hair (i.e. bleaching treatments reduce drug concentration), and therefore these hair treatments should be taken into account for interpretation.

As a consequence, all the appropriate information should be obtained and well documented.[16] In DFC cases, this information usually includes:

- a summary of the case, including
  - date
  - circumstances
  - type and length of time of the reported clinical effect(s) (i.e. an amnesia over a 6-hour period)
- question(s) to be answered by the analysis
- suspected date of drug intake
- suspected drug(s)
- any voluntary drug intake or treatment, and any noticeable cosmetic treatment
- date of hair sampling.

3.2 Hair Collection

The sample collection of hair can perhaps sometimes be considered to be an easy action. Collecting head hair is less intrusive than other biological collections, and does not require specialist facilities: it is not necessary for the collection to be carried out by a nurse, doctor or biologist. In addition, drugs are relatively stable in hair and the conditions for storing hair do not require a refrigerator or freezer.

Nevertheless, owing to the specific nature of testing, the hair sample should preferably be collected by laboratory staff. In many cases, this recommendation is not applicable due to practical difficulties (i.e. a victim a long way away from the laboratory). If this is not possible, a written collection protocol should be provided to the sampling operator.

It is usual to collect head hair from the area at the back of the head, called the vertex posterior. Compared with other areas of the head, this area presents restricted variability in the hair growth rate; the number of hairs in the anagen phase is more constant and the hair growth is less subject to age-related and sex-related influences. In addition, owing to hairstyling, hair collection in this area is often preferable for esthetical reasons.[18] Indeed, concerns are often raised in relation to leaving a visible "bald patch" after hair collection, particularly when small children or individuals with baldness or thinning hair are concerned. In such cases, the collection of several smaller hair samples from multiple sites, focusing around the vertex posterior, is acceptable.

The amount of hair needed for analysis is a "lock of hair" or a pencil-sized thickness of hair. Hair collection should be sufficient in order to carry out the analysis, as well as to repeat the analysis or to allow a confirmation test by another laboratory.

In DFC cases, it is usual to collect four strands of about 100 hairs: usually, one strand will be used for the specific screening for drugs involved in DFC, one for an eventual test for drugs of abuse, one more for an eventual test for GHB, while the last strand is reserved for a potential counter-analysis.[13]

In practice, a tuft of hair with a diameter of about 2 to 3 mm is previously isolated by a piece of string, and then carefully cut as close as possible to the scalp. A previously decontaminated pair of scissors (using a water-based detergent and/or a solvent) should be used for the operation, and, in the same way, the collector should wear gloves during the sampling procedure.

The hair sample should be aligned and the location root-tip must be identified and secured using a cord or aluminum foil.

The collected hair sample can be stored at room temperature in an appropriately labeled paper envelope, wrapped in aluminum foil. Like Pragst,[16] we recommend avoiding direct storage in plastic bags or plastic tubes owing to the risk of contamination by softeners (i.e. plasticizers), since plastic can potentially extract lipophilic substances from the hair, and because of the risk of a plastic tube being broken during shipping or storage maneuvers. A registered mail or courier service is recommended to ensure chain of custody to be despatched with the sample to the laboratory.

Hair samples should be stored at room temperature, in a dry and dark environment and away from direct sunlight.[18] It is of note that:

- hair samples should not be stored at low temperatures (refrigerator or freezer) as swelling may occur in such conditions and reduce the drug concentrations in hair,
- hair samples that are wet at the collection time must be dried before storage.

Generally speaking, regarding sample identity, avoidance of sample mix-up and data security, the same requirements established for other biological samples have to be satisfied and chain of custody procedures should be observed.[16] In practice, a standard hair collection kit containing the following components should be provided to the collector[15]:

- chain-of-custody form
- aluminum foil and an envelope for collection
- security seals
- evidence bag
- labeled transportation envelope
- datasheet about the sample and the case
  - identity of the victim (together with the identity of the collector)
  - date and site of collection (on the head)
  - brief summary of the case including at least the suspected date of the offense
  - hair length and color
  - any voluntary drug intake or treatment
  - any obvious cosmetic treatment
  - any other information of importance
- instructions for collection of a hair sample[15]
  - "cut 4 locks of hair close to the scalp from the vertex posterior region and align the hair identifying the root end
  - fold the aluminium foil lengthways and avoid folding in the middle as this will kink the hair making it difficult to handle
  - place the foil-wrapped hair sample within the collection envelope, seal, initial and date
  - place the completed chain of custody form, the datasheet and sealed collection envelope into the labelled transportation envelope and send to the laboratory for analysis."

3.3 Decontamination

The washing of a hair sample prior to analysis is necessary for two reasons: first, to remove the residues of hair care products (i.e. wax, shampoo, hair sprays, etc.) as well as sweat, sebum and dust regularly present on hair that may interfere with the analysis (i.e. by increasing the analytical noise, decreasing the extraction recovery, etc.); second, to remove the potential external contaminations by drugs of interest so as to subsequently avoid the risk of a false-positive result.

Nevertheless, in the literature, there is no consensual, standardized and/or validated washing procedure to assess the selection and removal of external contamination while, at the same time, guaranteeing not to remove (extract) the incorporated (following a real intake) drugs.

In a simple way, it is established that the organic solvent (acetone, dichloromethane, etc.) will preferably remove the surface contamination, whereas the aqueous solutions as well as methanol will promote a real extraction of the incorporated drugs by swelling the hair. The recommendations of the SoHT about this washing step are to have a procedure for washing hair including both the use of an organic solvent and an aqueous solution. It is strongly recommended to investigate to what extent the washing procedure removes surface contamination, and to plan additional clean-up procedures in the case of hair samples heavily soiled with body fluids.[18]

Historically, the first methods for benzodiazepine determination in hair involved decontamination of hair twice with dichloromethane or methylene chloride.[19,20,21] Then, Yegles et al. proposed to use water and acetone[22] while Kronstrand et al. proposed to wash the hair once with isopropanol, three times with phosphate buffer, and once again with isopropanol.[23]

More recently, the tendency is a washing bath twice with methylene chloride[5] or dichloromethane,[7] sometimes followed by water and/methanol baths,[24] a twice water and twice ethanol washing bath,[25] a twice water and twice dichloromethane washing bath,[26] etc. Table 8.1 summarizes some decontamination procedures found in the literature.

It is usual to keep the decontamination baths for further analysis in order to appreciate the risk of external contamination. Nevertheless, some authors consider that it is not necessary to perform analysis in the washings because the likelihood of benzodiazepine contamination from an external source was very low.[26] We do not subscribe to this appreciation, especially in cases of offenses relating to children.

To summarize, standardized decontamination washing procedures that will successfully remove external contamination without actively removing the drugs actually incorporated into the hair are not currently available. As a consequence, the possible role of external contamination must be considered when interpreting findings.[15]

After this decontamination step, hair samples are usually dried at room temperature. Nevertheless, some authors proposed to use an oven (i.e. 45°C, for 2 hours) for this drying step.[25,38]

3.4 Segmentation

The segmentation strategy depends on the case history, and especially on the delay between the offense(s) and the hair collection. Owing to the concept of absence of migration along the hair shaft, a single spot of exposure must be present in the hair segment corresponding to the date of the alleged offense. As the mean growth rate of human scalp hair is approximately 1 cm/month (range from 0.7 to 1.4 cm/month with a mean of about 1 cm/month accepted by the scientific community), the length of the hair section of interest must be calculated accordingly.

The usual recommendation is to analyze hair collected 4 to 6 weeks after the offense. As a consequence, sectional analysis of three 2-cm-long segments is usually considered to be satisfactory to have the hair shaft including

TABLE 8.1 Proposed Decontamination Procedures in the Literature

Ref.	Hair Decontamination Procedure
21	Hair samples were decontaminated twice with 5 ml of methylene chloride, for 2 min, at room temperature
22	Decontamination bath in warm water (5 min) and twice with acetone (1 min)
27	None
28	Decontamination using 1 mL of 0.1% sodium dodecyl sulfate for 1 min under ultrasonication, and three 1 min distilled water baths under ultrasonication
23	Decontamination with 2 mL of isopropanol, three times with 2 mL of 0.01 M phosphate buffer (pH 6.0), and finally with 2 mL of isopropanol, for 15 min each time in a heated water bath (37°C) with an orbital shaker
7	Hair samples were decontaminated twice with dichloromethane
5	Hair samples were decontaminated twice with methylene chloride (5 mL for 2 min)
24	Hair samples were decontaminated twice with dichloromethane, once with water, and once with methanol, 15 min each, under ultrasonication
25	Decontamination using water (5 mL), distilled and then deionized, and ethanol (3 mL)
26	Decontamination with 1 mL of 0.1% sodium dodecyl sulfate, 2 × 1 mL of deionized water, and then 2 × 1 mL dichloromethane, 10 min each, under ultrasonication
29	Decontamination with 1 mL of 0.1% aqueous sodium dodecyl sulfate, 2 × 1 mL deionized water and 2 × 1 mL dichloromethane, 10 min each, under ultrasonication
30	Decontamination baths[4] with methanol
31	Hair samples were decontaminated twice with distilled water, and methanol
32	Decontamination with 2 mL of iso-octane followed by 2 mL of acetone
33	Decontamination using 2 mL methanol, 2 mL distilled water and 2 mL methanol (twice)
34	Decontamination with 10 mL of a 10% (w/v) aqueous solution of sodium dodecyl sulfate, 10 mL of water (twice) and 10 mL of acetone for 3 min each
35	Decontamination with water and two times with acetone, 1 min each
36	Decontamination with dichlormethane and methanol
37	Hair samples were decontaminated twice with dichloromethane (3 mL, vortex mixed for 3 min)
38	Three consecutive 2 mL dichloromethane baths, for 2 min each
39	None
40	Decontamination using 0.1% sodium dodecylsulfate, water, methanol and water (three times)

the spot of exposure: administration of a single dose would be confirmed by the presence of the drug in the proximal segment (root), with no detection in the other segments. This approach is now internationally accepted by the active scientists involved in the field of hair analysis in DFC cases.[13]

Nevertheless, such an approach requires respecting the two following sampling commitments:

- the hair must be cut as close as possible to the scalp
- the individual hair in the strand retains the position it originally had beside the other hairs.

In addition, Kintz[42] assumes, on the basis of the literature evaluation and data obtained from the author's 20-year experience of drug testing in hair, a theory to validate the concept of single exposure in authentic forensic cases where the drug is detected in two or three consecutive segments in some cases (about one case out of 10 examinations in the daily experience of the author). The author proposed several explanations:

- There is substantial variability in the area over which an incorporated drug can be distributed in the hair shaft and in the rate of axial distribution of the drug along the hair shaft and, consecutively, a small concentration of the drug, as compared with the concentration in the proximal segment, can be measured in the second segment, as a result of an irregular movement.
- Drugs and metabolites are incorporated into hair during formation of the hair shaft via diffusion from sweat and other secretions, and the presence of confounding interferences in the hair matrix or changes in the hair structure due to cosmetic treatments might mislead the final result of hair analysis.

The author proposes, in order to qualify for a single exposure, to consider that the highest drug concentration must be detected in the segment corresponding to the period of the alleged offense and that this measured concentration must be at least three times higher than the ones measured in the previous or following segments.[42]

Nevertheless, in spite of these difficulties, the principle of segmental analysis in DFC cases remains fundamental. For instance, Chèze et al.[7] confirmed in more than 100 cases the value of segmental analyses.

Finally, it is of note that in the case of suspicion of administration of gamma hydroxybutyrate (GHB), hair should be segmented into very short segments (1−2 mm) in order to reveal an eventual elevation of the GHB concentration in the hair segment (corresponding to a period of a few days) consistent with the approximate timeframe of the offense. Indeed, GHB is an endogenous compound present in low concentrations in the body but it is also widely available and associated with the club scene and in cases of DFSA. Consecutively, GHB is generally detected in hair using a GC-MS/MS method at low concentrations,[43] and the presence of GHB alone is insufficient to confirm exogenous administration.[44,4]

In summary, the elaboration of the segmentation strategy of hair is of importance with major potential consequences on the interpretation of the findings.

On the basis of the elaborated segmentation strategy, the section of hair should be cut with a pair of scissors previously cleaned using a water-based detergent and/or a solvent (i.e. methanol).

Subsequently, the hair should be cut into smaller pieces or milled to a powder, and then typically 10 to 50 mg of hair accurately weighed prior to analysis. Table 8.2 summarizes the choice made by several authors between

TABLE 8.2 Sample Homogeneity Procedure and Hair Quantity Needed for Analysis Found in Literature

Ref.	Pulverization in a Ball Mill	Cut in Small Pieces	Quantity of Hair
21	✓		50 mg
41	✓		30 mg
27	✓		50 mg
28		✓	10 mg
7	✓	✓	20 mg
5		✓	20 mg
24	✓		20 mg
25		✓	50 mg
26		✓	10 mg
30		✓	10 mg
32		✓	50 mg
33		✓	10 mg
31		✓	30 mg
34	✓		50 mg
37		✓	100 mg
36		✓	20 mg
38	✓		50 mg
35		✓	20 mg
40		✓	45 mg
39		✓	20 mg

pulverization in a ball mill or cutting into small segments, together with the hair quantity needed for analysis.

The two approaches for this "homogenization step" are found in the literature. The proposition of a direct extraction of drugs from hair without this "homogenization step" is infrequent.[23]

In fact, the choice between the hair being powdered in a ball mill or finely cut with scissors can depend on the quantities available.[7]

The use of a ball mill will improve sample homogeneity. Nevertheless, owing to the significant loss of hair sample (of particular concern, especially when the majority of hair samples submitted for analysis are limited in volume), this method is limited to preparing larger volumes of hair. In addition, this is not a practical method for preparing numerous individual hair samples or segments as the ball mill requires widespread clean-up procedures between each sample.

The recommendations of the SoHT[18] are based on the notion of the importance of the hair sample being homogeneous and that the portion taken for analysis is a representative sample: "hair samples that have been washed and dried should be cut into smaller pieces or milled to a powder, and then typically 10–50 mg of hair accurately weighed prior to analysis."

In summary, cutting the hair into small pieces of 2–3 mm in length using a pair of scissors is undoubtedly the most efficient method for hair preparation; even so an alternative micropulverized extraction procedure for small sample volumes has been proposed.[45,46]

3.5 Extraction of Drugs from Hair Matrix and Clean-up

The analysis of hair involves an initial pretreatment step to release the drugs from within the hair matrix prior to clean-up using liquid–liquid or solid-phase extraction. It is of note that direct analysis using immunological screening can directly be performed following this extraction step in some hair analysis cases (i.e. drugs of abuse): this analytical approach using immunological screening is not convenient for DFC cases.

Just before or at the time of this extraction step, it is usual to add the internal standard(s) to the hair sample. In our opinion, the use of deuterated internal standards should be the rule. For instance, prazepam is used as an internal standard in analytical screening methods for benzodiazepines in hair as it is known to be totally and quickly metabolized ("first-pass" dealkylation by the liver) in nordiazepam and oxazepam.[25] However, prazepam was recently detected in the hair of a 10-year-old child[47] and in one of our personal DFC cases (personal unpublished data) relating to a victim with a regular prazepam treatment (3 × 10 mg tablets per day). In fact, the presence in hair of a parent compound which is not usually detected in blood, or in urine, is not incongruous, as attested by the presence of heroin in addicts' hair in spite of its very fast degradation (less than 5 minutes) in monoacetyl-6 morphine in blood.[48]

The choice of deuterated internal standards is conducted by the nature and the identity of the tested psychotropic drugs. It is obvious that the multiplicity of the used deuterated internal standards should take into account efficiency/cost considerations. Table 8.3 presents a selection of internal standards used in methods dedicated to analysis of benzodiazepines and related compounds in hair.

A variety of drugs extracted from hair matrix and clean-up conditions have been reported for benzodiazepines, and a selection of these is listed in Table 8.4.

TABLE 8.3 A Selection of Deuterated Internal Standards Used in Analytical Methods for Benzodiazepines and Related Compounds in Hair

Ref.	Used Internal Standard(s)
21	Prazepam-d5
41	Oxazepam-d5, diazepam-d5, nordazepam-d5, lorazepam-d4
27	Diazepam-d5
28	1-Hydroxymethyltriazolam-d4
23	Diazepam-d5, nordazepam- d5, oxazepam-d5, flunitrazepam-d7, clonazepam-d4, 7-aminoflunitrazepam-d7, alprazolam-d5, 7-aminoclonazepam-d4
7	7-Aminoclonazepam-d4, 7-aminoflunitrazepam-d7, clonazepam-d4
5	Diazepam-d5
24	7-Aminoclonazepam-d4, 7-aminoflunitrazepam-d7, clonazepam-d4, flunitrazepam-d7, alprazolam-d5, temazepam-d5, desalkylflurazepam-d4, oxazepam-d5, nordiazepam-d5, triazolam-d4, lorazepam-d4, prazepam-d5, diazepam-d5
26	7-Aminoflunitrazepam-d7, flunitrazepam-d7, oxazepam-d5, lorazepam-d4, temazepam-d5, diazepam-d5, nordiazepam-d5
30	Diazepam-d5
32	7-Aminoflunitrazepam-d7, α-hydroxytriazolam-d7, nordiazepam-d5, nitrazepam-d5
33	Diazepam-d5
31	Diazepam-d5, lorazepam-d4
38	Alprazolam-d5, diazepam-d5, flunitrazepam-d7, oxazepam-d5, zopiclone-d4
35	Alprazolam-d5, alpha-hydroxyalprazolam-d5, diazepam-d5, nordazepam-d5, oxazepam-d5, 7-aminoflunitrazepam- d7, flunitrazepam-d7, lorazepam-d4
39	Diazepam-d5

TABLE 8.4 A Selection of Extraction of Drugs from Hair Matrix and Clean-up Conditions Reported in the Literature

Ref.	Extraction	Clean-up
21	Soerensen buffer (pH 7.6)	Liquid–liquid extraction (diethyl ether-chloroform)
41	Actetate buffer (pH = 4) + beta-glucuronidase/arylsulfatase for 2 h at 40°C	Solid-phase extraction (Chromabond C18ec columns)
27	Methanol (3 mL) under ultrasonication for 1 h	Solid-phase extraction (mixed-mode isolute HCX columns)
28	Dichloromethane/methanol/ammonium hydroxide, under ultrasonication for 1 h	None
23	200 mg sodium dithiotreitol and 100 mg of proteinase K dissolved in 60 mL of 0.25 M tris buffer at pH 8.0	Solid-phase extraction (BondElut Certify columns)
7	Soerensen buffer (pH 7.6) 14 h at 56°C	Liquid–liquid extraction (dichloromethane/ether)
5	Phosphate buffer (pH 8.4), overnight	Liquid–liquid extraction (methylene chloride/diethylether)
24	Methanol at 45°C for 2 h with orbital shaking	Liquid–liquid extraction (saturated ammonium chloride buffer + 1-chlorobutane)
25	Trifluoroacetic acid + methanol, 18 h at room temperature	Liquid–liquid extraction (phosphate buffer/dichloromethane)
26	Methanol/ammonium hydroxide, overnight	Solid-phase extraction (mixed-mode cation exchange-hydrophobic phase extraction columns)
30	Methanol/acetonitrile/ammonium formate, at 37°C for 18 h	None
32	Phosphate buffer (pH 8.4), overnight	Liquid–liquid extraction (methylene chloride/diethylether)
33	Methanol at 38°C for 16 h	None
31	Methanol at 38°C for 16 h	Solid-phase extraction (Clean Screen column)
34	Water/acetonitrile/trifluoroacetic acid, using a 5 min simultaneous pulverization/extraction step	None
37	Methanol at 55°C for 15 h	None

(Continued)

TABLE 8.4 (Continued)

Ref.	Extraction	Clean-up
36	Phosphate buffer (pH 8.4), under ultrasonication for 1 h	Liquid–liquid extraction (dichloromethane-diethylether)
38	Acetonitrile at 50°C overnight.	Liquid–liquid extraction (hexane: ethyl acetate) + solid-phase extraction (Strata-X cartridges)
35	Methanol/acetonitrile/H₂O/ammonium formate, for 18 h at 37°C	None
40	Microwave-assisted extraction (MAE)	None
39	Methanol/acetonitrile/formiate buffer (pH 3), 18 h in an orbital shaker	None

It is obvious that the efficiency of the extraction method is compromised in the case of unsuitable extraction procedures, not targeted to specific drugs, being used. In DFC cases, the release of the incorporated drugs from the hair matrix is regularly achieved through incubation of the hair in solutions that remove drugs without damaging the hair: methanol, buffered solutions or trifluoroacetic acid. Nevertheless, a digestion of the hair can be used for this extraction step: i.e. Kronstand et al. proposed the use of dithiotreitol and proteinase K to hydrolyze hair protein.[23] Wietecha-Posłuszny et al. proposed a preparation of human hair samples using microwave irradiation for the purpose of determination of six benzodiazepines.[40]

In order to make the appropriate choice out of the different possibilities, the chemical structure of the drug and its sensitivity to agents used for this extraction step must be taken into account. Indeed, it is important to consider the potential deleterious effect on the drugs when choosing the extraction procedure, especially in the case of benzodiazepine. In particular, it is imperative to take special care with the temperature owing to the risk of *in vitro* degradation of these substances.

Following the extraction step, the extract requires a further clean-up using the same techniques employed for blood or urine, namely liquid–liquid extraction or solid-phase extraction.

All these considerations about the extraction of drugs from hair matrix and clean-up are summarized in the recommendations of the SoHT: "Laboratories introducing new hair testing methodologies must investigate the efficiency of different incubation conditions to optimise their in-house extraction procedures, while minimising hydrolysis of labile drugs"[18].

3.6 Detection and Quantification

In DFC cases, instrumental methods used in hair analysis must be suitable for unambiguous drug identification (and quantitation): separation and detection of the psychotropic drugs are systematically achieved using chromatographic methods coupled to mass spectrometry. Although standard bench-top single quadrupole systems have sufficient sensitivity for some hair testing applications, this is not the case for drugs incorporated into hair at very low concentrations. As a consequence, in DFC cases (where concentrations in the picogram per milligram range are generally detected after a single intake), the trend is to replace GC-MS methods by LC-MS/MS or by LC-HRMS (i.e. time of flight or Orbitrap).

Table 8.5 summarizes chromatographic columns and devices used for detection found in the literature.

TABLE 8.5 Chromatographic Columns and Devices Used for Detection Proposed in the Literature

Ref.	Chromatographic Column	Analytical Method (Device Used for Detection)
21	HP5-MS capillary column (30 m × 0.25 mm, 0.25 µm)	GC-MS (HP 5989 B)
41	HP-Ultra 2 capillary column (12 m × 0.2 mm, 0.33 µm)	GC-MS (HP 5971)
27	HP-5MS capillary column (30 m × 0.25 mm, 0.25 µm)	GC-MS (HP 5973)
28	Mightysil RP-18 column (100 × 20 mm, 3 µm)	LC-MS (Finnigan MAT LCQ ion trap mass spectrometer)
23	Zorbax phenyl column (50 × 2.1 mm, 3 µm)	LC-MS/MS (AB Sciex API 2000)
7	Uptisphere ODB column (150 × 2 mm, 5 µm)	LC-MS/MS (Quantum TSQ, ThermoElectron)
5	XTerra MS C18 column (100 × 2.1 mm, 3.5 µm)	LC-MS/MS (Micromass Quattro Micro, Waters)
24	XTerra MS C18 column (100 × 2.1 mm, 3.5 µm)	LC-MS/MS (Micromass Quattro Premier, Waters)
25	Luna phenyl hexyl column (50 × 2 mm, 3 µm)	LC-MS/MS (API 2000, AB Sciex)
26	Gemini C18 column (150 × 2 mm, 5 µm)	LC-MS/MS (LCQ Deca XP Plus ion trap MS)

(Continued)

TABLE 8.5 (Continued)

Ref.	Chromatographic Column	Analytical Method (Device Used for Detection)
30	Acquity HSS T3 C18 column (100 × 2.1 mm, 1.8 μm)	LC-HRMS (Micromass LCT Premier XE, Waters)
32	Luna C18 column (150 × 1 mm, 5 μm)	LC-HRMS (LTQ-Orbitrap, Thermo Fisher Scientific)
33	Zorbax Eclipse XDB-C18 column (150 × 4.6 mm, 5 μm)	LC-MS/MS (API 3200 Qtrap, AB Sciex)
31	HP5-MS capillary column (30 m × 0.25 mm, 0.25 μm)	GC-MS (5973, Agilent)
34	Atlantis T3 column (150 × 2.1 mm, 3 μm)	LC-HRMS (LTQ-Orbitrap, Thermo Fisher Scientific)
37	Synergi Fusion-RP column (150 × 2 mm, 4 μm)	LC-MS/MS (API 4000, AB Sciex)
36	Hypersil gold column (100 × 2.1 mm, 3 μm)	LC-MS/MS (API 4000 Qtrap, AB Sciex)
38	Atlantis T3 column (100 × 2.1 mm, 3 μm)	LC-MS/MS (Micromass Quattro Micro, Waters
35	Zorbax Eclipse plus C18 column (100 × 2.1 mm, 3.5 μm)	LC-HRMS (6530 Accurate-Mass LC-QTOF-MS, Agilent)
40	Acclaim column (250 × 4.6 mm, 5 μm)	LC-HRMS (MicrOTOF-QII, Bruker)
39	Silica T3 column (150 × 2.1 mm, 1.8 μm)	LC-HRMS (6540 Accurate-Mass LC-QTOF-MS, Agilent)

The main issues for the choice of technical solution for detection and quantification that must be considered are whether or not the method will have sufficient sensitivity for low drug levels in hair, and whether the target analytes are specific.[18] For this purpose, Table 8.6 presents LODs and LOQs obtained in some published methods dedicated to benzodiazepine analysis in DFC cases.

For identification using LC-MS/MS, Villain et al.[5] used two precursor ion/product ion transitions for each drug. Chèze et al.[7] used three transitions, while Laloup et al.[24] proposed screening using one transition and then further confirmation of the identity of the compounds through a second injection of positive samples, monitoring two transitions per compound. Kronstand et al.[23] proposed to use only one transition. In our opinion, the specificity is questionable for LC-MS/MS analyses performed in the selected reaction-monitoring mode and involving a large number of compounds with only one

TABLE 8.6 LODs and LOQs in Some Published Methods

	Chèze 2005		Villain 2005		Vogliardi 2011		Salomone 2011		Morini 2012		Lendoiro 2012		Rust 2012		Broecker 2012	
Ref.	7		5		32		37		36		38		49		35	
	LOD	LOQ	LOD	LOQ	LOD	LOQ	LOD	LOQ	LOD	LOQ	LOD	LOQ	LOD	LOQ	LOD	LOQ
7-aminoclonazepam	2	10	–	5	5	10	–	–	0.1	0.3	–	–	–	10	–	–
7-aminoflunitrazepam	2	5	–	2	2	5	–	–	0.1	0.3	–	–	–	3.3	5	6
7-aminonitrazepam	–	–	–	–	2	5	–	–	–	–	–	–	–	–	–	–
Alprazolam	0.5	2	–	1	5	10	1.8	5.9	0.1	0.3	5	10	–	1.6	5	7
Bromazepam	2	5	–	2	5	10	2	6.7	1	3	5	20	–	–	2	4
Clobazam	1	2	–	2	2	5	–	–	0.3	1	–	–	–	–	–	–
Clonazepam	0.5	2	–	–	5	10	0.6	2	0.3	1.5	10	20	–	10	–	–
Clotiazepam	–	–	–	–	0.5	1	–	–	–	–	–	–	–	–	–	–
Chlordiazepoxide	–	–	–	–	1	2	–	–	–	–	–	–	–	–	–	–
Delorazpam	–	–	–	–	10	10	–	–	–	–	–	–	–	–	–	–
Diazepam	1	2	–	1	1	5	0.5	1.7	0.1	0.3	2	5	–	1.6	1	3
Estazolam	–	–	–	–	2	5	–	–	–	–	–	–	–	–	–	–

(Continued)

TABLE 8.6 (Continued)

Ref.	Chèze 2005 — 7		Villain 2005 — 5		Vogliardi 2011 — 32		Salomone 2011 — 37		Morini 2012 — 36		Lendoiro 2012 — 38		Rust 2012 — 49		Broecker 2012 — 35	
	LOD	LOQ	LOD	LOQ	LOD	LOQ	LOD	LOQ	LOD	LOQ	LOD	LOQ	LOD	LOQ	LOD	LOQ
Etizolam	–	–	–	–	1	2	–	–	–	–	–	–	–	–	–	–
Flunitrazepam	1	2	–	–	2	5	4	13	0.1	0.3	2	5	–	10	4	6
Flurazepam	–	–	–	–	2	2	–	–	–	–	–	–	–	–	–	–
α-hydroxyalprazolam	–	–	–	–	5	10	–	–	–	–	–	–	–	–	–	–
2-hydroxyethylflurazepam	–	–	–	–	1	2	–	–	–	–	–	–	–	–	–	–
Ketamine	–	–	–	–	–	–	0.2	0.7	–	–	2	5	–	–	–	–
Loprazolam	2	5	–	–	–	–	–	–	–	–	–	–	–	–	4	5
Lorazepam	2	5	–	5	5	10	3.2	11	1	5	2	5	–	10	–	–
Lormetazepam	1	5	–	1	2	5	2.4	7.9	0.3	1.5	2	5	–	3.3	–	–
LSD	–	–	–	–	–	–	–	–	–	–	0.2	0.5	–	–	–	–
Methadone	–	–	–	–	–	–	–	–	–	–	2	20	–	–	–	–
Midazolam	1	5	–	0.5	2	5	–	–	0.1	0.3	–	–	–	3.3	–	–

Nitrazepam	–	–	–	–	5	10	–	–	–	–	–	–	–	–	–	–
Nordazepam	1	5	–	2	1	2	1.2	4	0.3	1	2	5	–	3.3	2	4
Oxazepam	1	5	–	1	2	5	–	–	1	5	10	20	–	10	1	3
Pinazepam	–	–	–	–	1	5	–	–	–	–	–	–	–	–	–	–
Prazepam	2	5	–	–	2	5	–	–	0.3	1	–	–	–	0.6	–	–
Scopolamine	–	–	–	–	–	–	0.7	2.3	–	–	2	5	–	–	–	–
Temazepam	1	5	–	1	2	5	–	–	0.3	1	–	–	–	3.3	–	–
Tetrazepam	10	–	–	5	–	–	–	–	–	–	10	20	–	–	–	–
Triazolam	0.5	2	–	0.5	2	5	0.7	2.3	0.1	0.5	5	10	–	3.3	–	–
α-hydroxytriazolam	–	–	–	–	2	5	–	–	–	–	–	–	–	–	–	–
Zolpidem	1	5	–	0.5	–	–	0.2	0.7	0.1	0.3	2	5	–	1.6	–	–
Zopiclone	1	5	–	–	–	–	0.9	3	–	–	5	10	–	10	–	–

transition per compound. Furthermore, verification of the relative abundances between the selected transitions with respect to those calculated in the spiked calibrator sample(s) with concentrations closest to the calculated concentration and of the relative retention times should be the rule. In addition, owing to the risk of false-positive results, especially in the case of the presence of metabolites of phenothiazines and antidepressants, some fragments (for example, at m/z 58, 86 or 100) are not specific enough and should be avoided for compounds with amino side chains.[50]

Using the LC-HRMS method, identification is based on the accurate mass, isotopic pattern and retention time of sample components, from which the atomic formula is calculated and searched against a database of relevant compounds, preferably using dedicated software. In spite of a) the small number of publications using the LC-HRMS method for hair analysis in DFC cases, and b) the high cost of this technology (time of flight or Orbitrap), it is obvious that high resolution mass spectrometry offers higher mass precision, which greatly facilitates identification of unknown compounds, and apparently shows the best performance in comparative studies for drug screening assays in other matrices.[51]

3.7 Quality Assurance

Accrediting methods for the analysis of drugs in hair is challenging owing to several problems: difficulties and the cost of obtaining certified reference material, lack of dedicated guidelines, etc.[52] Nevertheless, implementation of quality assurance is recognized as a fundamental principle for all testing laboratories, obviously including drug testing laboratories. In this way, accreditation to the international standard ISO/IEC 17025 is an industry requirement. Nevertheless, a recent study highlighted that only a few forensic laboratories are currently accredited to ISO/IEC 17025 in Europe.[52,53] The cost is the main barrier facing laboratories wishing to introduce accreditation, as the entire accreditation process requires significant financial commitment: additional staff resources, purchasing consumables to carry out additional validation parameters in accordance with ISO/IEC 17025, costs of the annual audit, etc.[15]

3.8 Quality Controls

Ideally, quality control samples should be prepared from real hair samples collected from known drug users, and both negative and positive hair quality controls must be analyzed with each analytical batch of case samples.[18] As external quality controls are expensive, many laboratories prepare their own in-house controls.[54,55] Purchasing additional proficiency testing scheme samples to use for quality controls is one acceptable option and several suppliers and distributors provide this service (ACQ Science GmbH, Medichem

Diagnostica, LGC Standards).[15] But it is of note that these proficiency testing schemes mainly concern DOA, and rarely psychotropic drugs involved in DFC (i.e. benzodiazepines).

3.9 Proficiency Testing Schemes

The SoHT has published recommendations for good practice in hair testing and encourages the participation in proficiency testing schemes that use authentic hair samples. This society has conducted its own annual proficiency testing programs since 2001 and the results are published on its website (www.soht.org). The Gesellschaft für Toxikologische und Forensische Chemie (GTFCh) proposes the same approach including real hair samples as well as spiked ones. Recently, a new proficiency testing scheme has been proposed by LGC Standard: it includes benzodiazepines, but only in spiked hair samples.

3.10 Method Validation

Several ISO documents are available to provide guidance (http://www.iso.org) with validation requirements together with publications specifically targeted for forensic and clinical toxicology method validation.[56−58] According to these guidelines, suggestions for a validation scheme could be:

- inter- and intra-assay precision and accuracy assaying at five (including low and high) concentrations relative to calibration range: analysis of seven spiked hair samples at each concentration
- detection limit (LOD) defined as the lowest concentration giving a response of at least three times the average of the baseline noise
- quantification limit (LOQ) defined as the lowest concentration that could be measured with an intra-assay precision cost variance percent and relative bias less than 20%
- linearity assessed by analyzing five replicates for each calibration level on seven different days
- relative standard deviation (RSD) and bias calculated for inter- and intra-assay studies with, for acceptance, both parameters simultaneously lower than 25% for the limit of quantification and lower than 20% for the other concentrations in both studies
- for LC-MS/MS methods, ion suppression phenomena studied following the experimental system previously proposed by Antignac et al.[59] Briefly, a standard solution containing the compounds of interest (at 100 µg/L) was continuously and directly infused into the mass spectrometer interface. A simultaneous LC flow containing either a pure mobile phase or a blank biological extract (hair from 10 non-drug consumers were sampled) was introduced through a tee. Evolution of the signal of the transitions at the retention times of the corresponding compounds of interest was subsequently studied to evaluate presence and intensity of ion suppression phenomena.

4. INTERPRETATION OF RESULTS

Various sources of individual variability, including genetic polymorphisms, metabolic disorders, diet, use of cosmetics and environmental exposure, are likely to represent more important causes of bias and incorrect reporting in hair analysis than insufficient sensitivity and specificity.[4]

According to Pragst[60] and in our own experience of hair analysis, the most serious pitfalls of hair analysis are not in the practical performance but in the interpretation of results.

Pragst has fully described and also documented the parameters that can impact the findings in hair.[16,60]

As already described, the analytical findings of drugs in hair can originate from four general routes. Systemic circulation as the endogenous pathway, absorption or transfer to the keratinized hair from perspiration (sweat, sebum, transdermal excretion) as the endogenous–exogenous pathway, absorption by the external environment (e.g. pollution, hair treatments, pharmaceutical formulation) as the exogenous pathway, and unintentional systemic absorption by respiration or transdermal absorption.[61]

Thus, determining a single or repeated exposure and the timeframe of exposure is not always obvious.

To a lesser extent, sample preparation before extraction (cutting or grinding), as well as the stage of incubation (hydrolysis or not) and the choice of solvents, will impact the extraction yield and induce some differences in the measured concentrations in real cases.[62]

Regarding the small quantity of hair samples available in DFC cases, the laboratories often cut the hair instead of grinding it, because of hair loss during the grinding process. A new faster extraction process on micropulverized hair allows reliable identification and quantification on 2.5 mg of hair sample, using high resolution mass spectrometry.[34]

However, the costs of such analyses could be decreased only by a high throughput.

Studies on real cases that could improve the processes of extraction are lacking on this domain. Therefore, it should be advisable that harmonized procedures are adopted in order to allow inter-laboratory comparisons in DFC cases. Before this occurs, some authors recommend to all the laboratories to have their own databases for interpreting drug concentrations in hair.[63]

Either way, it is advisable that analytical hair results for DFC cases are linked to blood and/or urine concentrations sampled close to the time event, in order to confirm the results and to prove unequivocally that exposure was very close to the time of the alleged offense to ensure that the best information is obtained for the court. Sometimes, circumstances such as a delayed complaint mean that only hair analysis can be useful. However, in DFC cases, hair analysis remains a convincing element if other elements of the investigation confirm the facts.

A good knowledge of the case and collaboration with the police involved in the investigation are essential to handle this type of file case effectively. The aim of the toxicologist is then to advise that the hypothesis raised by the investigation is supported or not by the analytical findings.

4.1 Interpretation of Concentrations in Hair—Single or Repeated Exposure

There are no cut-offs employed in hair testing for single exposure/intake. The SoHT has proposed cut-off values for drugs of abuse and alcohol markers in hair to enable identification of chronic use but this approach is not valuable for hair interpretation in the case of DFC. For DFC, low amounts of the drug in hair can prove the single exposure, if the drug is not detected in other segments. For this reason, the analysis of different segments of the hair shaft must be the rule, and the interpretation of hair concentrations of the involved substances must be based on the experience on healthy volunteers, and detected or reported values in the case of known treatment. When the complainant has not reported the incident for several months, or when the police require hair analysis a long time after the offense, or where there are concerns about contamination or chemical treatment, axillary, torso or leg hairs or nails can provide some valuable information. In these cases, quantitative analysis could be useful.[25,64−66] Indeed, even if the interpretation on the period of exposure will be of very low precision, the presence of a drug at a low picogram per milligram range in that kind of sample may be indicative of a low dose intake. In accordance with the enquiry, and the clinical symptoms observed during the offense, it can be a convincing element in DFC cases.

We report in Table 8.7 our main internal data needed for the interpretation of concentrations in hair in cases of DFC, based on 10 years' experience of analysis by liquid chromatography-triple quadrupole tandem mass spectrometry. Hair was cut into small pieces (1 to 2 mm) and incubated into water-based buffer before extraction.

Some molecules are detected with great difficulties due to their low active dosage or to their poor binding in hair. Moreover, some major metabolites (e.g. norclobazam or lorazepam glucuronide) may be more deposited in hair than the given active molecule itself.

It is important at this stage to stress that a single exposure in a DFC case may be in the toxic range in blood, so that hair concentrations could be much more elevated that those reported for single exposure of a therapeutic dose in the literature. The toxicologist must be aware of this when interpreting hair concentrations.

TABLE 8.7 Internal Data on Hair Concentration Ranges According to the Alleged Drug Use of the Most Frequently Encountered Drugs in DFC Cases in France (by LC-MS/MS Triple Quadrupole and 2-cm Segment Length)

Drug or Metabolite	Drug Use	nb Specimens	Concentrations in Hair (pg/mg)		Comments/Details
			Range	Mean	
Aceprometazine	S	n = 1	8	–	1 tab, 10 mg
Alimemazine	S	n = 1	7	–	1 tab, 5 mg
	R	n = 1	280–898	634	7 mg/day
		n = 1	170		–
Alprazolam	S	n = 3	<1	–	1 tab, 0.25 mg
		n = 8	<1–3		–
	O	n = 12	2–35	10.7	Pubic hair
		n = 3	17–22	18.7	
	R	n = 1	27–62	33	Abuse?
		n = 1	1349		
Amitriptyline	S	n = 1	37	–	1 tab, 25 mg
	R	n = 2	48–156	87.5	
Bromazepam	S	n = 8	2.0–19	8	
	O	n = 11	10–304	94	
	R	n = 5	479–1600	1180	4 tab/day
		n = 1	3139	–	

(Continued)

	DFC		<1		Pubic hair, in jail
Buprenorphine					
Cetirizine as levocetirizine	S	n = 1	23	–	1 tab, 5 mg levocetirizine
Cetirizine as hydroxyzine metabolite	S	n = 2	<5	–	1 tab, 25 mg hydroxyzine
	O	n = 3	34–76	49	
	R	n = 2	97–598	307	
Chlorphenamine	S	n = 1	9	–	1 tab, 4 mg
Clobazam	S	n = 1	<LOD (1 pg/mg)	–	1 tab, 5 mg
(Clonazepam) 7-aminoclonazepam	S	n = 9	1.3–15	7	1 tab, 2 mg
	O	n = 4	17–157	67	
	R	n = 9	133–1300	403	
Cyamemazine	S	n = 1	55	–	1 tab, 25 mg
		n = 4	19–58		
Diazepam	S	n = 1	<LOD (2 pg/mg)	–	1 tab, 2 mg
	O	n = 6	1.8–50	19	
	R	n = 2	194–378	–	
Diphenhydramine	S	n = 1	34	–	1 tab, 90 mg
		n = 1	396		2 tab, 180 mg
Doxylamine	S	n = 1	17	–	2 tabs, 30 mg, blond hair

TABLE 8.7 (Continued)

Drug or Metabolite	Drug Use	nb Specimens	Concentrations in Hair (pg/mg)		Comments/Details
			Range	Mean	
Estazolam	O	n = 4	51–597	244	
	R	n = 6	1696–4359	2866	
Fluoxetine	S	n = 1	3	–	1 tab, 2 mg
	R	n = 2	967–1730	–	
Flunitrazepam	S	n = 5	–	–	
7-aminoflunitrazepam			0.5–5	3	
	O	n = 3	–	–	
			4.2–52	21	
Haloperidol	R	n = 1	4050	–	
Hydroxyzine	S	n = 1	16	–	1 tab, 25 mg
		n = 2	35–84		1 tab, 25 mg?
	O	n = 4	108–219	157	
	R	n = 5	331–5687	1402	
Ketamine	O	n = 1	8	–	Sniff
	R	n = 1	30–64	–	Multidrug abuse
Levomepromazine	R	n = 1	667	–	

Loprazolam	S	n = 1	3	–	1 tab, 1 mg
	DFC	n = 2	<5	–	
Lorazepam	S	n = 1	<LOD (2 pg/mg)	–	1 tab, 2.5 mg
	DFSA	n = 4	0.6–15.9	6.6	
	O	n = 1	4	–	
	R	n = 6	10–88	25	
Lormetazepam	S	n = 1	<LOD (1 pg/mg)	–	1 tab, 1 mg
	O	n = 6	2–12	6	
Loxapine	S	n = 1	6	–	1 tab, 25 mg
	R	n = 2	155–799	–	
Midazolam	O	n = 3	79–753	394	Resuscitation attempts
Niaprazine	S	n = 1	542	–	10 mL, 30 mg
	R	n = 6	4120–46,900	22,600	Children younger than 5.5 years old
Nitrazepam 7-aminonitrazepam	S	n = 1	2 17	–	1 tab, 5 mg
Nordiazepam	S	n = 1	4.5	–	1 tab, 7.5 mg of chlordiazepoxide
		n = 1	7		{1/2} tab, 5 mg of prazepam
		n = 1	1.5		1 tab, 10 mg of prazepam

(Continued)

TABLE 8.7 (Continued)

Drug or Metabolite	Drug Use	nb Specimens	Concentrations in Hair (pg/mg)		Comments/Details
			Range	Mean	
	DFC	n = 7	<1–164	55	
	O	n = 3	55–128	83	
	R	n = 1	557	–	Librax® 5 mg
		n = 1	243	–	Valium® 2 mg
		n = 6	250–654	439	
Oxazepam	S	n = 1	1	–	1 tab, 10 mg
	R	n = 1	1358	–	
Oxomemazine	S	n = 1	51	–	10 mL, 3.3 mg
		n = 1	14		
	R	n = 2	151–164	–	About 12 mg
	O	n = 1	925	–	
Paroxetine	R	n = 1	20,465	–	
Prazepam	S	n = 1	<LOD (1 pg/mg)	–	1 tab, 10 mg
					See nordiazepam
	R	n = 1	416→1000	–	
Temazepam	S	n = 1	0.5	–	1 tab, 10 mg
		n = 1	2.5		1 tab, 20 mg

		n	Range	Value	Notes
	O	n = 3	<1–27	—	
	R	n = 3	20–76	40	20 mg/day
Tetrazepam	S	n = 3	60–129	87	1 tab, 50 mg
		n = 1	6.6–14.5	—	—
	O	n = 1	168	—	4 tabs, 200 mg
		n = 1	68–37	—	—
	R	n = 1	525	—	
Tramadol	O	n = 1	239	—	5 tabs, 187.5 mg
Triazolam	S	n = 1	1.3	—	
Zolpidem	S	n = 17	1.2–19	7	1 tab, 10 mg
	DFC	n = 4	2.2–163	84	Beard hair
		n = 1	2.3	—	
	O	n = 25	34.5–333	162	
	R	n = 3	542–743	619	1 tab (10 mg)/day
	A	n = 8	3500–9200	—	10 to 30 tab/day
		n = 3	16,400–22,100	—	About 70 tab/day, Asiatic
Zopiclone	S	n = 4	17–36	23.3	1 tab/month
	DFC	n = 1	59–174	—	
	O	n = 2	198–348	—	

(Continued)

TABLE 8.7 (Continued)

Drug or Metabolite	Drug Use	nb Specimens	Concentrations in Hair (pg/mg)		Comments/Details
			Range	Mean	
	R	n = 3	815–1396	–	Several tab/day
GHB	S		<1–15 ng/mg	–	66
	R	n = 3	54–110 ng/mg	–	
		n = 1	62 ng/mg		
		n = 1	105 ng/mg		
4-Methylethylcathinone	S	n = 1	741	–	
	O	n = 1	2303	–	
	R	n = 1	163,000	–	7 inj. twice per month
Mephedrone	S	n = 1	300	–	Axillary hair

S: Single intake of a therapeutic dose (one or two tablets).
O: Occasional intake of therapeutic doses (several times per month).
R: Regular intake of therapeutic doses (daily or so).
A: Abuse of the drug.

4.2 Interpreting GHB in Hair

Detection of GHB in biological fluids is problematic due to its short residual time in the body (less than 12 hours in urine). Hair analysis is therefore a useful tool to investigate GHB administration in DFC cases. However, the interpretation of GHB concentrations in hair is tricky. Levels of GHB in hair are often quite low from endogenous incorporation, and the ingestion of GHB will result in an increased GHB concentration corresponding to the approximate time period of the offense. However, a large range of GHB levels in the general population is reported (range: $<0.5-12$ ng/mg[43] and $0.31-8.4$ ng/mg[66]) particularly at the hair root (owing to the impregnation of hair by sweat and sebum). Such concentrations can raise difficulties in interpreting GHB hair concentrations of a suspected case of isolated exposure to the drug. The regular abuse of GHB leads to concentrations far above the endogenous GHB levels (five to 10 times higher) and is not difficult to interpret. When an isolated exposure is suspected, the analyst should detect a peak concentration of GHB from the baseline of the individual GHB pattern on the period corresponding to the time of the offense. However, according to the dose ingested and the individual variability due to diet, seasons, stress, etc., the peak concentration of GHB in hair could be undistinguishable enough from the baseline and thus not convincing enough to be reported without another element in the case file.

Because of the variability of GHB baseline coupled to the variability of hair growth rate in each individual, as stressed by Scott[4] and Kintz,[42] late hair sampling for GHB is an issue and we do not recommend performing GHB hair analysis (sampling) more than about 3−4 months after the alleged offense.

4.3 Interpretation of Time Exposure

Interpreting the time exposure period is the most difficult task. Incorporation rate is the first pitfall. As reported by Negrusz et al.,[67] there is a large variability of drug incorporation rate between individuals. The ingestion of a single dose of clonazepam by 10 healthy volunteers appeared in hair between 3 and 28 days after ingestion. It is therefore not reasonable to determine a precise timeframe from the hair analysis, like a week or a day, even if the court would be in favor of this. Segmental analysis of hair cut close to the scalp can, however, provide an approximate historical profile of drugs exposure, and is useful when a single exposure has occurred.

Another variable is the hair's growth rate depending on individuals, seasons and area of the scalp. It is widely admitted that the steadiest growth rate is located at the vertex posterior, and sampling should be done in this area.[68] If the sampling is not done in this area, it should be noted because unexpected results may arise.

The mean hair growth rate is about 1 cm ± 0.2 cm per month; however, the range of established hair growth rate is from 0.6 to 3.4 cm/month.[69] Thus, the longer the time elapsed after the offense, the wider the uncertainty of the hair pattern. When months have passed, the amount of the drug in hair is spread along the hair shaft and makes any precise interpretation of time exposure difficult. It could be hard to detect a single therapeutic drug intake if sampling is done more than 6 months after the alleged offense.

In addition, we have observed that in some cases, notably when the victim has been exposed to a high single dose, the drug could be detected in the near segments. In our own daily experience, the measured concentrations do not exceed about 10% of the main concentration detected and could be considered as not significant even if they are above the LOQ. It is not clear if it is due to some controversial axial diffusion or to incorporation by sweat or sebum at the time of intoxication, or also to the variability of hair growth or incorporation rate. According to Pragst,[16] alterations of the drug distribution along the hair sample may result from a variety of causes: slowly growing strands, catagen and telogen hair, and delayed incorporation from tissues cause an extension of the drug zone in proximal direction, whereas fast growing strands and incorporation from sweat or sebum lead to an extension of the drug zone in the distal direction. The degree to which these effects influence hair drug distribution depends on the individual (large portion of telogen hair), the pharmacokinetics of the drug (high excretion rate in sweat or sebum) and the occasion of drug use (extreme sweating during a rave party, for example). Thus, there is no axial migration within the hair; therefore, proximal hair must be drug free after several months of abstinence.

Kintz considered that the highest drug concentration must be detected in the segment corresponding to the period of the alleged event and that the measured concentration be at least three times higher than the ones measured in the previous or following segments.[42]

4.4 Natural Hair Color and Cosmetic Hair Treatment

Natural hair color could also be an issue when interpreting hair results, since melanocytes and pigmentation play an important role in the incorporation of basic drugs into hair.[16] We carried out an internal experiment on a healthy volunteer with salt-and-pepper-colored hair after a single intake of a dose of zolpidem. The quantification of zolpidem performed on separated white and brown hair of the same strand showed concentrations of 0.4 pg/mg in white hair and 39.7 pg/mg in brown hair. However, the binding of a number of drugs and metabolites is not solely influenced by melanin content.

Another issue is aggressive cosmetic hair treatments. Dying may interfere with the analytes or the analysis, while bleaching or caustic treatment damages the hair fiber and may lead to an elimination of the drugs in hair. A decrease of 1−90% of the original drug concentration may occur.[70−72,22]

The sun's UV rays can also damage the hair by bleaching out the pigments found therein, and by the degradation of proteins.[73] This kind of damage is more subtle and takes significantly more time than chemical cosmetic treatment, but is nonetheless just as damaging to the hair with prolonged exposure. Therefore, elimination of drugs from the hair may occur, as well as direct degradation of drugs, like cannabis[74] or LSD, if sensitive to UV light.

4.5 Contamination

Hair drug contamination or passive exposure is widely developed in the literature regarding illicit drugs, notably cocaine or methadone. With regard to DFC cases, the problem is usually avoided, considering the route of intake of the drugs used and the low doses. However, in some cases misinterpretation can emerge. This could be due to an important sweat/sebum contamination of hair, for instance after a long stay in hospital without hair washing—some DFC cases occur while staying in hospital—or in the case of very curly short black hair. It could also be due to contamination of hair by blood or bio-fluids in DFC postmortem cases. We report a case where the corpse of the victim was found many years after the offense, and traces of 7-aminoflunitrazepam were found in postmortem fluid and also along the hair shaft. In this DFC case, the first interpretation of the drug hair pattern was a regular intake of a low dose of flunitrazepam. The study was carried out at Toxlab to investigate the possibility of external contamination of hair by 7-aminoflunitrazepam present in the blood. Ten strands of hair from a healthy volunteer were soaked in a whole blood solution of 7-aminoflunitrazepam at 100 ng/mL during 7, 14 and 30 days. Three temperatures were tested: +4°C, ambient and +37°C. The results are reported in Table 8.8.

TABLE 8.8 7-Aminoflunitrazepam Concentrations (pg/mg) in Hair after Incubation in Spiked Blood

Time	Incubation at +4°C	Incubation at Ambient Temp.	Incubation at +37°C
T0	<LOD	<LOD	<LOD
T + 7 days	221	484	187
T + 14 days	346	705	282
T + 30 days	525	777	323

These results clearly show an important hair contamination, when soaked in blood containing drugs, whatever the temperature of incubation. Kintz[75] and Paterson[76] confirm our results and report hair contamination cases concerning 6-acetylmorphine, MDMA, cyamemazine, morphine and buprenorphine. This phenomenon was also previously described by El Mahjoub et al.[77] with hair soaked with standard solutions of clonazepam, flunitrazepam, midazolam, diazepam, oxazepam and methylclonazepam, and incorporation rates ranging from 6.5 to 18.7%.

Thus, homogeneous low concentrations along the hair shaft after segmental analysis could be indicative of external contamination that may have arisen not only from direct contamination by the drug but also via contamination with body fluids at postmortem or from sweat produced close to the time of the offense.[78,79]

This phenomenon must be kept in mind in the case of postmortem DFC cases, particularly if the body was not found immediately after death or if sampling shows that hair is wet or might have been soaked in blood or fluid residues at autopsy, for example. This underlines, once again, all the precautions to be taken during the interpretation of a hair result.

5. CONCLUSION

Segmental hair analysis might provide good retrospective information about drug intake, and also inform about the frequency of drug exposure in DFC cases. However, the interpretation of hair results is an issue, must always be made with care and should only be done by experienced staff.

The UNODC (United Nations Office on Drugs and Crime) guidelines for the forensic analysis of DFSA and other criminal acts[79] states the minimum required performance limits (MRPL) in urine for the most frequently encountered drugs in DFC, in order to ensure that all laboratories report the presence of the substances in a uniform way. At this time, there is no equivalent table for hair analysis.

Substances which should be targeted first (not exhaustive) in DFC and DFSA analysis and their suggested MRPL in hair are listed in Table 8.9.

We hope that in the near future, the multiresidue analysis by full scan LC-HRMS, for instance, essential in a broad drug screening of unknown analytes, will be available in many laboratories dealing with hair analysis.[34] It will particularly help to face the emerging phenomenon of designer drugs, cathinones and the use of spices that may raise difficulties in solving DFC cases by hair analysis.[80]

TABLE 8.9 Substances which should be First Targeted (Not Exhaustive) in DFC Analysis and their Suggested Minimum Required Performance Limit in Hair

Molecules	Suggested MRPL in Hair (pg/mg)
Aceprometazine	5
Alimemazine	5
Alprazolam	1
Bromazepam	2
Buprenorphine	1
Clobazam	1
Clonazepam	1
7-Aminoclonazepam	1
Cyamemazine	10
Diazepam	<2 (see nordiazepam)
Diphenhydramine	10
Doxylamine	10
Estazolam	1
Flunitrazepam	1
7-Aminoflunitrazepam	1
Haloperidol	10
Hydroxyzine	10
Ketamine	2
Levomepromazine	10
Loprazolam	2
Lorazepam	<2
Lormetazepam	<1
Meprobamate	10
Methadone	20
Midazolam	1
Niaprazine	10
Nitrazepam	1
7-Aminonitrazepam	5

(Continued)

TABLE 8.9 (Continued)

Molecules	Suggested MRPL in Hair (pg/mg)
Nordiazepam	1–2
Oxazepam	1
Oxomemazine	10
Prazepam	<1 (see nordiazepam)
Temazepam	0.5
Tetrazepam	5
Tramadol	10
Triazolam	1
Zolpidem	1
Zopiclone	1
GHB	1

REFERENCES

1. Gaulier JM, Fonteau F, Jouanel E, Lachâtre G. Rape drugs: practical, pharmacological and analytical aspects. *Ann Bio Clin* 2004;**62**:529–38.
2. Chèze M, Muckensturm A, Hoizey G, Pépin G, Deveaux M. A tendency for re-offending in drug-facilitated crime. *Forensic Sci Int* 2010;**196**:14–7.
3. Pecoraro V, Astore IPL. Measurement of hair growth under physiological conditions. In: Happle CE, editor. *Hair and hair disease*. Berlin: Springer; 1990. p. 237.
4. Scott KS. The use of hair as a toxicological tool in DFC casework. *Sci Justice* 2009;**49**:250–3.
5. Villain M, Concheiro M, Cirimele V, Kintz P. Screening method for benzodiazepines and hypnotics in hair at pg/mg level by liquid chromatography-mass spectrometry/mass spectrometry. *J Chromatogr B* 2005;**825**:72–8.
6. Kintz P, Villain M, Ludes B. Testing for the undetectable in drug-facilitated sexual assault using hair analyzed by tandem mass spectrometry as evidence. *Ther Drug Monit* 2004;**26**:211–4.
7. Chèze M, Duffort G, Deveaux M, Pépin G. Hair analysis by liquid chromatography-tandem mass spectrometry in toxicological investigation of drug-facilitated crimes: report of 128 cases over the period June 2003–May 2004 in metropolitan Paris. *Forensic Sci Int* 2005;**153**:3–10.
8. Kintz P, Villain M, Cirimele V. Hair analysis for drug detection. *Ther Drug Monit* 2006;**28**:442–6.
9. Xiang P, Sun Q, Shen B, Chen P, Liu W, Shen M. Segmental hair analysis using liquid chromatography-tandem mass spectrometry after a single dose of benzodiazepines. *Forensic Sci Int* 2011;**204**:19–26.

10. Société Française de Toxicologie Analytique. Consensus. Soumission chimique: prise en charge toxicologique. *Ann Toxicol Anal* 2003;**15**:239−42.

11. LeBeau M, Andollo W, Lee Hearn W, Baselt R, Cone F, Finkle D, et al. Recommendations for toxicological investigations of drug-facilitated sexual assaults. *J Forensic Sci* 1999;**44**:227−30.

12. ElSohly MA, Salamone SJ. Prevalence of drugs used in cases of alleged sexual Assault. *J Anal Toxicol* 1999;**23**:141−6.

13. Kintz P. Bioanalytical procedures for detection of chemical agents in hair in the case of drug-facilitated crimes. *Anal Bioanal Chem* 2007;**388**:1467−74.

14. Gaulier JM, Sauvage FL, Pauthier H, Saint-Marcoux F, Marquet P, Lachâtre G. Identification of acepromazine in hair: an illustration of the difficulties encountered in investigating drug-facilitated crimes. *J Forensic Sci* 2008;**53**:755−9.

15. Cooper GA. Hair testing is taking root. *Ann Clin Biochem* 2011;**48**:516−30.

16. Pragst F, Balikova MA. State of the art in hair analysis for detection of drug and alcohol abuse. *Clin Chim Acta* 2006;**370**:17−49.

17. Tsanaclis L, Kingston R, Wicks J. Testing for alcohol use in hair: is ethyl glucuronide (EtG) stable in hair? *Ann Toxicol Anal* 2009;**21**:67−71.

18. Cooper GA, Kronstrand R, Kintz P, Society of Hair Testing. Society of Hair Testing guidelines for drug testing in hair. *Forensic Sci Int* 2012;**218**:20−4.

19. Cirimele V, Kintz P, Mangin P. Detection and quantification of lorazepam in human hair by GC-MS/NCI in a case of traffic accident. *Int J Legal Med* 1996;**108**:265−7.

20. Cirimele V, Kintz P, Staub C, Mangin P. Testing human hair for flunitrazepam and 7-amino-flunitrazepam by GC/MS-NCI. *Forensic Sci Int* 1997;**84**:189−200.

21. Cirimele V, Kintz P, Ludes B. Screening for forensically relevant benzodiazepines in human hair by gas chromatography-negative ion chemical ionization-mass spectrometry. *J Chromatogr B Biomed Sci Appl* 1997;**700**:119−29.

22. Yegles M, Marson Y, Wennig R. Influence of bleaching on stability of benzodiazepines in hair. *Forensic Sci Int* 2000;**107**:87−92.

23. Kronstrand R, Nyström I, Josefsson M, Hodgins S. Segmental ion spray LC-MS-MS analysis of benzodiazepines in hair of psychiatric patients. *J Anal Toxicol* 2002;**26**:479−84.

24. Laloup M, Ramirez Fernandez Mdel M, De Boeck G, Wood M, Maes V, Samyn N. Validation of a liquid chromatography-tandem mass spectrometry method for the simultaneous determination of 26 benzodiazepines and metabolites, zolpidem and zopiclone, in blood, urine, and hair. *J Anal Toxicol* 2005;**29**:616−26.

25. Irving RC, Dickson SJ. The detection of sedatives in hair and nail samples using tandem LC-MS-MS. *Forensic Sci Int* 2007;**166**:58−67.

26. Miller EI, Wylie FM, Oliver JS. Detection of benzodiazepines in hair using ELISA and LC-ESI-MS-MS. *J Anal Toxicol* 2006;**30**:441−8.

27. Negrusz A, Moore CM, Kern JL, Janicak PG, Strong MJ, Levy NA. Quantitation of clonazepam and its major metabolite 7-aminoclonazepam in hair. *J Anal Toxicol* 2000;**24**:614−20.

28. Toyo'oka T, Kanbori M, Kumaki Y, Nakahara Y. Determination of triazolam involving its hydroxy metabolites in hair shaft and hair root by reversed-phase liquid chromatography with electrospray ionization mass spectrometry and application to human hair analysis. *Anal Biochem* 2001;**295**:172−9.

29. Anderson RA, Ariffin MM, Cormack PA, Miller EI. Comparison of molecularly imprinted solid-phase extraction (MISPE) with classical solid-phase extraction (SPE) for the detection of benzodiazepines in post-mortem hair samples. *Forensic Sci Int* 2008;**174**:40−6.

30. Nielsen MK, Johansen SS, Dalsgaard PW, Linnet K. Simultaneous screening and quantification of 52 common pharmaceuticals and drugs of abuse in hair using UPLC-TOF-MS. *Forensic Sci Int* 2010;**196**:85–92.

31. Lee S, Han E, In S, Choi H, Chung H, Chung. Determination of illegally abused sedative-hypnotics in hair samples from drug offenders. *J Anal Toxicol* 2011;**35**:312–5.

32. Vogliardi S, Favretto D, Tucci M, Stocchero G, Ferrara SD. Simultaneous LC-HRMS determination of 28 benzodiazepines and metabolites in hair. *Anal Bioanal Chem* 2011;**400**:51–67.

33. Kim J, Lee S, In S, Choi H, Chung H. Validation of a simultaneous analytical method for the detection of 27 benzodiazepines and metabolites and zolpidem in hair using LC-MS/MS and its application to human and rat hair. *J Chromatogr B* 2011;**879**:878–86.

34. Favretto D, Vogliardi S, Stocchero G, Nalesso A, Tucci M, Ferrara SD. High performance liquid chromatography-high resolution mass spectrometry and micropulverized extraction for the quantification of amphetamines, cocaine, opioids, benzodiazepines, antidepressants and hallucinogens in 2.5 mg hair samples. *J Chromatogr A* 2011;**1218**:6583–95.

35. Broecker S, Herre S, Pragst F. General unknown screening in hair by liquid chromatography-hybrid quadrupole time-of-flight mass spectrometry (LC-QTOF-MS). *Forensic Sci Int* 2012;**218**:68–81.

36. Morini L, Vignali C, Polla M, Sponta A, Groppi A. Comparison of extraction procedures for benzodiazepines determination in hair by LC-MS/MS. *Forensic Sci Int* 2012;**218**:53–6.

37. Salomone A, Gerace E, Di Corcia D, Martra G, Petrarulo M, Vincenti M. Hair analysis of drugs involved in drug-facilitated sexual assault and detection of zolpidem in a suspected case. *Int J Legal Med* 2012;**126**:451–9.

38. Lendoiro E, Quintela O, de Castro A, Cruz A, López-Rivadulla M, Concheiro M. Target screening and confirmation of 35 licit and illicit drugs and metabolites in hair by LC-MSMS. *Forensic Sci Int* 2012;**217**:207–15.

39. Kronstrand R, Forsman M, Roman M. A screening method for 30 drugs in hair using ultrahigh-performance liquid chromatography time-of-flight mass spectrometry. *Ther Drug Monit* 2013;**35**:288–95.

40. Wietecha-Posłuszny R, Woźniakiewicz M, Garbacik A, Chęsy P, Kościelniak P. Application of microwave irradiation to fast and efficient isolation of benzodiazepines from human hair. *J Chromatogr A* 2013;**1278**:22–8.

41. Yegles M, Mersch F, Wennig R. Detection of benzodiazepines and other psychotropic drugs in human hair by GC/MS. *Forensic Sci Int* 1997;**84**:211–8.

42. Kintz P. Issues about axial diffusion during segmental hair analysis. *Ther Drug Monit* 2013;**35**:408–10.

43. Kintz P, Cirimele V, Jamey C, Ludes B. Testing for GHB in hair by GC/MS/MS after a single exposure. Application to document sexual assault. *J Forensic Sci* 2003;**48**:195–200.

44. Kintz P, Villain M, Cirimele V. Chemical abuse in the elderly: evidence from hair analysis. *Ther Drug Monit* 2008;**30**:207–11.

45. Miyaguchi H, Kakuta M, Iwata YT, Matsuda H, Tazawa H, Kimura H, et al. Development of a micropulverized extraction method for rapid toxicological analysis of methamphetamine in hair. *J Chromatogr A* 2007;**1163**:43–8.

46. Miyaguchi H, Takahashi H, Ohashi T, Mawatari K, Iwata YT, Inoue H, et al. Rapid analysis of methamphetamine in hair by micropulverized extraction and microchip-based competitive ELISA. *Forensic Sci Int* 2009;**184**:1–5.

47. Humbert L, Wiart JF, Binoche A, Cornez R, Allorge D, Lhermitte M. Respiratory depression after methadone ingestion and polyintoxication discovery of a chronic or multiple addictions in a 10-year-old boy by a segmental hair analysis. Ann Toxicol Anal 2010;22:123−8.

48. Kintz P, Bundeli P, Brenneisen R, Ludes B. Dose-concentration relationships in hair from subjects in a controlled heroin-maintenance program. J Anal Toxicol 1998;22:231−6.

49. Rust KY, Baumgartner MR, Meggiolaro N, Kraemer T. Detection and validated quantification of 21 benzodiazepines and 3 "z-drugs" in human hair by LC-MS/MS. Forensic Sci Int 2012;215:64−72.

50. Sauvage FL, Gaulier JM, Lachâtre G, Marquet P. Pitfalls and prevention strategies for liquid chromatography-tandem mass spectrometry in the selected reaction-monitoring mode for drug analysis. Clin Chem 2008;54:1519−27.

51. Marquet P. LC-MS vs. GC-MS, online extraction systems, advantages of technology for drug screening assays. Methods Mol Biol 2012;902:15−27.

52. Society of Hair Testing, Cooper G, Moeller M, Kronstrand R. Current status of accreditation for drug testing in hair. Forensic Sci Int 2008;176:9−12.

53. Malkoc E, Neuteboom W. The current status of forensic science laboratory accreditation in Europe. Forensic Sci Int 2007;167:121−6.

54. Lee S, Park Y, Yang W, Han E, Choe S, In S, et al. Development of a reference material using methamphetamine abusers' hair samples for the determination of methamphetamine and amphetamine in hair. J Chromatogr B 2008;865:33−9.

55. Lee S, Park Y, Yang W, Han E, Choe S, Lim M, et al. Estimation of the measurement uncertainty of methamphetamine and amphetamine in hair analysis. Forensic Sci Int 2009;185:59−66.

56. Peters FT, Maurer HH. Bioanalytical method validation and its implications for forensic and clinical toxicology—a review. Accredit Qual Assur 2002;7:441−9.

57. Peters FT, Drummer OH, Musshoff F. Validation of new methods. Forensic Sci Int 2007;165:216−24.

58. Musshoff F, Madea B. New trends in hair analysis and scientific demands on validation and technical notes. Forensic Sci Int 2007;165:204−15.

59. Antignac JP, de Wasch K, Monteau F, De Brabander H, Andre F, Le Bizec B. The ion suppression phenomenon in liquid chromatography-mass spectrometry and its consequences in the field of residue analysis. Anal Chim Acta 2005;529:129−36.

60. Pragst F. Physiology of hair growth and its consequences on hair analysis for drugs. Chicago (IL): Oral communication—Congress of the Society of Hair Testing; 2004.

61. Potsch L, Skoop G, Moeller MR. Biochemical approach on the conservation of drug molecules during hair fiber formation. Forensic Sci Int 1997;84:25−35.

62. Eser HP, Potsch L, Skopp G. Influence of sample preparation on analytical results: drug analysis [GC-MS] on hair snippets versus hair powder using various extraction methods. Forensic Sci Int 1997;81:271−9.

63. Musshoff F, Madea B. Analytical pitfalls in hair testing. Anal Bioanal Chem 2007;388:1475−94.

64. Hang C, Ping X, Min S. Long-term follow-up analysis of zolpidem in fingernails after a single oral dose. Anal Bioanal Chem 2013;405:7281−9.

65. Villain M, Chèze M, Dumestre V, Ludes B, Kintz P. Hair to document drug-facilitated crimes: four cases involving bromazepam. J Anal Toxicol 2004;28:516−9.

66. Goullé JP, Chèze M, Pépin G. Determination of endogenous levels of GHB in human hair. Are there possibilities for the identification of GHB administration through hair analysis in cases of drug-facilitated sexual assault? *J Anal Toxicol* 2003;**27**:574−80.

67. Negrusz A, Bowen AM, Moore CM, Dowd SM, Strong MJ, Janiack PG. Deposition of 7-aminoclonazepam in hair following a single dose of Klonopin. *J Anal Toxicol* 2002;**26**:471−8.

68. Society of Hair Testing. Recommendations for hair testing in forensic cases. *Forensic Sci Int* 2004;**145**:83−4.

69. Harkley MR. Anatomy and physiology of hair. *Forensic Sci Int* 1993;**63**:9−18.

70. Skopp G, Pötsch L, Moeller MR. On cosmetically treated hair—aspects and pitfalls of interpretation. *Forensic Sci Int* 1997;**84**:43−52.

71. Cirimele V, Kintz P, Mangin P. Drug concentration in human hair after bleaching. *J Anal Toxicol* 1995;**19**:331−2.

72. Jurado C, Kintz P, Menéndez M, Repetto M. Influence of the cosmetic treatment of hair on drug testing. *Int J Leg Med* 1997;**110**:159−63.

73. Santos Nogeira AC, Joekes I. Hair color changes and protein damage caused by ultraviolet radiation. *J Photochem Photobiol B* 2004;**74**:109−17.

74. Skopp G, Pötsch L, Mauden M. Stability of cannabinoids in hair samples exposed to sunlight. *Clin Chem* 2000;**46**:1846−8.

75. Kintz P. Segmental hair analysis can demonstrate external contamination in post-mortem cases. *Forensic Sci Int* 2012;**215**:73−6.

76. Paterson S, Lee S, Cordero R. Analysis of hair after contamination with blood containing 6-acetylmorphine and blood containing morphine. *Forensic Sci Int* 2011;**210**:129−32.

77. El Mahjoub A, Staub C. Determination of benzodiazepines in human hair by on-line high-performance liquid chromatography using a restricted access extraction column. *Forensic Sci Int* 2001;**123**:17−25.

78. Kintz P. Interpretation of hair findings in children after methadone poisoning. *Forensic Sci Int* 2010;**196**:1−3.

79. United Nations Office on Drugs and Crime. *Guidelines for the forensic analysis of drugs facilitating sexual assault and other criminal acts.* United Nations Publication; 2011.

80. Vincenti M, Salomone A, Gerace E, Pirro V. Application of mass spectrometry to hair analysis for forensic toxicological investigations. *Mass Spectrom. Rev.* 2013;**32**:312−32.

Chapter 9

Case Reports in Drug-Facilitated Crimes

From A for Alprazolam to Z for Zopiclone

Véronique Dumestre-Toulet and Hélène Eysseric-Guérin

1. INTRODUCTION

Drug-facilitated crimes (DFCs) are not a new phenomenon but rather an age-old practice. However, reports of DFCs have significantly increased since the mid-1990s. In the last few years, considerable information about DFCs (rape, sexual assault, robbery, sedation of elderly persons) has been collected.

To all intents and purposes, the drug acts as the offender's weapon; so many jurisdictions require analytical proof of its presence, which helps substantiate the alleged victim's claim. Blood and urine are the conventional specimens to document drug exposure. However, in cases of DFC, hair sampling is a useful complement to these analyses as segmentation of the hair allows differentiation of a single exposure from chronic use of a drug. Moreover, due to the long delays that are frequently encountered between the event and the matter being reported to the police, hair can often be the only matrix capable of providing corroborative evidence of a committed crime.

Data from literature were scarce before 2005, but numerous case reports have been published recently allowing a better interpretation of measured concentrations.

In this chapter, an attempt has been made to collect cases reported up to now in the literature by conducting a bibliographic research. It is hoped these cases will be as complete as possible without claiming to be exhaustive.

Toxicological Aspects of Drug-Facilitated Crimes. DOI: http://dx.doi.org/10.1016/B978-0-12-416748-3.00009-8

2. METHODS

A literature search for articles on "drug-facilitated crimes" and "drug-facilitated sexual assault" (DFSA) cited in the Analytical Abstracts and Medline databases was performed between June and September 2013 to produce citations. A similar request for articles on "soumission chimique" was performed with the search engine from the "Annales de Toxicologie Analytique" website. Moreover, abstract books from the last meetings of the International Association of Forensic Toxicologists (TIAFT) and the Société Française de Toxicologie Analytique (SFTA) were reviewed for the same keywords.

We looked for: compounds, gender and age of the victims, case history, described symptoms, delay before sampling, blood, urinary and hair (segmented head hair, leg hair and pubic hair) concentrations and some hair characteristics. We excluded cases without compound quantitation.

Data corresponding to more than 200 DFC case reports are presented in Table 9.1. The systematic review also revealed significant studies on healthy volunteers with administration of a single dose of a drug. Data corresponding to these controlled studies are presented in Table 9.2. The aim was to produce useful tools for the interpretation of concentrations measured in DFC of blood, urine and hair specimens.

TABLE 9.1 Case Reports

Gender and Age	History, Symptoms and Comments	Delay Before Sampling	[C] Blood ng/mL or precised	[C] Urine ng/mL or precised	Hair: Color [C] pg/mg or precised	Ref.
Acepromazine						
F, 29 y	Sexual assault. Found tied to a table. Forced to drink an unknown beverage identified later as Vetranquil®. Memory lapses, sedation	8 h (blood) 1.5 m (hair)	ND		brown hair 31	1
Alimemazine (trimiprazine)						
1 F, 80 y	Mistreatment in a retirement home Sedation—repetitive exposure				colored hair 8/21	2
F, 15 m	Drugs in a feedbottle given by a nanny Sedation—repetitive exposure	2 m			1400/2200/700	3
3 F, 79 to 95 y	Mistreatment in a retirement home Sedation—repetitive exposure				990 to 3600/ 860 to 3600/ 1490	4
M, 7 y F, 13 y	Given by the stepmother at least 3 months Drowsiness, ataxia, sedation, muscular weakness—repetitive exposure				M: light brown hair: 126/127 F: brown hair: 339/199/23/ ND	5
Alprazolam (A)/7 Hydroxyalprazolam (OHA)						
F, 12 y	Abused several months, once per week, by her father	m			4.9/2.4	6

(Continued)

TABLE 9.1 (Continued)

Gender and Age	History, Symptoms and Comments	Delay Before Sampling	[C] Blood ng/mL or precised	[C] Urine ng/mL or precised	Hair: Color [C] pg/mg or precised	Ref.
F, 16 y	Sequestered and battered for prostitution Drug in dinners Sedation, impairment, memory lapses	m			bleach hair 3.1*/0.8/0.4/ 0.4	6
M, 51 y	Robbery by his nurse Sedation				gray hair 71/85/8.5/13/ <LOQ	7
2 M, 34, 49 y	Sexual assault				M1: 10 M2: 90/15/160	8
F, 8 y	Xanax given by a stepfather Sedation, incoherent	22 h	3.5	A: 11, OHA: 125		9
4 victims	Sexual assault			A: ND to 71 OHA: 23.4 to 388		10
Atropine (A)/Scopolamine (S)						
2 F, 7 y	*Datura* given by the parents Sedation, deceased in a fire		F1: A: 32, S: 4.4 F2: A: 7.5, S: 0.8			11
Bromazepam/3-OH-bromazepam (OHB)						
F, 39 y	Trouble with her husband. Drank a coffee Deep sleeping 24 h	24 h (blood) 1 m (hair)	51		10.3*/ND/ND	12

F, 25 y	Abused in a highway station. Forced to absorb a tablet. Sleep	18 h (blood) 3 w (hair)	151		5.7*/0.9/ND	12
M	Robbery and sexual assault. Forced to absorb an unknown mixture	6 h (fluids) 19 w (hair)	10.4	18	pubic hair: 4.1	12
F, 25 y	Sexual assault	6 w			15*/7/6/2	12
2 F, 80–96 y	Mistreatment in a retirement home Sedation—repetitive exposure				gray or colored hair F1: 361 F2: 2900	2
M, 37 y	Robbery after a cup of coffee with a woman Sedation—loss of memory	11 h	8			13
F >70 y	Mistreatment in a retirement home Sedation—repetitive exposure				gray hair 26	14
F, 20 y	Have a drink in a bar with friends Tiredness, incoherent behavior, irritability	3 d (urine) 3 w (hair)		11.8 OHB: 41.8	6.7/ND/ND	15
Buprenorphine (B)/Norbuprenorphine (NB)						
M, 14 y	Sexual assault Found dead in a pedophile's home		B: 1.1 NB: 0.2	B: 9.1 NB: 9.6	B: 23	13
Carbamazepine						
F, 80 y	Mistreatment in a retirement home Sedation—repetitive exposure				gray hair 4.9/9.8	2

(Continued)

TABLE 9.1 (Continued)

Gender and Age	History, Symptoms and Comments	Delay Before Sampling	[C] Blood ng/mL or precised	[C] Urine ng/mL or precised	Hair: Color [C] pg/mg or precised	Ref.
Chloroform						
F, 13 y	Sexual assault—deceased		834 µg/mL	9.7 µg/mL		16
Clobazam						
F, 6 y	Given by the mother				6280	13
F, 85 y	Mistreatment in a retirement home Sedation—repetitive exposure				white hair 270/301	2
Clonazepam (C)/7NH2 clonazepam (AC)						
M, 63 y	Robbery after drinking a coffee offered by two men	13 h (fluids) 8 w (hair)	C: 12.4 AC: 11.4	C: 14.7 AC: 332	hair: C: 1.9, AC: 41.2 pubic hair: C: <LOQ, AC: 19.2	17
22 M and F	Credit card robbery after drinking a whiskey/Coke—quickly sleeping	20–144 h (fluids) 3 w–18 m (hair)	C: <1 to 9.5 (n = 5) AC: <1 to 9 (n = 5)	C: <1 to 14 (n = 5) AC: 16 to 165 (n = 5)	C: 4 to 9.5 (n = 2) AC: 3 to 47.5 (n = 3)	18
M, 71 y	Robbery by a young woman after drinking fruit juices several times—sedation, memory lapses—repetitive exposure	1 m			AC: 91	7
F	Sexual assault after a dinner Sedation, incoherent, euphoria	13–18 h	C: 50 AC: 30	AC: 650		11

F, 27 y	Sexual assault after a fruit juice given by an anesthetist—sedation, memory lapses	24 h	C: 34 AC: <LOQ	C: 3.3 AC: 82		19
M, 40 y	Robbery after have a drink in a gay nightclub of Pigalle—deep sleeping	few h		C: 17.8, AC: 561.7	axillary hair: AC: 3.2	15
M, 49 y	Sexual assault				C: 20/20/ND AC: 40/80/30	8
5 victims	Sexual assault			AC: 2.6 to 651		10
2 victims V1, V2	Sexual assault	18 h (blood) 5 w (hair)	C: 0.22, 1.05 AC: 15.34, 20.6		black hair V1: C: 11.93*/1.31/1.63 AC: 33.47*/<LOQ/ND V2: C: 15.47*/5.31/ND AC: 45.3*/ND/ND	20
F <25 y	Drink a herb tea with a friend Sedation	24 h	C: 42.4 AC: 28.4	C: 28.5 AC: 16.4		21
F	Context of divorce—rape by her husband Sedation—memory lapses	28 h (blood) 1 m (hair)	C: 115 AC: 2980	C: 17 AC: 35		22
2 M, 15, 16 y	Sexual assault after sniffing a white powder Fell asleep—awoke in a bed with a man	72 h (fluids) 1 m (hair)	M1: AC: 7 M2: AC: 10	M1: AC: 58 M2: AC: 233	M1: brown hair: AC: 141 M2: black hair: AC: 336	23
F, 21 y	Confined for 12 days—raped by three men				AC: 1/35/ND	24

(Continued)

TABLE 9.1 (Continued)

Gender and Age	History, Symptoms and Comments	Delay Before Sampling	[C] Blood ng/mL or precised	[C] Urine ng/mL or precised	Hair: Color [C] pg/mg or precised	Ref.
	Sedation, incoherent, memory lapses					
Clozapine						
F, 18 m	Munchausen syndrome by proxy (mother) Deceased—repetitive exposure	exhumation 10 m after death			3200	25
Cyamemazine						
F, 36 y	Rape after drinking a bottle of wine with a business customer- Sedation	6 m			100*	3
22 M and F	Credit card robbery after drinking a whiskey/Coke—deep sleeping	20–144 h (fluids) 3 w–18 m (hair)	<1 to 1.6 (n = 5)	<1 to 229 (n = 5)	37 to 66 (n = 3)	18
2 F, 80–90 y	Mistreatment in a retirement home Sedation—repetitive exposure				white or gray hair 28 to 189	2
Diazepam (D)/Nordiazepam (N)/Oxazepam (O)						
F >70 y	Mistreatment in a retirement home Sedation—repetitive exposure				gray hair 81	14
F, 41 y	Sexual assault while at work after drinking a fruit juice with her employer	17 m			black hair (African) 9.6	26
M, 59 y	Robbery				D: 50, N: 120	8

F, 13 y	Kidnapped during 4 h. Two men put a cloth soaked in a solvent over her mouth. Unconscious several hours	4 h	D: 20 N: <LOQ		27
F, 29 y	Rape by a gynecologist after injection of drugs—unconscious for several hours	30 h	D: 28 N: 8	D: + N: +	28
F >70 y	Mistreatment in a retirement home Sedation—repetitive exposure			gray hair N: 213	14
F, 8 y	Nordaz® given by stepfather Sedation, incoherent	22 h	N:5	N: 3 O: 23	9
M, 14 y	Sexual assault Found dead in a pedophile's home		N: 2810 O: 390	N: 5230 O: 80	13
4 F, 80–96 y	Mistreatment in a retirement home Sedation—repetitive exposure			white, gray or colored hair O: 26 to 153	2
Digoxine					
7 victims	Sedation before murder (massacre of Solar Temple—Vercors/France)		Peripheral blood: 0.53 to 3.0 (n = 7) Central blood: 1.84 and 18.85 (n = 2)		29
Diphenhydramine					
F, 81 y	Mistreatment in a nursing home Sedation			white hair 683	7

(Continued)

TABLE 9.1 (Continued)

Gender and Age	History, Symptoms and Comments	Delay Before Sampling	[C] Blood ng/mL or precised	[C] Urine ng/mL or precised	Hair: Color [C] pg/mg or precised	Ref.
F, 9 y	Sexual assault Repetitive exposure	7 w			brown hair 37/39/33	30
F >70 y	Mistreatment in a retirement home Sedation—repetitive exposure				gray hair 40	14
Doxylamine						
F, 22 y	Rape after drinking at a party—sedation	4 m			40*	3
22 M and F	Credit card robbery after drinking a whiskey/ Coke—quickly sleeping	20–144 h (fluids) 3 w–18 m (hair)	<1 (n = 3)	1 to 72 (n = 5)	12 to 76 (n = 8)	18
F, 81 y	Mistreatment in a nursing home Sedation				white hair 152	7
F >70 y	Mistreatment in a retirement home Sedation—repetitive exposure				gray hair 65	14
Fentanyl						
F >70 y	Mistreatment in a retirement home Sedation—repetitive exposure				gray hair 11	14

Flunitrazepam (F)/7 NH2-flunitrazepam (AF)

7 victims	Sedation before murder (massacre of Solar Temple—Vercors/France)		Peripheral blood 2.2 to 5.0 (n=7)			29
M, 50 y	Credit card robbery Death after hypothermia		AF: 0.013			31
M, 18 y	Robbery after two drinks in a nightclub	84 h (fluids) 6 w (hair)	F <0.20 AF: 0.20		F <LOQ AF: 4.2	17
F	Sequestered and raped for one week	2.5 m			AF: 31.7*/2/ND	32
M, 42 y	Robbery after a drink in a party Sedation—loss of memory				AF: 31.7*	24
22 M and F	Credit card robbery after drinking a whiskey/Coke—deep sleep	20–144 h (fluids) 3 w–18 m (hair)	F <1 to 3 (n=3) AF <1 to 3.2 (n=4)	F <1 to 1.7 (n=3) AF: 6.2 to 145 (n=5)	AF: 1.5 to 3 (n=2)	18
M, 64 y	Given by his wife in the evening soup to decrease libido—dead by respiratory depression repetitive exposure				AF: 78	7
3 M, 30 y	After drinking a free beverage Sedation—loss of memory		AF: 5.8 to 6.2	AF: + (n=2)	AF: 19 (n=1)	11
M, 49 y	Offender in a sexual assault				F: 30/30/10 AF: 210/290/20	8
M, 42 y	Sexual assault by a woman after drinking an alcoholic beverage Unconscious 4 h—loss of memory	21 d			AF: 5.2*/ND	5

(Continued)

TABLE 9.1 (Continued)

Gender and Age	History, Symptoms and Comments	Delay Before Sampling	[C] Blood ng/mL or precised	[C] Urine ng/mL or precised	Hair: Color [C] pg/mg or precised	Ref.
Gamma-Valerolactone (GHV)						
F, 29 y	Sexual assault after drinking in a bar Muscular weakness, "blackouts"	10–11 h		GHV: 3 µg/mL		33
GHB						
F <20 y	After drinking a Ti'Punch at a party Deep sleeping	some w			1.8/1.8/5.5*/ 1.8/1.8 ng/mg	11
F, 48 y	Alleged sexual assault after a sports drink containing relaxing health product Unconsciousness for about 4 hours	12 h		26.9 µg/mL		34
F, 29 y	Sexual assault	7 d			black hair 0.17/0.17/5.3*/ 4.3* ng/mg	35
F, 19 y	Sexual assault after drinking a soft drink Loss of memory	1 m			2.4/2.7*/0.7/ 0.7 ng/mg	6
2 victims	Not precised				0.6/2.6/0.6/ 0.6 ng/mg 0.9/3.5/0.9 ng/ mg	36
F, 24 y	Sexual assault filmed by her boyfriend during studying abroad Confused, nausea, headaches	1 m after return to home			5*/4*/3*/4*/1/ 1 ng/mg	37

Glibenclamide					
M, 30 y	After drinking several beers with his brother Hypoglycemia, vegetative coma and death Repetitive exposure	hospital admission	41	23/31	38
Haloperidol					
M, 8 y	Munchausen syndrome by proxy	hospital admission	39	1574	39
2 F, 80 to 96 y	Mistreatment in a retirement home Sedation—repetitive exposure			gray or colored hair 5 to 31	2
Hydroxyzine					
F <25 y	Drinking a herb tea with a friend—sedation	24 h	5.8	40.9	21
Ketamine (K)/Norketamine (NK)					
F, 29 y	Rape by a gynecologist after injection of drug unconscious for several hours		K: 2 NK: 6	K: + NK: +	28
Lorazepam					
M, 37 y	Robbery after a cup of coffee with a woman Sedation—loss of memory	11 h	10		13
F, 25 y	Sexual assault after eating a strawberry tartlet	18 h (fluids) 2 m (hair)	16	1041	18
F, 23 y	Offense?—unconscious 3 h	1 m	32	8*/ND/ND	6
M, 58 y	Drinking with a man after an unusual encounter via the internet	19 h	14	10	22

(Continued)

TABLE 9.1 (Continued)

Gender and Age	History, Symptoms and Comments	Delay Before Sampling	[C] Blood ng/mL or precised	[C] Urine ng/mL or precised	Hair: Color [C] pg/mg or precised	Ref.
	Sedation—loss of memory			(2200 after hydrolyze)		
F <25 y	Drinking a herb tea with a friend—sedation	24 h	86.4		15.9	21
Lormetazepam						
F, 27 y	Abused by her ex-husband Sedation, impairment	4 m			bleached and colored hair 1.2*	32
M	Jewel robbery after a dinner with his family Sedation	24 h		+	0.91	21
LSD						
F <30 y	Sexual assault after a coffee with three men Euphoria—incoherent	<24 h	0.45	0.12	ND	11
M, 23 y	Drug abuser sexually assaulted in a night club after drinking a beverage Tiredness, loss of memory	many h	0.1	0.42		40
MDMA (M)/MDA						
F, 20 y	Sexual assault after drinking in a nightclub Sedation, euphoria, loss of memory	36 h (fluids) 5 w (hair)	M <0.1 MDA <0.1	M: 1.2 MDA <0.1	brown hair M: 602* MDA: 42*	41

2 M, 9 F 17 to 26 y	Various crimes or sexual assaults Anterograde amnesia	2–44 h (fluids) 4–6 m (hair)	M: 0.1 to 475 (n = 5) MDA: 0.1 to 2 (n = 4)	M: 1.2 to 90 (n = 5) MDA: 0.1 to 4 (n = 4)	M: 16 to 2700* (n = 8) MDA: 16 to 400* (n = 7)	42
F, 22 y	Sexual assault after an alcoholic drink Dizziness, weakness, incapacity to resist	8–12 h	M: 90 MDA: 13	M: +		43
3,4-Methylenedioxypyrovalerone (MDPV)						
M	Victim of a robbery		MDPV: 52			44
Meprobamate						
14 F, 80 to 96 y	Mistreatment in a retirement home Sedation—repetitive exposure				white, gray or colored hair 0.089 to 50 ng/mg	2
Methadone (MTD)/EDDP						
6 victims	Children admitted to hospital unconscious Repetitive exposure				MTD: 50 to 770 (n = 6) EDDP: 10 to 60 (n = 3)	45
Mianserine						
3 F, 80 to 96 y	Mistreatment in a retirement home Sedation—repetitive exposure				white, gray or colored hair 227 to 528	2
Midazolam						
2 victims F # 20 y	Mutilations, rapes during many months or years repetitive exposure				F1: 50/200 F2: 130/170	46

(Continued)

TABLE 9.1 (Continued)

Gender and Age	History, Symptoms and Comments	Delay Before Sampling	[C] Blood ng/mL or precised	[C] Urine ng/mL or precised	Hair: Color [C] pg/mg or precised	Ref.
M, 73 y	Robbery of jewels and money after drinking a coffee in a hotel—comatose 3 days				150*	46
Morphine						
F, 24 y	Sexual assault filmed by her boyfriend during studying abroad Confused, nausea, headaches	1 m after return to home			1*/1*/1*/ND/ ND/ND ng/mg	37
Niaprazine						
F, 15 m	Drugs in a feedbottle given by a nanny Sedation—repetitive exposure	2 m			11.4/16.3/ 3.2 ng/mg	3
6 victims 0.5 to 5 y	Nopron® given by a nanny Sedation, convulsions—repetitive exposure				4.12 to 46.9 (n = 6)	11
2 F, 1 M <12 y	Nopron® given by a stepfather Sedation—repetitive exposure				F1: 382*/21/21 F2: 315*/<10/ <10 M1: 3461/2642	47
Nitrazepam						
Victim	Sexual assault			18.3		10
Paroxetine						
2 F, 80 to 96 y	Mistreatment in a retirement home Sedation—repetitive exposure				white or colored hair F1: 18 F2: 568	2

Pethidine					
F >70 y	Mistreatment in a retirement home Sedation—repetitive exposure			gray hair 714	14
Pholcodine					
F	Sexual assault after a dinner Sedation, incoherent, euphoria	13–18 h	35	2500	11
Promazine					
M, 87 y	Living in a retirement home Behavior inconsistent, incoherent speech Repetitive exposure			white hair 9/2/6	7
Risperidone					
F, 90 y	Mistreatment in a retirement home Sedation—repetitive exposure			900/1080	4
Scopolamine (S) Codeine (C)					
3 victims	Children			S: 0.3 to 1.1 C: 89 to 540	48
Solvents: benzene (B)/Toluene (T)/Xylene (X)					
F, 13 y	Sexual assault	4 h	B: 7.6 µg/mL T: 24.8 µg/mL X: 0.6 µg/mL		27

(Continued)

TABLE 9.1 (Continued)

Gender and Age	History, Symptoms and Comments	Delay Before Sampling	[C] Blood ng/mL or precised	[C] Urine ng/mL or precised	Hair: Color [C] pg/mg or precised	Ref.
Tetrahydrozoline						
2 F, 16 y, 19 y	Sexual assault after drinking eye drops mixed with alcoholic beverage Vomiting, unconscious, feel weird, gray out	7 h 23 h		F1: 1.48 F2: 108		49
F, 19 y	Sexual assault after drinking a vodka-cranberry juice with a man after a movie Groggy, vomiting, unconscious	20 h		114		50
F, 31 y	Kidnapping 2 weeks in a resort Robbery, sodomy and rape after an injection Vomiting, unconscious, loss of memory			150		50
M, 6 y	Eye drops given by mother Drowsiness, sedation, muscular weakness	18–20 h		257		51
Tetrazepam						
6 victims	Sedation before murder (massacre of Solar Temple—Vercors/ France)		Peripheral blood 50 to 680 (n = 6)			29
F, 15 y	Rape after drinking a glass of alcohol with friends Sedation, loss of memory	18 m			220*	52
Thiopental (T)/Pentobarbital (P)						
F, 61 y	Sexual assault in a medical unit after injection of thiopental in her perfusion Unconscious	1 m			hair: T: 300*/ND, P: 400*/ND pubic hair:	53

				T: 250, P: 400	
Tiapride					
5 F, 80 to 96 y	Mistreatment in a retirement home Sedation—repetitive exposure			white, gray or colored hair 0.012 to 50 ng/mg	2
4 F, 79 to 95 y	Mistreatment in a retirement home Sedation—repetitive exposure			F1: 22.7/7.5 ng/mg F2: 1.5/0.35 ng/mg F3: 0.028/ 0.04 ng/mg F4: 0.026/ 0.012 ng/mg	4
Tramadol					
F >70 y	Mistreatment in a retirement home Sedation—repetitive exposure			gray hair 3.57 ng/mg	14
Triazolam (T)/Hydrox/triazolam (OHT)					
M, 49 y	Offender in a sexual assault			T: ND/10/ <LOQ	8
3 victims	Sexual assault		OHT: 204 to 522 (n = 3)		10
F, 58 y	Robbery at home after drinking a coffee with a Japanese compatriot—sleepy 24 h	61 h (fluids) 15 d (hair)	ND	OHT: 2.6 black hair (Asiatic) 1.3*/ND/ND	54

(Continued)

TABLE 9.1 (Continued)

Gender and Age	History, Symptoms and Comments	Delay Before Sampling	[C] Blood ng/mL or precised	[C] Urine ng/mL or precised	Hair: Color [C] pg/mg or precised	Ref.
Valproic acid						
F, 8 y	Depakine® given by stepfather Sedation, incoherent	22 h	140 µg/mL			9
Zolpidem						
F, 19 y	Sexual assault Sedation, loss of memory		39			13
F, 27 y	Sexual assault after eating a strawberry tartlet	1.5 m			19	18
22 victims	Credit card robbery after drinking a whiskey/Coke Deep sleeping	20–144 h (fluids) 3 w–18 m (hair)	<1 to 5.3 (n = 3)	1 to 20 (n = 3)	hair: 8 to 81 (n = 12) pubic hair: <2 (n = 3)	18
6 F, 80 to 96 y	Mistreatment in a retirement home Sedation—repetitive exposure				white, gray or colored hair 6.8 to 2000	2
F, 28 y	Victim forced into drug abuse				black hair (Asiatic) 70/70/20/220	8
F, 23 y	Sexual assault after a party at home Deep sleeping—loss of memory	6 d (fluids) 7 w (hair)	0.016	0.032	blond hair 0.10/0.75*/ND	55

F, 21 y	Sexual assault after drinking a coffee with a male nurse in a hospital Deep sleeping, loss of memory	15 d		4.4*/ND	56
F, 26 y	Sexual assault while at work after drinking several bitter coffees Unconscious, loss of memory Episodic exposures	5 m		2.8/ND/ND/ 1.6/0.9	26
F, 35 y	Sexual assault by husband who replaced contents of capsules with Stilnox® tablets Sleepy, loss of memory, dizziness	11 h	47		57
F >70 y	Mistreatment in a retirement home Sedation—repetitive exposure			gray hair 21	14
Zopiclone					
3 victims M and F >50 y	Robbery after a bitter coffee or cake with a 60 year old man at a train station	<9 h (blood) 3.5 m (hair)	51 to 152	leg hair: 13 (n = 1) pubic hair: 20 (n = 1)	18
5 victims M and F >50 y	Robbery after drinking a bitter coffee or cake with a 60 year old man at an airport Deep sleeping	<9 h (blood); 3 w–8 m (hair)	56 (n = 1) 331 (n = 1)	15 to 42 (n = 5)	18
F, 28 y	After drinking a beverage with a man Deep sleeping	24 h	ND 670	13	11

(Continued)

TABLE 9.1 (Continued)

Gender and Age	History, Symptoms and Comments	Delay Before Sampling	[C] Blood ng/mL or precised	[C] Urine ng/mL or precised	Hair: Color [C] pg/mg or precised	Ref.
F, 16 y	Sexual assault Sedated, alleged event 6 days after	9 w			4.2*/1/ND	58
M, 50 y	Inappropriate behavior with female students—alcohol +++ Loss of memory—repetitive exposure	4 w			21.3/21.5	58
M <25 y	Robbery, 1 cup of Imovane given by two women in a fruit juice—sedation, loss of memory				9*	59
F >70 y	Mistreatment in a retirement home Sedation—repetitive exposure				gray hair 135	14

*: period of the offense.
x/x/x/x: segment 1 (proximal)/segment 2/segment 3/etc.
M: male, F: female.
y: years, m: months, w: weeks, d: days.
ND: not detected.

TABLE 9.2 Controlled Studies

Number (Gender; Age)	Dose	Delay Before Sampling	Hair: Color [C] pg/mg or precised	References
Bromazepam/3-OH-bromazepam (OHB)				
2 (1 F, 1 M)	6 mg oral		0.8 and 4.7	12
6	3 to 12 mg		2.8 to 12	21
2	6 mg oral	3 to 5 w	1.3 and 2.5	60
1	6 mg oral		3.5	31
Clonazepam (C)/7NH2 clonazepam (AC)				
6	1 to 4 mg		AC: 2 to 12	21
2	2 mg oral	3 to 5 w	AC: 12 and 36	60
2	2 mg oral	3 w	AC: traces and 4.8	61
1	2 mg oral		AC: 22	31
Codeine				
9 (6 F, 3 M)	100 mg oral	1, 2, 3 and 4 w	up to 0.57	62
Diazepam (D)/Nordiazepam (N)				
3 from 6 (4 F, 2 M; 27 to 38 y)	10 mg oral	3 w	D: 2.3 to 6 N: traces to 5.7	63
Estazolam				
14	1 to 6 mg oral	1 m	0.56 to 2.60	64
Flunitrazepam (F)/7NH2-flunitrazepam (AF)				
10 (21 to 49 y)	2 mg oral	1 to 28 d	F: 0.5 to 2.3 AF: 0.5 to 8	65
1	1 mg oral	3 to 5 w	AF: 3.5	60
1	3 mg oral		2.0	31
GHB				
1	25 mg/kg oral		*Increase of 30 %/basal level*	66

(Continued)

TABLE 9.2 (Continued)

Number (Gender; Age)	Dose	Delay Before Sampling	Hair: Color [C] pg/mg or precised	References
1	25 mg/kg oral		Basal [C]: 3.0 Exposure period [C]: 5.1 *Increase of 170 %/basal level*	36
Glibenclamide				
1 (M, 44 y)	5 mg oral	1 m	5	38
1 (M)	20 mg/d oral during 1 y		650	38
Ketamine (K)/Norketamine (NK)				
4	10 mg oral	1 to 16 w	K: up to 19 NK: up to 18.7	67
Lorazepam				
2	2.5 mg oral	3 to 5 w	ND	60
1	1 mg oral		0.5 to 1	68
Selegeline				
10	15 mg oral		Amphetamine and metamphetamine: up to 120	69
Tetrazepam (T)/Diazepam (D) *like T metabolite*				
2 (1 F, 1 M)	50 mg oral	4 w	123 and 176	70
3 from 6 (4 F, 2 M; 27 to 38 y)	50 mg oral	3 w	T: 17.3 to 59.7	63
1 (F; 27 y)	25 mg/d oral during 1 w	3 w	T: 454/13 D: 10.7/ND	63
Zolpidem				
3	10 mg oral	3 to 5 w	1.8; 2.2 and 9.8	56

(*Continued*)

TABLE 9.2 (Continued)

Number (Gender; Age)	Dose	Delay Before Sampling	Hair: Color [C] pg/mg or precised	References
15	5 to 20 mg		1.2 to 19	21
2	10 mg oral	3 to 5 w	1.2 and 7.5	60
20 (12 F, 8 M; 21 to 44 y)	10 mg oral	1 m	135 to 554.6	71
Zopiclone				
2	7.5 mg oral	3 to 5 w	5.4 and 9.0	58
2	7.5 mg/d oral several m	3 to 5 w	37 and 66	58
2	7.5 mg oral	3 to 5 w	1.7 and 5.3	60

x/x/x/x: segment 1 (proximal)/segment 2/segment 3/etc.
M: male, F: female.
y: years, m: months, w: weeks, d: days.
ND: not detected.

3. DISCUSSION

More than 200 case reports concerning about 320 victims are listed in Table 9.1.

Case reports concern approximately 50 substances, essentially psychotropic compounds:

- Benzodiazepines drugs: 120 victims (alprazolam, bromazepam, clobazam, clonazepam (40 victims), diazepam, nordiazepam, oxazepam, flunitrazepam, lorazepam, lormetazepam, midazolam, nitrazepam, tetrazepam, triazolam).
- Neuroleptics and antipsychotic compounds: 54 victims (alimemazine/trimeprazine and niaprazine for the elderly and children, cyamemazine, clozapine, haloperidol, tiapride, risperidone, etc.).
- Hypnotics: zolpidem (36 victims) and zopiclone (13 victims).
- Antihistamine agents: 34 victims (diphenhydramine, doxylamine, tetrahydrozoline, etc.).
- Other sedatives: 16 victims (meprobamate, hydroxyzine and acepromazine).

- Drugs of abuse such as MDMA (3,4-methylenedioxy-N-methylamphetamine) (11 victims) or LSD (lysergic acid diethylamide).
- Opiate substitutes: methadone and buprenorphine (six victims).
- Anesthetics: ketamine and GHB (six victims), and midazolam.
- Scopolamine with atropine (*Datura*) or with codeine (Feminax®) in two case reports concerning six young victims.

However, some unusual substances such as glibenclamide, a hypoglycemic agent, digoxine, a cardiotropic agent, or solvents (benzene, xylene, toluene, chloroform) can be observed.

Gender is indicated in 64% of the case reports and 141 (78%) victims were women.

Age of the victims ranges from a few months to 96 years and confirms that DFC concerns children as well as the elderly.

Case histories and symptoms described in Table 9.1 confirm that most of the used substances possess amnesic properties. The victims are therefore less able to accurately remember the circumstances of the offense. Substances are generally short acting and impair an individual rapidly. Due to their low dosage, surreptitious administration into coffee, soda, alcoholic beverages and cakes, for example, is simple and often described by the victims.

The majority of the cases presented in the Table 9.1 contain hair analyses (84%). Blood and urine analyses provide short-term information (2−4 days for most drugs) of an individual's drug exposure, whereas long-term histories (weeks to months, depending on the length of the hair shaft) are accessible through hair analysis. It is especially useful in situations where collection relates to an event that occurred several weeks or months earlier. This can be observed in cases of DFCs with a lack of immediate reporting because of late complaints to the police, and blood and urine collection was achieved while compounds were already eliminated or in too low concentrations to be detected.

Tandem mass spectrometry appears to be a prerequisite for detection at very low concentrations (pg/mg) in hair. LC-MS/MS (liquid chromatography, tandem mass spectrometry) methods are performed in 80% of the case reports listed in Table 9.1, while GC-MS (gas chromatography-mass spectrometry) methods are used in 13% of the case reports (drugs of abuse, solvents, tetrahydrozoline, GHB and gamma-valerolactone in blood specimens). The GC-MS/MS method is necessary to perform GHB analysis in hair specimens.

This is particularly important for endogen compounds such as GHB. GHB exposure is demonstrated in hair analysis by comparing the concentrations along the hair shaft. Basal GHB concentration is five times less than GHB concentration in the segment corresponding to the time of the assault.[6,11,34−37]

A few cases listed in Table 9.1 do not report hair analyses. Sometimes, it is not possible to have hair specimens 3 weeks or more after the offense.

For each DFC case, the concentrations measured have to be compared with data available after administration of a single dose to obtain a suitable interpretation and to evaluate the amount of drug that could have been administered.

When it comes to interpreting drug concentrations in conventional specimens (blood and urine), it is relatively easy to use pharmacological studies. This aspect is described in Chapter 3.

By contrast, there is a lack of data for hair concentrations, as Kintz pointed out.[72] Bibliographic data on controlled studies are presented in Table 9.2. These concern few compounds compared to the data listed in Table 9.1 and these studies were often conducted by the same authors. However, the value of the concept of minimal detectable dosage in human hair is essential for interpretation.[72]

Even if hair analysis in DFC has been accepted in the forensic community, there is a lack of consensus among the active investigators on how to interpret the results of hair analysis.

4. CONCLUSION

DFC is a general term that includes the rape, sexual assault, robbery, money extortion or maltreatment of vulnerable people under the influence of psychotropic substances. It concerns mostly young people (especially women for DFSA), but also the elderly, children and mental health patients. This phenomenon has developed over the last 20 years or so, but for a long period, the lack of good analytical performance has led to a poor level of evidence. DFC has been now highlighted by an increase in reports worldwide.

Blood and urine are the conventional specimens to document drug exposure but the case reports presented in this chapter clearly indicate that the value of hair analysis is steadily gaining recognition.

In the last 15 years, the development of very sensitive chromatographic equipment such as LC-MS/MS or GC-MS/MS, which allows detection of a very low amount of xenobiotics in hair, was especially useful to document a single exposure to a drug.

Segmental hair analysis is a useful complement to blood and urine analysis to increase the window of detection of a DFC, and to differentiate a single exposure from chronic use. But, some issues concerning axial diffusion are to be considered for interpretation particularly in the case of young and elderly people.[73]

REFERENCES

1. Gaulier JM, Sauvage FL, Pauthier H, Saint-Marcoux F, Marquet P, Lachatre G. Identification of acepromazine in hair: an illustration of the difficulties encountered in investigating drug-facilitated crimes. *J Forensic Sci* 2008;**53**:755−9.
2. Dumestre-Toulet V, Laborie Charvier F, and Eyquem A. Mistreatment of older people in a retirement home: evidence of chemical abuse through hair analysis. In: *Proceedings of the 2011 TIAFT/SOFT International Meeting*, San Francisco, CA, 25−30 September 2011. p. 241.
3. Duffort G, Deveaux M, Cheze M, Pepin G. Neuroleptiques et anti-histaminiques: des molécules à ne pas négliger dans l'exploration de la soumission chimique. *Ann Toxicol Anal* 2006;**18**:174−5.
4. Raul JS, Jamey C, Tracqui A, Geraut A, Ludes B. Tiapride et vieilles dentelles: une observation inusitée de soumission chimique. *Ann Toxicol Anal* 2005;**17**:140−1.
5. Kintz P, Villain M, Cirimele V. Determination of trimeprazine-facilitated sedation in children by hair analysis. *J Anal Toxicol* 2006;**30**:400−2.
6. Kintz P, Villain M, Ludes B. Testing for the undetectable in drug-facilitated sexual assault using hair analyzed by tandem mass spectrometry as evidence. *Ther Drug Monit* 2004;**26**:211−4.
7. Kintz P, Villain M, Cirimele V. Chemical abuse in the elderly: evidence from hair analysis. *Ther Drug Monit* 2008;**30**:207−11.
8. Kim J, In S, Choi H, Lee S. Illegal use of benzodiazepines and/or zolpidem proved by hair analysis. *J Forensic Sci* 2013;**58**:548−51.
9. Lemaire-Hurtel AS, Durand-Maugard C, Devolder C, Grassin Delyle S, Hary L, Masson H, et al. Soumission chimique chez l'enfant: à propos d'un cas chez une fillette de 8 ans diagnostiqué en milieu hospitalier. *Ann Toxicol Anal* 2008;**20**:211−5.
10. Elsohly MA, Gul W, Elsohly KM, Avula B, Khan IA. LC-MS-(TOF) analysis method for benzodiazepines in urine samples from alleged drug-facilitated sexual assault victims. *J Anal Toxicol* 2006;**30**:524−38.
11. Pepin G, Cheze M, Duffort G, Vayssette F. De l'intérêt des cheveux et de la spectrométrie de masse tandem pour la soumission chimique: à propos de neuf cas. *Ann Toxicol Anal* 2002;**14**:395−406.
12. Villain M, Cheze M, Dumestre V, Ludes B, Kintz P. Hair to document drug-facilitated crimes: four cases involving bromazepam. *J Anal Toxicol* 2004;**28**:516−9.
13. Kintz P, Cirimele V, Villain M, Tracqui A, Ludes B. Soumission chimique: approches pratiques en toxicologie médico-légale. *Ann Toxicol Anal* 2002;**14**:361−4.
14. Kintz P, Villain M, Salquebre G, Cirimele V. Maltraitance chimique sur personne âgée. Pas de limite à l'arme chimique. *Ann Toxicol Anal* 2007;**19**:182.
15. Cheze M, Villain M, Pepin G. Determination of bromazepam, clonazepam and metabolites after a single intake in urine and hair by LC-MS/MS. Application to forensic cases of drug facilitated crimes. *Forensic Sci Int* 2004;**145**:123−30.
16. Gaillard Y, Masson-Seyer MF, Giroud M, Roussot JF, Prevosto JM. A case of drug-facilitated sexual assault leading to death by chloroform poisoning. *Int J Legal Med* 2006;**120**:241−5.
17. Cheze M, Duffort G, Deveaux M, Pepin G. Hair analysis by liquid chromatography-tandem mass spectrometry in toxicological investigation of drug-facilitated crimes: report of 128 cases over the period June 2003−May 2004 in metropolitan Paris. *Forensic Sci Int* 2005;**153**:3−10.

18. Cheze M, Muckensturm A, Hoizey G, Pepin G, Deveaux M. A tendency for re-offending in drug-facilitated crime. *Forensic Sci Int* 2010;**196**:14–7.

19. Villain M, Dumestre-Toulet V, Ludes B, Kintz P. Soumission chimique au clonazépam: caractérisation formelle par chromatographie en phase gazeuse couplée à la spectrométrie de masse tandem (CPG-SM/SM). *Ann Toxicol Anal* 2003;**15**:229–31.

20. Xiang P, Sun Q, Shen B, Chen P, Liu W, Shen M. Segmental hair analysis using liquid chromatography-tandem mass spectrometry after a single dose of benzodiazepines. *Forensic Sci Int* 2011;**204**:19–26.

21. Cheze M, Pepin G, Deveaux M. La soumission chimique: des analyses ultra-performantes. *Ann Toxicol Anal* 2005;**17**:141–2.

22. Alvarez JC, Abe E, Duverneuil C, Mathieu B, Bourokba N. Conjoint, médecin traitant: des personnes au-dessus de tout soupçon? *Ann Toxicol Anal* 2007;**19**:180–1.

23. Dumestre-Toulet V, Eyquem A, Villain M, Kintz P. La cocaïne n'en était pas: une soumission chimique originale. *Ann Toxicol Anal* 2007;**19**:153–6.

24. Villain M. Applications of hair in drug-facilitated crime evidence. In: Kintz P, editor. *Analytical and practical aspects of drug testing in hair*. Boca Raton: CRC Press; 2007. p. 255–72.

25. Bartsch C, Risse M, Schütz H, Weigand N, Weiler G. Munchausen syndrome by proxy (MSBP): an extreme form of child abuse with a special forensic challenge. *Forensic Sci Int* 2003;**137**:147–51.

26. Salomone A, Gerace E, Di Corcia D, Martra G, Petrarulo M, Vincenti M. Hair analysis of drugs involved in drug-facilitated sexual assault and detection of zolpidem in a suspected case. *Int J Legal Med* 2012;**126**:451–9.

27. Martínez MA, Ballesteros S. An unusual case of drug-facilitated sexual assault using aromatic solvents. *J Anal Toxicol* 2006;**30**:449–53.

28. Di Fazio V, Wille S, and Samyn N. Drug facilitated sexual assault by use of ketamine and diazepam by a gynaecologist. In: *Proceedings of the 21ème congrès annuel de la Société Française de Toxicologie Analytique, 51ème congrès de la Société de Toxicologie Clinique*; 2013, Saint Malo—11 au 14 juin. p. 27.

29. Eysseric H, Marka C, Bessard J, Jourdil N, Barret L. Les 16 victimes du Vercors dans l'affaire de l'Ordre du Temple Solaire: aspects toxicologiques. *Toxicorama* 1999;**11**:199.

30. Kintz P, Evans J, Villain M, Salquebre G, Cirimele V. Hair analysis for diphenhydramine after surreptitious administration to a child. *Forensic Sci Int* 2007;**173**:171–4.

31. Pepin G. Analytical, toxicological and forensic aspects of drug-facilitated crimes: 10 years of experience. *Ann Pharm Fr* 2010;**68**:61–75.

32. Villain M, Cirimele V, Kintz P. Soumission chimique. Recherche des benzodiazepines et hypnotiques dans les cheveux par LC-MS/MS. *Ann Toxicol Anal* 2005;**17**:33–42.

33. Andresen-Streichert H, Jungen H, Gehl A, Müller A, Iwersen-Bergmann S. Uptake of gamma-valerolactone: detection of gamma-hydroxyvaleric acid in human urine samples. *J Anal Toxicol* 2013;**37**:250–4.

34. Stillwell ME. Drug-facilitated sexual assault involving gamma-hydroxybutyric acid. *J Forensic Sci* 2002;**47**:1133–4.

35. Goulle JP, Cheze M, Pepin G. Determination of endogenous levels of GHB in human hair. Are there possibilities for the identification of GHB administration through hair analysis in cases of drug-facilitated sexual assault? *J Anal Toxicol* 2003;**27**:574–80.

36. Cirimele V, Baumgartner M, Vallet E, Duez M. Interprétation des concentrations de GHB mesurées dans les cheveux. *Ann Toxicol Anal* 2010;**22**:161–4.

37. Rossi R, Lancia M, Gambelunghe C, Oliva A, Fucci N. Identification of GHB and mor-phine in hair in a case of drug-facilitated sexual assault. *Forensic Sci Int* 2009;**186**:e9—11.

38. Villain M, Tournoud C, Flesch F, Cirimele V, Kintz P. Hair to document exposure to glib-enclamide. *J Chromatogr B: Analyt Technol Biomed Life Sci* 2006;**842**:111—5.

39. Fonseca S, Dias M. Munchausen by proxy with haloperidol: a case report. In: *Proceedings of the 2013 TIAFT International Meeting*, Funchal, Madeira, Portugal, 2—6 September 2013. p. 140.

40. Richeval C, Wiart JF, Humbert L, Lhermitte M. Screening for psycho-active drugs in case drug facilitated crimes: a case involving LSD. In: *Proceedings of the 2011 TIAFT/SOFT International Meeting*; 2008, San Francisco, CA, 25—30 September 2011. p. 144.

41. Sastre C, Cheze M, Baillif-Couniou V, Deveaux M, Pepin G, Leonetti G, Pelissier-Alicot AL. Amnésie antérograde consécutive à l'absorption de MDMA et d'alcool: à propos d'un cas. *Ann Toxicol Anal* 2012;**24**:23—7.

42. Deveaux M, Hoizey G, Cheze M, Muckensturm A, Pelissier-Alicot AL, Pepin G. Findings of MDMA and MDA in hair, blood and urine by LCESI-MS/MS: report of 11 drug facili-tated crime cases with anterograde amnesia. In: *Proceedings of the 2011 TIAFT/SOFT International Meeting*; 2011, San Francisco, CA, 25—30 September 2011. p. 017.

43. Eiden C, Cathala P, Fabresse N, Galea Y, Mathieu-Daude JC, Baccino E, Peyriere H. A case of drug-facilitated sexual assault involving 3,4-methylenedioxy-methylampheta-mine. *J Psychoactive Drugs* 2013;**45**:94—7.

44. Marinetti LJ, Antonides HM. Analysis of synthetic cathinones commonly found in bath salts in human performance and postmortem toxicology: method development, drug distri-bution and interpretation of results. *J Anal Toxicol* 2013;**37**:135—46.

45. Kintz P, Evans J, Villain M, Cirimele V. Interpretation of hair findings in children after methadone poisoning. *Forensic Sci Int* 2010;**196**:51—4.

46. Sibille P, Milan N, Ricordel I. Midazolam drug-facilitated crimes: three recent observations in hair. *Ann Toxicol Anal* 2008;**20**:S1—16.

47. Villain M, Vallet E, Cirimele V, Kintz P. Mise en évidence d'une soumission chimique à la niaprazine chez des enfants par analyse des cheveux en CL-SM/SM. *Ann Toxicol Anal* 2008;**20**:85—7.

48. Pujol ML, Villain M, Salquebre G, Vallet E, Cirimele V, Kintz P. Scopolamine: un nou-veau cas de soumission médicamenteuse sur des enfants. *Ann Toxicol Anal* 2006;**18**:207—12.

49. Stillwell ME, Saady JJ. Use of tetrahydrozoline for chemical submission. *Forensic Sci Int* 2012;**221**:e12—6.

50. Spiller HA, Siewert DJ. Drug-facilitated sexual assault using tetrahydrozoline. *J Forensic Sci* 2012;**57**:835—8.

51. Kintz P, Mccleary N, Gaulier JM. A US-France collaboration to document a drug-facilitated crime using tetrahydrozoline (Visine®). *TIAFT Bull* 2013;**43**:41—3.

52. Aknouche F, Besnard T, Buti R, Duval HP. Drug facilitated crime using tetrazepam. *TIAFT Bull* 2010;**40**:49.

53. Frison G, Favretto D, Tedeschi L, Ferrara SD. Detection of thiopental and pentobarbital in head and pubic hair in a case of drug-facilitated sexual assault. *Forensic Sci Int* 2003;**133**:171—4.

54. Cheze M, Lenoan A, Deveaux M, Pepin G. Simultaneous determination of 18 benzodia-zepines and their main metabolites in hair, blood and urine by LC-ESI-MS/MS.

Application to the determination of triazolam in a drug-facilitated crime. *Ann Toxicol Anal* 2008;**20**, S1−15.

55. Kintz P, Villain M, Dumestre-Toulet V, Ludes B. Drug-facilitated sexual assault and analytical toxicology: the role of LC-MS/MS. A case involving zolpidem. *J Clin Forensic Med* 2005;**12**:36−41.

56. Villain M, Cheze M, Tracqui A, Ludes B, Kintz P. Windows of detection of zolpidem in urine and hair: application to two drug facilitated sexual assaults. *Forensic Sci Int* 2004;**143**:157−61.

57. Maravelias C, Stefanidou M, Dona A, Athanaselis S, Spiliopoulou C. Drug-facilitated sexual assault provoked by the victim's religious beliefs: a case report. *Am J Forensic Med Pathol* 2009;**30**:384−5.

58. Villain M, Cheze M, Tracqui A, Ludes B, Kintz P. Testing for zopiclone in hair application to drug-facilitated crimes. *Forensic Sci Int* 2004;**145**:117−21.

59. Cheze M, Pepin G. Mise en évidence d'un cas de soumission chimique après prise d'un seul comprimé d'Imovane® par l'analyse séquentielle. Comparaison des différentes techniques HPLC/BD, HPLC/MS/MS à trappe d'ions, HPLC/MS/MS à triple quadripôle. *Ann Toxicol Anal* 2003;**15**:153.

60. Deveaux M, Cheze M, Pepin G. The role of liquid chromatography-tandem mass spectrometry (LC-MS/MS) to test blood and urine samples for the toxicological investigation of drug-facilitated crimes. *Ther Drug Monit* 2008;**30**:225−8.

61. Negrusz A, Moore CM, Kern JL, Janicak PG, Strong MJ, Levy NA. Quantitation of clonazepam and its major metabolite 7-aminoclonazepam in hair. *J Anal Toxicol* 2000;**24**:614−20.

62. Kronstrand R, Förstberg-Peterson S, Kågedal B, Ahlner J, Larson G. Codeine concentration in hair after oral administration is dependent on melanin content. *Clin Chem* 1999;**45**:1485−94.

63. Laloup M, Ramirez Fernandez M, Wood M, Maes V, De Boeck G, Vanbeckevoort Y, Samyn N. Detection of diazepam in urine, hair and preserved oral fluid samples with LC-MS-MS after single and repeated administration of Myolastan and Valium. *Anal Bioanal Chem* 2007;**388**:1545−56.

64. Xiang P, Sun Q, Shen B, Chen P, Liu W, Shen M. Segmental hair analysis using liquid chromatography-tandem mass spectrometry after a single dose of benzodiazepines. *Forensic Sci Int* 2011;**204**:19−26.

65. Negrusz A, Moore CM, Hinkel KB, Stockham TL, Verma M, Strong MJ, Janicak PG. Deposition of 7-aminoflunitrazepam and flunitrazepam in hair after a single dose of Rohypnol. *J Forensic Sci* 2001;**46**:1143−51.

66. Kintz P, Cirimele V, Jamey C, Ludes B. Testing for GHB in hair by GC/MS/MS after a single exposure. Application to document sexual assault. *J Forensic Sci* 2003;**48**:195−200.

67. Xiang P, Sun Q, Shen B, Shen M. Disposition of ketamine and norketamine in hair after a single dose. *Int J Legal Med* 2011;**125**:831−40.

68. Gaulier JM, Mercerolle M, Sauvage FL, Lamballais F, Lachatre G. Soumission chimique: des difficultés à chaque étape, illustrées par un cas de viol en réunion sous lorazepam. In: *Proceedings of the 18ème congrès annuel de la Société Française de Toxicologie Analytique*; 2010, Antibes Juan-Les-Pins—9 au 11 juin. p. 48.

69. Kronstrand R, Andersson MC, Ahlner J, Larson G. Incorporation of selegiline metabolites into hair after oral selegiline intake. *J Anal Toxicol* 2001;**25**:594−601.

70. Concheiro M, Villain M, Bouchet S, Ludes B, López-Rivadulla M, Kintz P. Windows of detection of tetrazepam in urine, oral fluid, beard, and hair, with a special focus on drug-facilitated crimes. *Ther Drug Monit* 2005;**27**:565–70.
71. Cui X, Xiang P, Zhang J, Shi Y, Shen B, Shen M. Segmental hair analysis after a single dose of zolpidem: comparison with a previous study. *J Anal Toxicol* 2013;**37**:1–7.
72. Kintz P. Value of the concept of minimal detectable dosage in human hair. *Forensic Sci Int* 2012;**218**:28–30.
73. Kintz P. Issues about axial diffusion during segmental hair analysis. *Ther Drug Monit* 2013;**5**:408–10.

Chapter 10

The Specific Problem of Children and Old People in Drug-Facilitated Crime Cases

Pascal Kintz

1. INTRODUCTION

The use of a drug to modify a person's behavior for criminal gain is not a recent phenomenon. However, the sudden increase in reports of drug-facilitated crimes, or DFC (sexual assaults, robbery, administration for sedation, etc.), has caused alarm in the general public. The drugs involved can be pharmaceuticals, drugs of abuse or more often ethanol. Most of these substances possess amnesic properties and therefore the victims are less able to accurately recall the circumstances under which the offense occurred. As they are generally short acting, these substances can rapidly impair an individual. Due to their low dosage, except for GHB, a surreptitious administration into beverages such as coffee, soft drinks (e.g. Cola) or even better alcoholic cocktails is relatively simple.[1]

To perform successful toxicological examinations, the analyst must follow some important rules[1]: obtain the corresponding biological specimens quickly (blood, urine and hair),[2] use sophisticated analytical techniques (GC-MS—gas chromatography-mass spectrometry—LC-MS/MS—liquid chromatography coupled with tandem mass spectrometry—headspace/GC-MS, accurate mass spectrometry), and[3] interpret of the findings correctly.

The narrow window of detection of GHB, 6 and 10 hours in blood and urine, respectively, is an example of the current limitation of these specimens to demonstrate exposure after late sampling. For all compounds involved in DFC, the detection times in blood and urine depend mainly on the dose and sensitivity of the method used. Prohibiting immunoassays and using only hyphenated techniques, substances can be found in blood from 6 hours to 3–4 days and in urine from 12 hours to up to 10 days.[2] Sampling blood or urine has low importance 48–72 hours after the offense has occurred.

Toxicological Aspects of Drug-Facilitated Crimes. DOI: http://dx.doi.org/10.1016/B978-0-12-416748-3.00010-4

To address a response to this important caveat, hair was suggested as a valuable specimen. While there are a lot of papers focused on the identification of drugs (mainly drugs of abuse) in hair following chronic use, those dealing with a controlled single dose are very scarce.[3]

When using hair analysis as a matrix during investigative analysis, it is important to know whether the analytical procedure was sensitive enough to identify traces of drugs; this is particularly so when the urine sample(s) of the subject was positive and the hair sample(s) was negative. It has been accepted in the forensic community that a negative hair result cannot exclude the administration of a particular drug, or one of its precursors, and the negative findings should not overrule a positive urine result. Nevertheless, negative hair findings can, on occasion, cast doubt on the positive urine analysis, resulting in substantial legal debate and various consequences for the subject.

The concept of minimal detectable dosage in hair is of interest to document the negative findings, but limited data are currently available in the scientific literature. Such data include cocaine, codeine, ketamine, some benzodiazepines and some unusual compounds.[3]

Until laboratories have sensitive enough methodologies to detect a single use of a drug, care should be taken to compare urine and hair findings.

This is even more complicated at the two scales of life, for both young people and the elderly. Immature enzymatic processes in children and renal or hepatic failure in aged subjects will influence the circulating drug blood concentrations and therefore the level of impairment. In some cases, what can be detected as a normal concentration for a healthy adult can be fatal for young or elderly people. Moreover, the physiology of hair, one of the three mandatory specimens in each DFC case, is different according to the age of the subject.

2. AGE AS A FACTOR OF INFLUENCE OF DRUG DISTRIBUTION

Changes in the rate but not the extent of drug absorption are usually observed with age. Factors that affect drug absorption (gastric pH and emptying, intestinal motility, blood flow) change with age. Gastric acid secretion does not approach adult levels until the age of 3 and gastric emptying and peristalsis is slow during the first months of life. Higher gastric pH, delayed gastric emptying and decreased intestinal motility and blood flow are observed in elderly individuals.[4]

Children are not "little adults" but rather immature individuals whose bodies and organ functions are in a continuing state of development. More particularly, the new-born infant has to adapt very rapidly to a new environment by going through a series of rapid and continuous anatomical and physiological changes. It is not surprising, therefore, that the pharmacokinetics and toxicity of most drugs vary considerably throughout the pediatric age range and may differ profoundly from findings in adults.[5]

Most drugs for children are administered orally. Oral preparations are cheaper to manufacture and are more acceptable to children. There are differences between adults and children in terms of drug distribution; body composition and protein binding are responsible for many of these differences. Water soluble drugs will have a greater volume of distribution in the neonate. Sometimes, the neonate may require a greater loading dose per kg compared to the older child to have a similar effect. Muscle and fat content as a proportion of total body mass is smaller in neonates compared to older children. Therefore, anesthetic drugs that redistribute to muscle and fat would be expected to have a prolonged clinical effect. Protein binding is altered during (approximately) the first 6 months of life. The effect of reduced quantity and quality of protein binding has a marked effect on the concentration of "free" active drug as well as its ability to cross membranes—it is of particular importance in those drugs that are highly protein bound, such as phenytoin, diazepam, bupivacaine, barbiturates, many antibiotics and theophylline. Other factors that alter distribution include regional blood flow and the maturation of the blood—brain barrier.

The metabolism of many drugs is dependent on the liver and its blood flow. Hepatic blood flow is reduced in the neonate and increases as a proportion of the cardiac output as the infant matures. The complex enzyme systems involved in drug metabolism mature at differing rates in the pediatric population. Many drugs undergo Phase I metabolism and are metabolized by enzymes of the cytochrome p450 system. The important gene families of these iso-enzymes are CYP1, CYP2 and CYP3. The enzymes of these families develop at very different rates. The development is also variable between individuals, which emphasizes the need to titrate drugs to effect or to concentration levels if available. As an example of this variability, the enzyme CYP2D6 is responsible for transforming codeine into its active form of morphine. The activity of this enzyme is very low in neonates and can take more than 5 years to develop to adult levels. In contrast, CYP3A4 has an important role in the metabolism of many drugs, e.g. midazolam, diazepam, paracetamol; however, it matures rapidly to adult levels in the first 6—12 months of life.

Renal efficiency in neonates is considerably reduced compared to adults. This is due to a combination of factors; incomplete glomerular development with immature glomerular filtration and tubular function, low renal perfusion pressure and inadequate osmotic load to produce full counter-current effects.

The pharmacokinetics of several drugs have been shown to be influenced by concurrent disease process, often observed in older people. The clearance of many drugs decreases in those individuals with chronic hepatic disease, such as cirrhosis. The volumes of distribution of some drugs are unaltered in hepatic disease while an increase is observed for other drugs, especially those bound to albumin. Renal disease such as uremia may result in decreased renal clearance of certain drugs. Further, respiratory diseases such as cystic fibrosis increase the renal clearance of some drugs.

Finally, elderly persons commonly receive two or more drugs concurrently. Multiple drug use may result in drug interactions that may end in decreased therapeutic efficacy or an increased risk of toxicity.[6]

Aging is characterized by a progressive loss of functional capacities of most if not all organs, a reduction in homeostatic mechanisms and a response to receptor stimulation. Also, loss of water content and an increase in fat content in the body are reported. Analysis of data revealed that the most important pharmacokinetic changes in old age include a decrease in the excretory capacity of the kidney more than the decline in the rate of hepatic drug metabolism. In the elderly, the central nervous system becomes vulnerable to agents that affect brain function (e.g. opioids, benzodiazepines and psychotropic drugs). Therefore, these drugs must be used very cautiously in this age group.[7] Use of hypnotics or sedatives in old age seems to be related to female gender. Also, among elderly users of hypnotics or sedatives, women appear to be more likely to use benzodiazepines and benzodiazepine-related drugs than men.[8] In general, recommendations for the pharmacotherapy of insomnia in elderly patients include using a reduced dosage. For some substances (e.g. zolpidem, zopiclone, zaleplon, temazepam and triazolam) the dosage is half that recommended for younger patients.[9] This has obvious consequences when interpreting blood concentrations in cases where old persons have been surreptitiously administered such a drug for the first time.

3. THE SPECIFIC PROBLEM FOR CHILDREN

From our experience, children are exposed to drugs in two major situations:

- to sedate them to keep them quiet
- to sedate them for the purposes of sexual assault

It seems that the former situation is underreported and only discovered by the authorities when the child is experiencing an overdose or even when death has occurred.

Excepting the lower amount of biological material in children versus adults, there is no specific analytical problem when processing samples from children. Obviously, the same procedure can be used. The issue is the interpretation of the findings with respect to the different pharmacological parameters. Although numerous controlled studies have been performed in adults, those dealing with children are very scarce, except for antiepileptic drugs. The following examples are from the author's daily practice and are presented to demonstrate how interpretation was difficult. Drugs involved in these cases belong to various pharmaceutical classes or are listed as drugs of abuse.

3.1 Tetrahydrozoline

Topical imidazolines are found in many over-the-counter eye and nose decongestants. These drugs have central and peripheral alpha-2 agonist activity. Significant clinical consequences (respiratory depression, hypotension and bradycardia) can occur from ingestions in young children, requiring intensive care management.[10] In addition, imidazolines have been used in DFSA[11] to induce comatose victims that are unable to fend off the perpetrator, with an effect similar to that of clonidine. Products with imidazoline components are numerous and include tetrahydrozoline, sold as Visine®. The medication relieves itching, burning and watery eyes due to pollen and dust. This drug is not available in France.

A 6-year-old boy was living in France with his mother, an American lady, recently divorced. She was unable to take care of him due to lack of interest. Drowsiness, ataxia, sedation, muscular weakness and marked somnolence were noted at school and during the weekend, when the boy was with his father. These symptoms were present at least for 2 months. The father refused a hair specimen to be collected but asked to achieve a general unknown screening procedure in urine for sedative drugs. The urine was collected about 18 to 20 hours after the child was in contact with the mother. The testing, done by LC-MS/MS, was returned negative. The possibility of using a product not marketed in France, and therefore not screened by the target LC-MS/MS method, was an issue. After discussion with an American colleague, a literature search about specific US drugs used in DFCs and the discovery of a Visine® container in the mother's bag, potential exposure to tetrahydrozoline was discussed. Therefore, the urine was tested a second time for this specific drug.

The boy's urine tested positive at 257 ng/mg, demonstrating exposure to tetrahydrozoline within the hours before collection (Figure 10.1).

Visine contains 0.05% tetrahydrozoline (500 µg/ml). Few data about urine concentrations in children are available in the literature. After administration of two drops directly into the conjunctival sac of each eye, 10 adult patients had detectable urine concentrations 24 hours post dosing (range: 13 to 210 ng/ml).[12] Stillwell and Saady[11] found 1481 ng/ml (7 hours after ingestion) and 108 ng/ml (23 hours after ingestion) in two cases of chemical submission. The measured concentration in the present case is therefore consistent with exposure to the drug for its sedative properties but remains difficult to interpret in the case of a child.

3.2 Niaprazine

Niaprazine, under the trade name Nopron, is largely used in France as a hypnotic agent for occasional insomnia in children. This compound is available without medical prescription. Three children (two girls and one boy) were

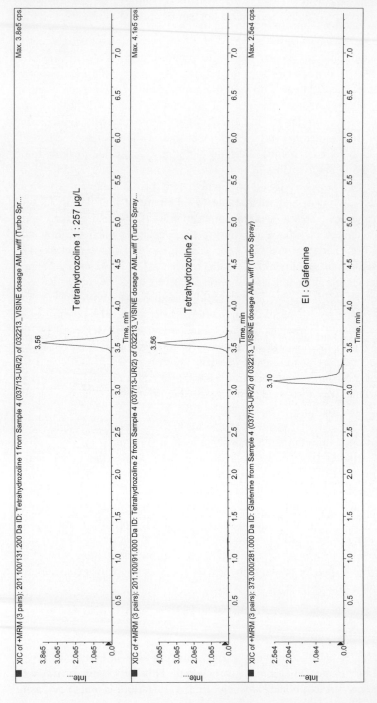

FIGURE 10.1 MRM chromatogram of the urine of a child poisoned with tetrahydrozoline. Concentration was 257 ng/ml.

repetitively sedated and assaulted by their father-in-law for several years. Niaprazine's liquid formulation is ideal for surreptitiously administering it in beverages. According to the request of the judge in charge of this case, the victims' hair was collected, segmented and screened for sedatives by LC-MS/MS.

Niaprazine was detected in the range 21 to 382, <LOQ to 315, 2642 to 3431 pg/mg for the three children, respectively. These concentrations could not be compared with previous results, due to a lack of literature. In particular, it was not possible to put any quantitative interpretation on the dosage that was administered to the children. It is, however, obvious that repetitive administrations have occurred but it is not possible to determine the number of exposures. Given the length of the hair, exposure to niaprazine should have occurred at least during the previous months. The surreptitious administration of niaprazine to obtain sedation was considered a DFC, even in an intra-familial situation. According to the French law, the drug can be considered as a chemical weapon.[13]

3.3 Alprazolam

Alprazolam (Xanax), a triazolobenzodiazepine derivative (1,4−benzodiazepine), is an antidepressant and anxiolytic agent. This drug is prescribed for the treatment of anxiety and panic disorder.

A 12-year-old girl claimed to have been repetitively assaulted (once per week) since she was 6 by her father and obliged to have oral sex. During the last 3 months of the period of the offense, to be more willing, she was sometimes administered half of a white tablet of Xanax 0.5 mg. Her father claimed to the police that he offered the drug on only three to four occasions during this time. The victim's hair was analyzed to document alprazolam exposure. Benzodiazepines and hypnotics were tested by LC-MS/MS and the first 2 cm segment was positive for alprazolam at a concentration of 4.9 pg/mg, the second (2 to 4 cm) positive at 2.4 pg/mg, whereas the last segment (4 to 6 cm) was alprazolam free. This appears to be consistent with few recent exposures to the drug.

In a second case, a 16-year-old adolescent met with friends of a relative that sequestered her in an apartment where she was physically abused and obliged to act as a prostitute. Several times at dinner she was given a drug that made her sedated. She noticed impairment associated with loss of memory. One day, she succeeded in running away and went to the police. Hair was collected and analyzed by LC-MS/MS. Despite bleached hair, alprazolam was identified in four consecutive 1-cm segments at 3.1, 0.8, 0.4 and 0.4 pg/mg, respectively.[14]

3.4 Buprenorphine

Under the trade name Subutex®, buprenorphine is largely used for the substitution management of opiate-dependent individuals, but can also be easily

found on the black market. A 14-year-old boy was found dead at the apartment of a well-known sex offender of minors. According to a police report,
this was not the first time the boy was seen around this apartment. A blister
of Subutex® was discovered at the scene. At the autopsy, no particular
morphological changes were noted, except for pulmonary and visceral
congestion. There was no evidence of violence and no needle mark was
found by the pathologist. Toxicological analyses, as achieved by LC-MS,
demonstrated both recent and repetitive buprenorphine exposure in combination with nordiazepam. Buprenorphine concentrations were 1.1 ng/ml and
23 pg/mg in blood and hair, respectively. Noruprenorphine concentration
was 0.2 ng/ml in blood and it was not detected in hair. Blood concentrations
were considered to correspond to therapeutic treatment in the case of a
heroin addict. The death of the boy was attributed to accidental asphyxia,
in a facilitated repetitive sexual abuse situation, due to the combination
of buprenorphine and benzodiazepines, even at therapeutic concentrations.
To make the boy vulnerable to sexual activity, he was administered a
mixture of buprenorphine and benzodiazepine. The aim of these drugs was
to induce sedation and to lower inhibitions. There was no intent to poison
the boy, even in the case of repetitive administrations. The use of buprenorphine as a sedative drug was not challenged by the perpetrator who was
charged for accidental homicide.[15]

3.5 Trimeprazine

Trimeprazine or alimemazine is largely used as an antipruritic agent but also
for insomnia, cough and oral premedication in pediatric day surgery. This
case involved repetitive sedation linked to the use of trimeprazine as a DFC
and subsequent impairment of two children. The children were living with
their stepmother. She was unable to take care of them due to lack of interest.
Drowsiness, ataxia, sedation, muscular weakness and marked somnolence
were noted in both children at school and during the weekend. These symptoms were present for at least 3 months. Due to the long delay between the
alleged crime and clinical examination, collection of blood or urine was of
little value. A strand of hair from each child was sampled about 2 months
after the first suspicion of administration and was cut into small segments. In
the hair of the two subjects, trimeprazine was detected at concentrations in
the range 23 to 339 pg/mg. Segmental analyses are presented in Table 10.1.
These concentrations could not be compared with previous results due to a
lack of literature. In particular, it was not possible to put any quantitative
interpretation on the dosage that was administered to the children. Given the
length of the boy's hair, exposure to trimeprazine should have occurred at
least during the previous 5 months. This is confirmed by the analysis of the
girl's hair. According to the police investigations, the window of potential
drug exposure was about 5 months, during the time the children were under

TABLE 10.1 Trimeprazine Concentrations after Segmental Analyses of the Hair of Both Children

Segment	Boy	Girl
1	126 pg/mg (0 to 2.5 cm)	339 pg/mg (0 to 2 cm)
2	127 pg/mg (2.5 to 5 cm)	199 pg/mg (2 to 4 cm)
3		23 pg/mg (4 to 6 cm)
4		Not detected (6 to 8 cm)

the responsibility of their stepmother. All symptoms of impairment disappeared after the children were placed with another family. The stepmother, who was the perpetrator in both cases, did not challenge the use of trimeprazine as a sedative drug.[16]

3.6 Diphenhydramine

Diphenhydramine was one of the first effective antihistamine agents discovered, its properties having been described in 1946. The compound is also used for its sedative and antiemetic effects. It is also a popular remedy for motion sickness and a common constituent of cough remedies. A wide variety of "over-the-counter" preparations exist in the form of tablets, capsules and elixirs to promote sleep and in the treatment of coughs, thus making it an easily accessible drug to the potential assailant. In addition, diphenhydramine's liquid formulations represent a suitable form for the surreptitious addition to beverages. After diphenhydramine exposure, subjective sedation, reduced sleep latencies and impairment in the performance of tasks requiring sustained attention were noticed.

This investigation began after a man left his phone number on the door of a train toilet asking young girls to contact him for sex. The police prompted a complex 10-month investigation that uncovered child abuse on eight victims. Among these victims, a 9-year-old girl was assaulted and the incident was filmed by two alleged assailants. Examination of mobile phones belonging to the suspects found references in text messages to "Nytol" and its use to subdue potential victims. Items recovered from the home of an accomplice were identified as Nytol®, a pharmaceutical tablet preparation with diphenhydramine as active ingredient. The child was not under medical prescription of the drug. A single strand of hair from the victim was obtained approximately 7 weeks after the alleged incident. It was brown in color and around 32 cm in length with no evidence of coloring or chemical treatment.

TABLE 10.2 Diphenhydramine Concentrations after Segmental Analysis of the Hair

Segment	Hair Concentrations
0 to 1 cm (13 mg)	37 pg/mg
1 to 3 cm (26 mg)	39 pg/mg
3 to 5 cm (28 mg)	33 pg/mg

It is obvious that LC-MS/MS is the method of choice for testing low levels of drug in hair due to its extraordinary sensitivity and specificity. The hair specimen supplied was very small and this only permitted 10−15 mg of hair per segment to be used; nevertheless the signal-to-noise ratio was considered as largely acceptable. The results of the segmental analyses are presented in Table 10.2. Diphenhydramine was detected in the range 33 to 39 pg/mg. The significance of these concentrations could not be determined due to a lack of data in the literature. In particular, it was not possible to put any quantitative interpretation on the dosage that was administered to the child. It is, however, obvious that repetitive administrations have occurred but it is not possible to determine the number of exposures. Given the length of the segment analyzed, exposure to diphenhydramine was expected to have occurred over a period of at least 5 months prior to the hair sample being obtained. This evidence was not challenged during the court trial.[17]

3.7 Carbamazepine

The scientific literature dealing with carbamazepine (an anti-epileptic drug but also an antidepressant with slight sedative properties) detection in hair is well documented. In various papers, the concentrations of carbamazepine in the hair of adult patients under daily therapy are >10 ng/mg.[18] At this time, nothing has been published about the detection of carbamazepine in the hair of children.

A recent case dealing with child custody has been noted, where the final outcome was difficult to establish. The following concentrations were measured by LC-MS/MS in the hair of a 21-month-old girl: 154 (0−1 cm), 198 (1−2 cm), 247 (2−3 cm) and 368 pg/mg (3−4 cm) after decontamination.

Obviously, the concentrations measured in the hair are much lower than those observed in patients under daily treatment. In that sense, exposures appear to be less frequent (low level of exposure), with a marked decrease in the more recent period. However, the girl was never prescribed carbamazepine and the mother, who was under carbamazepine therapy, denied any administration.

As a consequence, contamination was considered as an issue and interpretation of the results was a challenge that deserved particular attention. It was asked by the judge if this could result from a single exposure and at which period. There are many differences between the hair from children and those from adults: the hair from children is thinner and more porous, the ratio of anagen/catagen phases is not maintained, and the growth rate can be different, at some periods, from the usual 1 cm/month.

At least three possible interpretations of the measured carbamazepine concentrations were addressed: a) decrease in administration in the more recent period; b) increase of body weight due to physical development, so the same dosage will result in lower concentrations in hair; and c) sweat contamination from the mother at the time the girl was with her in bed, the older hair being in contact with the bedding for longer. In this case, it was impossible to conclude that the child was deliberately administered carbamazepine. The results of the analysis of hair could indicate that she was in an environment where carbamazepine was being used and where the drug was not being handled and stored with appropriate care. In view of these results it was concluded that a single determination should not be used firmly to categorize long-term exposure to a drug.

3.8 Glibenclamide and Munchausen's Syndrome by Proxy

Munchausen by proxy syndrome (MBPS) is a relatively rare form of child abuse that involves the exaggeration or fabrication of illnesses or symptoms by a parent or caregiver. Also known as "medical child abuse," MBPS was named after Baron von Munchausen, an eighteenth-century German dignitary known for making up stories about his travels and experiences in order to get attention. "By proxy" indicates that a parent or other adult, and not the child, is fabricating or exaggerating the infant's symptoms.

The adult deliberately misleads others (particularly medical professionals), and may go as far as to actually cause symptoms in the child through poisoning, medication or even suffocation. In most cases, the mother is responsible for causing the illness or symptoms. Typically, the cause is a need for attention and sympathy from doctors, nurses and other professionals. Some experts believe that it is not just attention that is gained from the child's "illness" that drives this behavior, but also the satisfaction in deceiving individuals who they consider to be more important and powerful than themselves. Because the parent or caregiver appears to be so caring and attentive, often no one suspects any wrongdoing. Diagnosis is made extremely difficult due to the ability of the parent or caregiver to manipulate doctors and induce symptoms in their child.

Often, the perpetrator is familiar with the medical profession and knowledgeable about how to induce illness or impairment in the child. Medical personnel often overlook the possibility of MBPS because it goes against the belief that parents and caregivers would never deliberately hurt their child. Most victims of MBPS are pre-schoolers (although there have been cases in children up to 16 years old), and there are equal numbers of boys and girls. Often, hospitalization is required. And because these children may be deemed a "medical mystery," hospital stays tend to be longer than usual. Whatever the cause, the child's symptoms decrease or completely disappear when the perpetrator is not present. According to experts, common conditions and symptoms that are created or fabricated by parents or caregivers with MBPS can include: failure to thrive, allergies, asthma, vomiting, diarrhea, seizures and infections. The long-term prognosis for these children depends on the degree of damage created by the illness or impairment and the amount of time it takes to recognize and diagnose MBPS. Some extreme cases have been reported in which children developed destructive skeletal changes, limps, mental retardation, brain damage and blindness from symptoms caused by the parent or caregiver. If the child lives long enough to comprehend what is happening, the psychological damage can be significant. The child may come to feel that he or she will only be loved when ill and may, therefore, help the parent try to deceive doctors, using self-abuse to avoid being abandoned. Therefore, some victims of MBPS are at risk of repeating the cycle of abuse.

If MBPS is suspected, healthcare providers are required by law to report their concerns. However, after a parent or caregiver is charged, the child's symptoms may increase as the person who is accused attempts to prove the presence of the illness. If the parent or caregiver repeatedly denies the charges, the child would likely be removed from the home and legal action would be taken on the child's behalf. In some cases, the parent or caregiver may deny the charges and move to another location, only to continue the behaviour. Even if the child is returned to the perpetrator's custody while protective services are involved, the child may continue to be a victim of abuse while the perpetrator avoids treatment and interventions.[19]

A 13-year-old girl was admitted to the emergency unit for coma and seizures after a stay with her mother. Blood glucose was 0.38 g/l. Blood screening for general unknowns revealed the presence of glibenclamide at 28 ng/ml. Glibenclamide is a potent, second-generation oral sulfonylurea antidiabetic agent widely used to lower glucose levels in patients with type II non-insulin-dependent diabetes mellitus. It acts mainly by stimulating endogenous insulin release from beta cells of the pancreas. The administration of glibenclamide by a parent (generally the mother) to a child has already been described.[20] Among the causes for recurrent hypoglycemic episodes in seemingly healthy patients, discriminating between sulfonylurea-induced hypoglycemia and insulinoma is of utmost importance because of medico-legal implications.

Several unnecessary laparotomies and partial pancreatectomies due of errone-
ous diagnosis of insulinoma involving patients with surreptitious sulfonylurea
exposure (inadvertent or factitious) have been reported. Therefore, toxicological analyses can be helpful. In the case of late sampling, blood or urine has little interest, and hair[21] must be considered as the best opportunity to document
exposure. The mother did not challenge the use of glibenclamide.

3.9 Methadone

With the exception of use in the treatment of opioid dependence, methadone
cannot be prescribed to children under 15 years of age. Low doses (1 mg/kg)
can be lethal to children, hence the presence of methadone in a household
(for use by parents, grandparents, etc.) with little or no respect for the safe
storage of the drug, poorly closed caps (even those with child-resistant caps)
and poor domestic hygiene conditions (e.g. contamination of dishes and uten-
sils). In cases of accidental or intentional administration, a lack of immediate
care when respiratory depression and/or intense sedation are observed can
prove fatal.

During recent years,[22] requests have been received to test for methadone
and EDDP, its major metabolite, in hair from children that were admitted to
hospital unconscious and where methadone had already been identified in a
body fluid (four cases) or where the children were deceased and evidence of
methadone overdosage had already been established (two cases).

Case 1: a boy was taken to hospital unconscious where a urine sample
was obtained and confirmed the presence of methadone. The police
requested testing of a hair sample for any evidence of previous methadone administration. A strand of hair 4 cm in length and blonde in color
was collected.

Case 2: parents were suspected of administering methadone to a
16-month-old child. A strand of hair 5 cm in length and blonde in color
was collected.

Case 3: this case involved a suggestion that methadone was administered
to a child over period of time. A strand of hair 4.5 cm in length and
blonde in color was collected. The hair tested positive for both heroin
and cocaine.

Case 4: a child was admitted to hospital after allegedly drinking some of
her mother's methadone. The investigators wanted know if the child had
been exposed to the drug on other occasions. A strand of hair 15 cm in
length and brown in color was collected.

Case 5: a 2-year-old child died of methadone overdose. A history of use
was required to assist the police in assessing if it was a one-off dose or if
it had been given on more than one occasion. A strand of hair 4 cm in
length and light brown in color was collected.

Case 6: a child (3 years old) was found dead at home. Both parents were reported to have been under methadone therapy. Analysis of cardiac blood tested positive for methadone at 0.24 mg/l. The police requested the testing of a hair sample to assess if there was any historical evidence that the mother or the father may have administered the drug to the child on more than one occasion. A strand of hair 4.5 cm in length and brown in color was collected.

After decontamination with dichloromethane and segmentation, the hair was cut into small pieces, incubated overnight at 40°C, liquid—liquid extracted and analyzed with LC-MS/MS, using two transitions per compound. The LOQ for both methadone and EDDP was 10 pg/mg. Individual data from each child are presented in Table 10.3. In all cases the methadone concentration was lower than 1 ng/mg. Although 20 mg of hair per segment was used, it must be considered that the amount available for analysis can be lower, particularly when other drugs of abuse have to be tested. This has consequences on the limit of quantitation and the identification of the metabolite EDDP, which is always at a lower concentration when compared to the parent drug. It must be also noted that hair from children is finer and more porous than hair from adults.

The relatively homogeneous concentrations of methadone along the hair lock in each specific case were surprising. In the past,[23] such a situation has been considered indicative of external contamination. Thus, the presence of homogeneous consecutive concentrations after segmental analysis in hair samples obtained from children known to have had methadone in their body close to the time of sampling may be considered indicative of potential contamination from an individual's body fluids or tissues.

The routine decontamination procedure of the laboratory involves two consecutive washes with 5 mL of dichloromethane for 5 minutes at room temperature, when about 200 mg of hair are processed. This procedure has been used for 20 years and is efficient for various compounds, including drugs of abuse, pharmaceuticals and doping. In cases involving dirty specimens (blood stains, vomit stains, ground, etc.), the specimens are pre-washed with warm water until a clear effluent is obtained, in addition to the 2 × 5 mL dichloromethane washes. In cases where there is some suspicion of external contamination, the second dichloromethane wash is analyzed and the ratio total concentration in hair (in ng) to concentration in wash is established. When this ratio is higher than 10, this indicates drug exposure as opposed to external contamination.

In the six cases, the last dichloromethane wash was negative for the target drugs. As hair damage or degradation promotes both contamination and incorporation via drug containing body fluids, a visual evaluation of the specimens was undertaken and this did not identify actual degradation.

The differentiation between drug use and external contamination has been frequently referred to as one of the limitations of drug testing in hair.

TABLE 10.3 Concentrations of Methadone and EDDP Measured in the Six Cases

Case	Segment	Methadone (ng/mg)	EDDP (ng/mg)
1	0–1 cm	0.05	<LOQ
	1–2 cm	0.07	<LOQ
	2–3 cm	0.07	<LOQ
	3–4 cm	0.08	<LOQ
2	0–1 cm	0.13	0.02
	1–2 cm	0.14	0.02
	2–3 cm	0.15	0.02
	3–5 cm	0.15	0.02
3	0–1.5 cm	0.08	0.02
	1.5–3 cm	0.07	0.01
	3–4.5 cm	0.09	0.03
4	0–2 cm	0.13	0.03
	2–4 cm	0.07	0.01
	4–6 cm	0.07	0.01
	6–8 cm	0.07	0.01
5	0–2 cm	0.53	<LOQ
	2–4 cm	0.58	<LOQ
6	0–1 cm	0.44	0.04
	1–2 cm	0.63	0.05
	2–3 cm	0.77	0.05
	3–4.5 cm	0.65	0.06

The detection of relevant metabolite(s) has been proposed to minimize the possibility of external contamination causing misinterpretation. Difficulty arises when a metabolite is not detected due either to the absence of specific metabolite or to low doses of the drug being used. Moreover, the presence of a metabolite cannot be considered as an absolute tool of discrimination, as the metabolite can also be present in the biological tissues, as is the case with EDDP.

In providing an interpretation of these findings, it can be proposed that potential explanations are:

- at the time of the incident the children were exposed to methadone (as the urine or blood were positive for methadone)
- the children were living in a household where methadone was being used
- the results of hair analysis may reflect the ingestion of methadone by the children on a fairly regular basis, although the frequency of the ingestion cannot be established
- the possibility that a significant proportion of the methadone and EDDP present in hair samples was the result of external contamination (sweat, body fluids during the course of the postmortem examination) cannot be excluded.

3.10 Zopiclone

Zopiclone is a hypnotic agent belonging to a class of hypnosedative drugs, the cyclopyrrolones, with a chemical structure unrelated to benzodiazepines. It is intended for once-nightly consumption at a dose of 7.5 mg. Despite its selective interaction with omega-1 receptors, several side effects, including visual disturbance and hallucinations, have been described. Moreover, impairment of psychomotor performance and effects on recent or remote recall can be both significant. Zopiclone is prescribed in the treatment of occasional insomnia in adults and does not have any official French market authorization for children. Zopiclone has been sold in France since 1987.

A number of off-label prescriptions have been described in adolescents but none in children. Mrs. X, 38 years old, called the emergency services explaining she had found her children lifeless in the bathtub. The paramedics found two children, G, 2 years old, and R, 5 years old, dead in a bathtub full of water. Suspicions quickly turned to the mother who rapidly confessed to have drugged her children with zopiclone, but denied any intention to kill them. Autopsies were performed 48 hours later and revealed lung and brain edema and a small amount of water in the lungs and stomach of the older child. No sign of abuse or injury in self-defense was noted. Samples were taken for conventional toxicological analysis. Drugs were determined by LC-MS/MS.

The results obtained from samples of the victims are presented in Table 10.4.

No reference values exist for zopiclone in children. The postmortem blood concentrations found in the victims corresponded to toxic concentrations in adults. The presence of very low concentrations of zopiclone in all segments of hair showed regular exposure of the two victims during the 8 months preceding the death. However, the children were never prescribed zopiclone and the mother denied any administration. As a consequence,

TABLE 10.4 Zopiclone Concentrations in Both Children's Specimens

| | Peripheral Blood (ng/mL) | Urines (ng/mL) | Hair (pg/mg) | |
			0 to 4 cm	4 to 8 cm
Victim G	260	1580	16	12
Victim R	174	946	45	40

contamination was considered an issue and interpretation of the results was a challenge that deserved particular attention. The mother was found responsible for her acts by expert psychiatrists and sentenced to 25 years' imprisonment.

3.11 Multi-Drug Exposure

In February 2008, UK police received a telephone call from the mother of a 9-year-old child, informing them that the child had not returned home from school. Extensive searching and enquiries resulted in the child being located 24 days later, at the home address of a friend of the child's mother. It was suspected that the child may have been administered drugs during the time period between disappearance in February and discovery in March. Numerous medications were recovered and seized during searches of both the mother's home address and the address where the child was discovered. Investigations revealed that the following medications were prescribed to the friend of the child's mother: amitriptyline hydrochloride; clonazepam; dihydrocodeine; temazepam; and tramadol. Meclozine (TRAVELeeze®)—an antihistamine with antiemetic action to prevent nausea and vomiting, particularly travel sickness—was also found at this address.

Initial analysis of a urine sample that was collected from the child shortly after his discovery, identified meclozine and a trace amount of temazepam (less than 10 ng/ml). This demonstrated recent ingestion of these drugs, i.e. ingestion within 48–72 hours of sample collection, and prompted the forensic toxicologist to request that hair samples be collected from the child as the urine result, in isolation, would offer little assistance in determining whether the child had ingested drugs at an earlier time during the period of captivity. The extended window of detection provided by the hair matrix could investigate this issue analytically and provide added value to the police investigation. The locks of hair were greater than 12, 15 and 18 cm in length, respectively, and were brown in color. The orientation of the hair samples had been maintained. It was requested that the hair samples be analyzed for a range of sedative and pharmaceutical/medicinal drugs by segmentation. All drugs were tested by LC-MS/MS.

The pattern of drug exposure is presented in Figure 10.2.

The presence of amitriptyline, temazepam, tramadol and dihydrocodeine in the hair samples demonstrated the ingestion of these drugs (knowingly or otherwise) by the child in the months leading up to discovery in March 2008. In this particular case, the results were unusual as the respective drug concentrations increased along the hair shaft, away from the scalp. This suggested dosing on more than one occasion prior to the time the child went missing. The presence of drugs in each hair segment did not necessarily mean that they were ingested during each representative time period. There is the possibility that the area of hair containing the drugs became more diffuse due to regular washing.[24] Based on the hair analysis results, it was likely that the child ingested the drugs on a number of occasions over an extended time period, possibly dating back more than 12 months prior to sample collection. The findings were not consistent with a single exposure/ingestion of these drugs. The increased concentration of the respective drugs in the 10 to 11 cm segments of hair and the 16 to 17 cm segments of hair supported the view that there was an increase in the amount of drug ingested at that time, i.e. an increase in the dosage and/or frequency of ingestion over this period. Accepting the variations in hair growth rate, these apparent "peaks" in drug concentration may have coincided with school vacation periods, i.e. Easter and summer breaks (case details shared by courtesy of Dr. Craig Chatterton).

The lack of published data on blood, urine and hair concentrations in children makes interpretation of analytical results problematic; one cannot simply apply the same interpretation (for adults) to the testing results of samples taken from children. Significantly fewer data are available concerning controlled laboratory studies on drug intake and subsequent pharmacological effects.

Given that child abuse is often observed in an intra-family context, only a few papers have been published regarding pediatric drug-facilitated observations.[25-29] In front of recent neuropsychological disturbances in a child, such an issue has to be considered. The quality of sampling, the use of ultra-sensitive and specific toxicological methods and a clinical—biological collaboration allow recognition of this form of delinquency, whose consequences are both medical and legal.

4. THE SPECIFIC PROBLEM FOR THE ELDERLY

Like other types of domestic violence, knowledge about abuse of the elderly until recently has been based on relatively few groups and thus was tenuous in nature. It appears that this specific problem is largely unreported and it is estimated, for example in the United States, that approximately 1% to 2% of

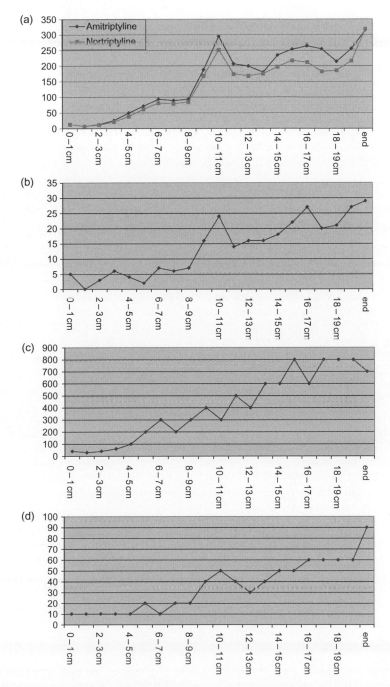

FIGURE 10.2   (a) Pattern of distribution of amitriptyline and nortriptyline; (b) pattern of distribution of temazepam; (c) pattern of distribution of tramadol; and (d) pattern of distribution of dihydrocodeine. All concentrations are in pg/mg.

elderly people living in their own homes are physically, emotionally, sexually and/or financially abused.[30] Abuse occurs across all socioeconomic, racial and religious groups.[31] It is considered that mental abuse and neglect are more frequent, but physical maltreatment such as beating, pushing, kicking and possibly sexual abuse is also reported. In addition, theft of money and property is noted.

Few reports deal with administration of drugs to the elderly for profit. Benzodiazepines, neuroleptics and opiates have been suggested,[32,33] but most sedatives or hypnotics can be used.[34] These intentional intoxications are generally committed with the aim of robbery.

4.1 Alprazolam

A 51-year-old man was admitted nine times to a local hospital over a period of months for drowsiness, ataxia, sedation, muscular weakness and marked somnolence. He was not under sedative treatment. The laboratory received a 7 cm hair lock with the request from a judge to screen for psychoactive pharmaceuticals. After segmentation and analysis, alprazolam, a benzodiazepine, was identified. The results are presented in Table 10.5. In this case, given the multiple admissions to the hospital, hair sections of 1 cm were considered a useful tool to establish the pattern of drug exposure. In comparison with other incidents,[14] the concentrations of alprazolam can be considered important, demonstrating multiple exposures. Segmentation was used as proof of repetitive administration of alprazolam as four 1 cm sections tested positive. Given the length of the segment analyzed, exposure to alprazolam

TABLE 10.5 Segmental Analysis of a Hair Strand Obtained from a Subject Admitted to the Hospital for Marked Somnolence. Analyses have Demonstrated Repetitive Surreptitious Administrations of Alprazolam during the Previous Months

Section (cm)	Alprazolam Concentration (pg/mg)
0 to 1	71
1 to 2	25
2 to 3	8
3 to 4	13
4 to 5	<LOQ (2 pg/mg)
5 to 6	<LOQ (2 pg/mg)
6 to 7	<LOQ (2 pg/mg)

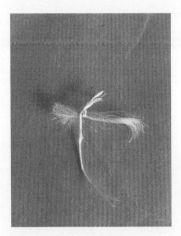

FIGURE 10.3   White hair strand of an elderly subject.

was expected to have occurred over a period of at least 4 months prior to the hair sample being obtained. This evidence was not challenged during the court trial. According to the police investigations, the window of potential drug exposure was about 4 months, during which the subject was living with a young woman. All symptoms of impairment disappeared after the woman was subsequently sentenced to jail. The aim of the drug administration was robbery and free use of the victim's home and hospitality.

4.2 Diazepam

A 76-year-old man was admitted to hospital for respiratory distress and walking difficulties. A urine screening indicated the presence of diazepam (124 ng/ml), nordiazepam (356 ng/ml) and oxazepam (67 ng/ml). However, he was not under benzodiazepine therapy. After information from the health authorities, the judge in charge of the case requested a hair test. A white strand of hair (Figure 10.3) was collected and segmented. Diazepam and its metabolite nordiazepam were identified in the two proximal segments (Table 10.6), corresponding to the time that a nurse was at his home for cleaning and providing food. All symptoms of impairment disappeared after the nurse was dismissed. The aim of drug administration was sedation and robbery.

4.3 Anti-Histamine Drugs

The white hair (3 cm) of a 81-year-old woman in a nursing home was obtained after her daughter noticed marked somnolence. She was not under sedative treatment. Hair analysis revealed the presence of diphenhydramine

TABLE 10.6 Segmental Analysis of a Hair Strand Obtained from a Subject Suffering of Severe Sedation and Alteration of Equilibrium

Segment	Diazepam	Nordiazepam
1	38 pg/mg	34 pg/mg
2	67 pg/mg	76 pg/mg
3	<LOQ	<LOQ
4	<LOQ	<LOQ

(683 pg/mg) and doxylamine (152 pg/mg), two anti-histamine drugs with sedative properties. Police and health authority investigations demonstrated that her registered nurse admitted giving the drugs to sedate the woman to reduce her workload. This case demonstrates that even with white hair, which contains no melanin, it is possible to identify drug exposure.

4.4 Clonazepam

A 71-year-old man was assaulted and robbed by a young woman. The offense occurred at his own home during a rendezvous arranged a few hours before through an erotic phone service. The woman prepared a mixture of juices and forced him to drink it. He rapidly fell asleep. Later in the investigation, the woman was found to have stayed in the home for about 1 week, abusing his hospitality. One day she requested the confidential number of his credit card, and disappeared with numerous personal items. The family noticed the unexplained disappearance of valuable possessions and sudden changes in his bank account. The man was without recollection of the events. On the request of the judge, head hair (3 cm) was collected 1 month later. 7-Aminoclonazepam was identified at 91 pg/mg, demonstrating repetitive exposure to clonazepam during the previous period, as a single exposure would produce a signal of 1 to 15 pg/mg.

4.5 Zolpidem

A 69-year-old man was admitted to hospital for marked somnolence and strange behavior. Besides his cardiac therapy, traces of zolpidem were found in urine (17 ng/ml). This drug was not part of his treatment. Once the result was presented to his wife, she admitted repetitive administration in the evening soup to decrease her husband's libido. The aim of this case is to emphasize the fact that surreptitious administration of a sedative can take place not only between strangers, but also between a married couple!

4.6 Promazine

An 87-year-old man living in an old people's home was found by his family to have inconsistent behavior, including totally incoherent speech. A 6 cm white hair lock was submitted to segmental analysis (3×2 cm section). Promazine, a neuroleptic with sedative properties, was detected at 9, 2 and 6 pg/mg. There were no data in the literature on promazine hair concentrations. In particular, it was not possible to put any quantitative interpretation on the dosage that was administered. It was, however, obvious that repetitive administrations had occurred but it was not possible to determine the number of exposures. Given the length of the man's hair and assuming a growth rate of 1 cm/month, exposure to promazine should have occurred at least during the previous 6 months. It was not possible to establish the origin of exposure to the drug.

4.7 Lorazepam

A 74-year-old man was robbed by two other men. The offense occurred at his own home, after having met the two men in a bar a few hours before. The perpetrators forced him to drink an unknown mixture and requested the confidential number of his credit card. Blood and urine sampled 8 hours after the offense revealed the presence of lorazepam at 9 and 16 ng/mL, respectively.

4.8 Morphine

If positive findings in hair can help in the characterization of chemical poisoning and therefore abuse of the elderly, negative findings can also be of importance, particularly with regard to neglect. Neglect can be defined as the refusal or failure to fulfill any part of a person's obligations or duties to an elder, including food/water, clothing, medicine, comfort and personal hygiene and safety. A 67-year-old man, suffering from cancer, was treated at home with morphine tablets. He was living alone, but was frequently visited by his younger son, an unemployed man. His older son, who was living overseas, visited his father and found him living in poor conditions, including malnutrition and poor personal hygiene. He also noticed abrupt changes in financial documents and unexplained withdrawals of large sums of money. The health authorities were informed and the public prosecutor requested medical investigations, including hair testing on a 4 cm grizzled lock. Irrespective of his treatment, morphine was not detected in hair (LOQ = 50 pg/mg). Later, the younger son admitted being addicted to morphine, having refined the anti-pain drug for his own abuse.

4.9 Multi-Drug Exposure

The victim, a 97-year-old woman, was found dead in a care home. It was an unexpected death, occurring under unknown circumstances. According to her family, who visited her the previous day, she was in good health. Her usual pharmaceutical treatment was zopiclone, one tablet at night. Postmortem blood analysis revealed the simultaneous presence of tramadol (1.82 mg/l), fentanyl (2.5 ng/ml), pethidine (22 ng/ml), midazolam (94 ng/ml) and free morphine (3 ng/ml). The analysis of a lock of hair, tested by LC-MS/MS, demonstrated the administration of numerous drugs, including diazepam (81 pg/mg), nordiazepam (213 pg/mg), bromazepam (26 pg/mg), zopiclone (137 pg/mg), zolpidem (21 pg/mg), temazepam (12 pg/mg), fentanyl (11 pg/mg), diphenhydramine (40 pg/mg), doxylamine (65 pg/mg), pethidine (714 pg/mg) and tramadol (3574 pg/mg). The care home (where 16 elderly persons were living) was inspected satisfactorily about 6 months before the death. However, in relation to this death, several other deaths were documented (Figure 10.4) and the owners of the care home were sentenced to jail.

Mistreatment of the elderly, whether it is abuse or neglect, can be classified as physical, psychological or financial/material. Several types of mistreatment may occur simultaneously. Very few data are available in the international literature.

Hair analysis may be especially useful when a history of drug use is difficult or impossible to obtain, notably when an elderly person is poisoned and the defense is one of the subject accidentally gaining access to a drug on a single occasion. The discrimination between a single exposure and long-term use can be documented by multi-sectional analysis.

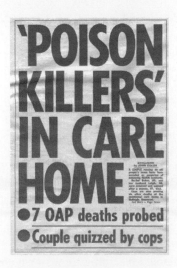

FIGURE 10.4   Copy of the heading of a newspaper.

The social context in which violence towards elderly people takes place remains crucial to the accurate identification of abuse. This includes a culture of violence in the family; a demented, debilitated, or depressed and socially isolated victim; and a perpetrator profile of mental illness, alcohol or drug abuse, or emotional and/or financial dependence on the victim.[35] Older people with learning disabilities may be viewed as potentially vulnerable and therefore in need of safeguarding. It may be worthwhile for administrators of violence programs to pay particular attention to substance exposure among their participants and in their community's environment, especially if older persons are involved.

Inappropriate and overprescribed medication is a practice in need of careful consideration with legal and ethical considerations. It can lead to people being chemically restrained and must only be used in exceptional situations.[36]

The most frequent types of elderly abuse are psychological and financial. Neglect is associated with current lifestyles. Physical and sexual abuse is considered infrequent, but possibly underdetected. Important risk factors are dysfunctional families, stressed and poorly trained caregivers, and hostile patients. Although the phenomenon of elderly abuse is well known, consensus guidelines for its detection and intervention still need to be defined, particularly with regard to drug screening. Obviously, this topic remains controversial, and the role of health authorities concerning the management of the elderly is under debate.[37]

Research into elder abuse is relatively recent. The forensic clinician has responsibilities to: a) the patient, with competent history taking and examination, b) interpret findings and recognize patterns of harm, and c) promulgate this issue in wider professional and public forums.[38]

5. CONCLUSION

It appears that the value of biological analysis for the identification of drugs in the specific context of DFC is steadily gaining recognition. Despite late sampling or even lack of collection of traditional biological fluids, such as blood and/or urine, results for hair testing allow exposure to a drug to be documented. Although there are still controversies about how to interpret the results, particularly concerning children and elderly persons, pure analytical work seems to have reached a plateau, having solved almost all of the problems.

In the case of DFCs, hair testing should be used to complement conventional blood and urine analysis as it increases the window of detection and permits differentiation, by segmentation, of long-term therapeutic use from a single exposure. However, the potential contamination by external sources of drugs remains the critical point when dealing with children. Several authors[39–41] have identified drugs in the hair of children from environmental contamination.

In the case of late crime declaration, positive hair findings are of paramount importance for a victim, in order to initiate, under suitable conditions, a psychological follow-up. It can also help in the discrimination of false reports of assault, for example in the case of revenge. These cases are often sensitive with little other forensic evidence. Tedious interpretations, concerning concomitant intake of hypnotics as a therapy for sleeping disorders, are avoided when investigations are done using hair in addition to blood and urine.

Overall, the interpretation of the analytical results remains difficult, because children are not "little adults" and numerous diseases can affect the distribution of drugs in elderly persons.

REFERENCES

1. Wells D. Drug administration and sexual assault: sex in a glass. *Sci Justice* 2001;**41**:197−9.
2. Verstraete A. Fenêtre de détection des xénobiotiques dans le sang, les urines, la salive et les cheveux. *Ann Toxicol Anal* 2002;**14**:390−4.
3. Kintz P. Value of the concept of minimal detectable dosage in human hair. *Forensic Sci Int* 2012;**218**:28−30.
4. Jenkins AJ. Pharmacokinetics: drug absorption, distribution, and elimination. In: Karch SB, editor. *Drug abuse handbook*. Boca Raton: CRC Press; 2007. p. 167.
5. Rylance G. Clinical pharmacology. Drugs in children. *Br Med J* 1981;**282**:50−1.
6. Hines LE, Murphy JE. Potentially harmful drug−drug interactions in the elderly: a review. *Am J Geriatr Pharmacother* 2011;**9**:364−77.
7. ElDesoky ES. Pharmacokinetic−pharmacodynamic crisis in the elderly. *Am J Ther* 2007;**14**:488−98.
8. Johnell K, Fastbom J. Gender and use of hypnotics or sedatives in old age: a nationwide register-based study. *Int J Clin Pharm* 2011;**33**:788−93.
9. Wortelboer U, Cohrs S, Rodenbeck A, Rüther E. Tolerability of hypnosedatives in older patients. *Drugs Aging* 2002;**19**:529−39.
10. Daggy A, Kaplan R, Roberge R, Akhtar J. Pediatric Visine (tetrahydrozoline) ingestion: case report and review of imidazoline toxicity. *Vet Hum Toxicol* 2003;**45**:210−2.
11. Stillwell ME, Saady JJ. Use of tetrahydrozoline for chemical submission. *Forensic Sci Int* 2012;**221**:e12−6.
12. Carr ME, Engebretsen KM, Ho B, Anderson CP. Tetrahydrozoline (Visine®) concentrations in serum and urine during therapeutic ocular dosing: a necessary first step in determining an overdose. *Clin Toxicol* 2011;**49**:810−4.
13. Villain M, Vallet E, Cirimele V, Kintz P. Mise en évidence d'une soumission chimique à le niaprazine chez des enfants par analyse des cheveux en CL-SM/SM. *Ann Toxicol Anal* 2008;**20**:85−8.
14. Kintz P, Villain M, Chèze M, Pépin G. Identification of alprazolam in hair in two cases of drug-facilitated incidents. *Forensic Sci Int* 2005;**153**:222−6.
15. Kintz P, Villain M, Tracqui A, Cirimele V, Ludes B. Buprenorphine as a drug-facilitated sexual abuse. A fatal case involving a 14-year old boy. *J Anal Toxicol* 2003;**27**:527−9.
16. Kintz P, Villain M, Cirimele V. Determination of trimeprazine-facilitated sedation in children by hair analysis. *J Anal Toxicol* 2006;**30**:400−2.

17. Kintz P, Evans J, Villain M, Salquebre G, Cirimele V. Hair analysis for diphenhydramine after surreptitious administration to a child. *Forensic Sci Int* 2007;**173**:171−4.

18. Kintz P, Marescaux C, Mangin P. Testing human hair for carbamazepine in epileptic patients: is hair investigation suitable for drug monitoring. *Human Exp Toxicol* 1995;**14**:812−5.

19. http://kidshealth.org/parent/general/sick/munchausen.html; seen 16 July 2013.

20. Caruso M, Bregani P, Natale B, D'Arcais A. Induced hypoglycemia. An unusual case of child battering. *Minerva Pediatr* 1989;**41**:525−8.

21. Villain M, Tournoud C, Flesch F, Cirimele V, Kintz P. Hair to document exposure to glibenclamide. *J Chromatogr B* 2006;**842**:111−5.

22. Kintz P, Evans J, Villain M, Cirimele V. Interpretation of hair findings in children after methadone poisoning. *Forensic Sci Int* 2010;**196**:51−4.

23. Kintz P. Segmental hair analysis can demonstrate external contamination in postmortem cases. *Forensic Sci Int* 2012;**215**:73−6.

24. Kintz P. Issues about axial diffusion during segmental hair analysis. *Ther Drug Monit* 2013;**35**:408−10.

25. Rey-Salmon C, Pépin G. Drug-facilitated crime and sexual abuse: a pediatric observation. *Arch Pediatr* 2007;**14**:1318−20.

26. Spiller HA, Rogers J, Sawyer TS. Drug facilitated sexual assault using an over-the-counter ocular solution containing tetrahydrozoline (Visine). *Leg Med* 2007;**9**:192−5.

27. Gavril AR, Kellog ND, Nair P. Value of follow-up examinations of children and adolescents evaluated for sexual abuse and assault. *Pediatrics* 2012;**129**:282−9.

28. Wood JN, Pecker LH, Russo ME, Henretig F, Christian CW. Evaluation and referral for child maltreatment in pediatric poisoning victims. *Child Abuse Negl* 2012;**36**:362−9.

29. Yin S. Malicious use of pharmaceuticals in children. *J Pediatr* 2010;**157**:832−6.

30. Dolan VF. Risk factors for elder abuse. *J Insur Med* 1999;**31**:13−20.

31. Paris BEC, Meier DE, Goldstein T. Elder abuse and neglect: how to recognize warning signs and intervene. *Geriatr* 1995;**50**:47−53.

32. Bredthauer D, Becker C, Eichner B. Factors relating to the use of physical restraints in psychogeriatrics care: a paradigm for elder abuse. *Z Gerontol Geriatr* 2005;**38**:10−8.

33. Stankova E, Gesheva M, Hubenova A. Age and criminal poisoning. *Przegl Lek* 2005;**62**:471−4.

34. Kintz P, Villain M, Cirimele V. Chemical abuse in the elderly: evidence from hair analysis. *Ther Drug Monit* 2008;**30**:207−11.

35. Murphy K, Waa S, Jaffer H, Sauter A, Chan A. A literature review of findings in physical elder abuse. *Can Assoc Radiol J* 2013;**64**:10−4.

36. Hughes R. Chemical restraint in nursing older people. *Nurs Older People* 2008;**20**:33−8.

37. Rich BA. Thinking the unthinkable: the clinician as perpetrator of elder abuse in patients in pain. *J Pain Palliat Care Pharmacother* 2004;**18**:63−74.

38. Fox AW. Elder abuse. *Med Sci Law* 2012;**52**:128−36.

39. Smith FP, Kidwell DA. Cocaine in hair, saliva, skin swabs, and urine of cocaine users' children. *Forensic Sci Int* 1996;**83**:179−89.

40. Joya X, Papaseit E, Civit E, Pellegrini M, Vall O, Garcia-Algar O, et al. Unsuspected exposure to cocaine in preschool children from a Mediterranean city detected by hair analysis. *Ther Drug Monit* 2009;**31**:391−5.

41. Bassindale T. Quantitative analysis of methamphetamine in hair of children removed from clandestine laboratories—evidence of passive exposure? *Forensic Sci Int* 2012;**219**: 179−82.

Chapter 11

Clinical Aspects of Drug-Facilitated Sexual Assault

A.L. Pelissier and J.S. Raul

Many drugs, alone or in combination, have the potential to be used to facilitate sexual assault, including alcohol, benzodiazepines, antihistamines, antidepressants, marijuana, cocaine, and gamma-hydroxybutyrate (GHB). Whether taken voluntarily or involuntarily, such drugs are often metabolized and excreted before the victim suspects that a sexual assault may have occurred. This contributes to the underreporting of drug-facilitated sexual assault (DFSA). During the last 20 years both the police and medical personnel have become more aware of drug-facilitated sexual assault. The use of chloral hydrate knock-out drops dates back to the 1800s, where they were used to facilitate robbery. DFSA is not a new phenomenon.[1,2]

Two different categories of victims are evident. The first category, which appears to be the most frequent, is the opportunistic DFSA, where the perpetrator takes advantage of someone already inebriated by voluntary ingestion of sufficient amounts of drugs or alcohol to become intoxicated. The second category is the proactive DFSA, with covert administration of drugs to an unsuspecting victim. In both cases, the potential victim has impaired consciousness and reduced ability to resist unwanted sexual advances.[3-6]

A British study combining laboratory data with information from police investigations found that less than 2% of the sedative drug findings could be attributed to proactive DFSA, whereas the vast majority of positive tests could be explained by voluntary intake.[7] In a study by Hagemann, among the 264 patients included, 155 (59%) tested positive for ethanol and/or drugs; 105 (40%) for ethanol only; and 50 (19%) for one or more drugs other than ethanol. In total, 57 patients (22%) were suspected of being the victims of proactive DFSA, but only five had findings of sedative drugs that could not be explained by self-reported voluntary intake. No case could unequivocally be attributed to proactive DFSA. Finally, patients testing positive for ethanol more often reported a public place of assault and a stranger assailant, and the higher the estimated blood alcohol concentration at the time of the assault,

Toxicological Aspects of Drug-Facilitated Crimes. DOI: http://dx.doi.org/10.1016/B978-0-12-416748-3.00011-6

the higher the frequency of suspecting proactive DFSA. As a conclusion, it can be said that voluntary drug and/or alcohol consumption increases the risk of being the victim of a sexual assault.[8]

The main clinical presentation of suspected DFSA is a "blank memory." The victim will then often expect that clinical examination and forensic tests will determine exactly what has happened. It is therefore of great importance to explain the limitations of both clinical examination and forensic testing. Especially in cases of DFSA, it is very rare to find injuries to the genital organs, anus, or mouth as well as injuries to the entire body. This is mainly because the victim is intoxicated and is not aware of the assault. Defense wounds are particularly rare. Therefore, if no evidence of sexual assault is found, this does not mean that nothing happened. Along with neuropsychiatric symptoms, which dominate the clinical picture, other symptoms can also be observed. Looking for these symptoms is important as it can sometimes give an indication of the drug used. Benzodiazepines can induce hypotonia and myorelaxation. The absorption of antihistaminic drugs (hydroxyzine, alimemazine, promethazine, diphenhydramine), or atropine, including *Datura*, and tri- or tetracyclic antidepressants, may cause anticholinergic syndrome characterized by delirium, dysarthria, mydriasis, tremor exacerbated by stress, restlessness, and clonic movements. There are also autonomic signs of mucosal dryness, urinary retention, constipation, and tachycardia. In most cases, patients do not exhibit all of these symptoms. The opiates can cause respiratory depression, bradycardia, and myosis.[9] Some drugs are also likely to cause visual disturbances (myosis, mydriasis, impaired accommodation), tachycardia, headache, nausea, vomiting, and dizziness.[10] Headaches have been reported after scopolamine exposure.[11] Abondo et al. reported a case of sexual assault involving MDMA (3,4-methylenedioxy-N-methylamphetamine) in which the victim described tachycardia, stiffness of the jaw and neck, and impression of swollen feet. She experienced pain in the lower back and groin as well as exaggerated sensibility (taste, touch, and smell).[12] Hyperthermia has also been described.[13] The clinician must be aware of these different clinical presentations. Along with these neurological signs, the victim will often talk about lower abdominal pain, genital, or anal irritation, vaginal discharge and it is mainly these gynecological signs that lead to the idea of a possible sexual assault. The victim being unable to recall what has happened due to drug or alcohol consumption will be suspicious and anxious about the possibility of having been raped. The clinician must question the victim to obtain a clear history of what happened up until the "blank" period and what happened after the victim regained consciousness. Some of the main questions focus on the victim's surroundings (was the victim alone at a time, did someone give him/her a drink...?) and on the first hours after the victim regained consciousness (where was he/she, was he/she dressed, what was he/she wearing, how was he/she taken to the hospital...?).

For clinicians caring for victims of sexual assault, it is important to recognize the possibility of DFSA. It is also important to provide the necessary therapeutic care and to address forensic issues, which may include evidence collection and documentation.

As the clinical presentation depends on the drugs used, different kinds of care may be necessary ranging from life support measures, to emergency contraception, to prophylaxis for sexually transmitted infections, and to psychosocial support, as well as managing injuries. It is of great importance to collect appropriate toxicological samples. Depending on the time of presentation, the types of forensic samples appropriate for toxicological examination after drug-facilitated sexual assault differ. Early after the assault mainly urine and blood samples need to be collected. For later presentations, hair samples may be used for drug identification.

Finally, consideration should also be given to performing a forensic medical examination to obtain DNA and other evidence, and addressing the different potential types of assault (e.g., penile penetration of the mouth, vagina, or anus; penetration with an object; or sexual touching). This could, however, cause distress to patients who may not have considered what sort of sexual acts might have taken place. Every effort should be made to preserve forensic evidence, and ideally the patient should not eat, drink, smoke, chew gum, or carry out oral hygiene until oral samples are taken, if indicated. Similarly, defecation, urination, and showering should be deferred until appropriate samples are obtained. The clinician should therefore always ask the victim about his/her behavior following the possibility of a sexual assault.

The specificity of DFSA through its clinical presentation and toxicological sampling must be well understood by all health professionals. When DFSA is suspected, victims of sexual assault should have easy and fast access to emergency health care with trained staff or sexual assault centers, and should be encouraged to seek immediate help. Toxicological screening should be routinely offered to achieve a comprehensive assessment in each individual case.

REFERENCES

1. Kintz P, Villain M, Ludes B. Testing for the undetectable in drug-facilitated sexual assault using hair analyzed by tandem mass spectrometry as evidence. Ther Drug Monit 2004;26:211–14.
2. Wells D. Drug administration and sexual assault: sex in a glass. Sci Justice 2001;41:197–9.
3. Du Mont J, Macdonald S, Rotbard N, Asllani E, Bainbridge D, Cohen MM. Factors associated with suspected drug-facilitated sexual assault. Can Med Assoc J 2009;180:513–19.
4. Gisladottir A, Gudmundsdottir B, Gudmundsdottir R, Jonsdottir E, Gudjonsdottir GR, Kristjansson M, et al. Increased attendance rates and altered characteristics of sexual violence. Acta Obstet Gynecol Scand 2012;91:134–42.

5. Nesvold H, Worm AM, Vala U, Agnarsdottir G. Different Nordic facilities for victims of sexual assault: a comparative study. *Acta Obstet Gynecol Scand* 2005;**84**:177–83.

6. Hurley M, Parker H, Wells DL. The epidemiology of drug facilitated sexual assault. *J Clin Forensic Med* 2006;**13**:181–5.

7. Scott-Ham M, Burton FC. Toxicological findings in cases of alleged drug facilitated sexual assault in the United Kingdom over a 3-year period. *J Clin Forensic Med* 2005;**12**:175–86.

8. Hagemann CT, Helland A, Spigest O, Espnes KA, Ormstad K, Schei B. Ethanol and drug findings in women consulting a sexual assault center- associations with clinical characteristics and suspicions of drug-facilitated sexual assault. *J Foren Leg Med* 2013;**20**:777–84.

9. Meehan TJ, Bryant SM, Aks SE. Drugs of abuse: the highs and lows of altered mental states in the emergency department. *Emerg Med Clin North Am* 2010;**28**:663–82.

10. Slaughter L. Involvement of drugs in sexual assault. *J Reprod Med* 2000;**45**:425–30.

11. Peatfield R, Villalon CM. Headache after exposure to "date rape drugs." *Springerplus* 2013;**2**:39.

12. Abondo M, Bouvet R, Baert A, Morel I, Le Gueut MA. Sexual assault and MDMA: the distinction between consciousness and awareness when it comes to consent. *Int J Legal Med* 2009;**123**:155–6.

13. Weir E. Raves: a review of the culture, the drugs and the prevention of harm. *CMAJ* 2000;**162**:1843–8.

Index

Note: Page numbers followed by "*f*" and "*t*" refer to figures and tables, respectively.

Printed and bound by CPI Group (UK) Ltd, Croydon, CR0 4YY

07/10/2024

01041904-0003